I0061432

# TO MAKE
# THE
# WOUNDED
# WHOLE

JUSTICE, POWER, AND POLITICS

*Coeditors*
Heather Ann Thompson
Rhonda Y. Williams

*Editorial Advisory Board*
Peniel E. Joseph
Daryl Maeda
Barbara Ransby
Vicki L. Ruiz
Marc Stein

The Justice, Power, and Politics series publishes new
works in history that explore the myriad struggles for
justice, battles for power, and shifts in politics that have
shaped the United States over time. Through the lenses
of justice, power, and politics, the series seeks to broaden
scholarly debates about America's past as well as to
inform public discussions about its future.

More information on the series, including a
complete list of books published, is available at
http://justicepowerandpolitics.com/.

# TO MAKE THE WOUNDED WHOLE

### THE AFRICAN AMERICAN STRUGGLE AGAINST HIV/AIDS

Dan Royles

The University of North Carolina Press | Chapel Hill

© 2020 Dan Royles
All rights reserved
Manufactured in the United States of America

Designed by April Leidig
Set in Minion by Copperline Book Services, Inc.

The University of North Carolina Press has been a
member of the Green Press Initiative since 2003.

Cover illustration: *Don't Love Your Partner to Death,* from an AIDS education poster
by Stephen John Phillips. Courtesy Rare Books and Special Collections, River Campus
Libraries, University of Rochester.

Library of Congress Cataloging-in-Publication Data
Names: Royles, Dan, author.
Title: To make the wounded whole : the African American struggle
against HIV/AIDS / Dan Royles.
Other titles: Justice, power, and politics.
Description: Chapel Hill : The University of North Carolina Press,
2020. | Series: Justice, power, and politics | Includes bibliographical
references and index.
Identifiers: LCCN 2020011785 | ISBN 9781469659503 (cloth : alk. paper) |
ISBN 9781469661339 (paperback : alk. paper) | ISBN 9781469659510 (ebook)
Subjects: LCSH: AIDS (Disease)—United States—History—20th century. |
AIDS activists—United States. | African Americans—Diseases. | African
Americans—Political activity.
Classification: LCC RA643.83 .R693 2020 | DDC 362.19697/9200973—dc23
LC record available at https://lccn.loc.gov/2020011785

Portions of chapter 1 previously appeared in Dan Royles, "'Don't We Die Too?':
The Politics of AIDS and Race in Philadelphia," in *Beyond the Politics of the Closet:
Gay Rights and the American State since the 1970s,* ed. Jonathan Bell (Philadelphia:
University of Pennsylvania Press, 2020), 100–117. © 2020 University of Pennsylvania
Press.

*To all those who break the silence*

# CONTENTS

# ILLUSTRATIONS

# TO MAKE
# THE
# WOUNDED
# WHOLE

# Introduction

## The AIDS Capital of the World

I N 1985 RESEARCHERS and reporters alike focused their attention on the city with the highest rate of AIDS diagnoses anywhere, a city that had become colloquially known as the "AIDS Capital of the World." This city was neither New York City nor San Francisco, nor was it to be found in Haiti, all places that had become identified with the new disease. The place with the highest per capita rate of the most fearsome epidemic on Earth was a small rural community in South Florida called Belle Glade. There, public health officials were baffled by the local epidemic, which looked altogether different from anything they had seen before.

THE BLACK SOIL IN THE FIELDS that surround Belle Glade, also known as "Muck City," is unbelievably rich. Since the draining of the Everglades began over a century ago, that soil has yielded countless bushels of potatoes, sweet corn, and string beans, along with tons of sugarcane. The soil is so rich because, for millennia, nearby Lake Okeechobee would overflow with heavy rains, depositing loamy black silt—the "muck" that gives Belle Glade its nickname—on the land where the town and its surrounding farms now sit. The soil is so rich, in fact, that it sometimes catches fire.[1]

For as long as Belle Glade has produced vegetables and sugar for the rest of the country, it has attracted migrant workers from other parts of the U.S. South and the Caribbean. These men and women are overworked and underpaid. Zora Neale Hurston described life there during the 1920s in *Their Eyes Were Watching God*, including the "hordes of workers [that] poured in" during picking season, "permanent transients with no attachments and tired looking men with their families and dogs in flivvers." During the 1930s, U.S. Sugar used the promise of good pay to lure Black[2] workers to its brand-new mill in nearby Clewiston. When they arrived, the migrants found themselves plunged into debt peonage, working under white overseers who promised a beating or worse to those who tried to escape. Some decades later, Belle Glade featured prominently in the 1960 CBS documentary *Harvest of Shame*, which exposed terrible working conditions for migrant farm laborers across the country. "We used to own our slaves," one farmer told reporters. "Now we just rent them."[3]

By the 1980s, conditions in Belle Glade had changed very little. If anything, they had gotten worse. Year-round Black residents crammed into the derelict apartment buildings, mobile homes, and shacks that dotted the old "colored town" in southwest Belle Glade. Their bodies bore scars from the field knives and machetes used to harvest lettuce, corn, and cane. During the cutting season, as many as ten thousand migrant workers flooded in from Haiti, Jamaica, and the Bahamas to work in the fields. In the midst of the sugarcane harvest, prostitution and drug use flourished. Injection drugs, popular in the early 1980s, gave way to crack cocaine as the decade wore on. A concurrent rise in rates of gonorrhea and syphilis pointed to crack's power to lower sexual inhibitions, as users sought out multiple partners and sometimes traded sex for the drug.[4] Not unlike the combustible soil that surrounded it, Belle Glade was fertile ground for HIV.

In the early 1980s, Dr. Ron Wiewora ran the town's public health clinic out of a trailer on Avenue D, which runs west to east through the middle of "colored town." By 1984 he noticed a growing number of residents seeking treatment for AIDS. He began keeping track of these patients and their connections to one another—whether they had shared needles or had been sexual partners. Around the same time, a pair of researchers from the Institute of Tropical Medicine in Miami were also homing in on Belle Glade. One of them, Dr. Mark Whiteside, treated a vegetable packer for cryptosporidiosis, a parasitic infection frequently seen in people with AIDS. The vegetable packer led Whiteside and his partner, Dr. Carolyn MacLeod, back to Belle Glade.

For Wiewora, Whiteside, and McLeod, the outbreak in Belle Glade didn't make any sense. Most of the reported AIDS cases in America were among gay men in big cities like New York, San Francisco, and Los Angeles. But about half of the Belle Glade cases were in women, and almost all of those diagnosed were straight. The small community's per capita AIDS rate was also five times higher than New York City's and seven times higher than San Francisco's.

Few of the patients they saw fit into the identified risk groups of gay men or intravenous drug users, so Whiteside and MacLeod looked for explanations that didn't involve sex or shared needles. They proposed that the disease might be tied in some way to poverty: to the rats that scurried through apartments and shacks, or to the human excrement that lined Belle Glade's streets and yards. Perhaps poverty and malnutrition made residents more susceptible to infection from mosquito bites, which didn't seem to be a factor anywhere else. Whiteside presented this theory in April 1985 at the First International

AIDS Conference in Atlanta. His theory—and Belle Glade—became a media sensation.[5]

It's easy to see why: Whiteside pointed to casual contact and the environment as vectors of transmission. The map of Belle Glade that he presented in Atlanta used stars to indicate where residents with AIDS had lived; it looked like the one that John Snow had created to trace an 1854 cholera outbreak in London to a single water pump on Broad Street, or like the maps of tuberculosis cases that Progressive Era reformers drew up to convince others of the links between poverty and disease. But both cholera and tuberculosis were much easier to spread than HTLV-III (later HIV), the newly discovered AIDS virus, was believed to be. If he was right, the deadly new disease would not confine itself to gay men or drug users, two groups that many Americans—consciously or not—saw as expendable.

Meanwhile, news reporters and TV cameras flooded to Belle Glade. As the town's dubious notoriety grew, the local economy took a major hit. Visitors driving through Belle Glade wore surgical masks and refused to stop at the town's fast food joints. High schools in the region balked at sending their sports teams to Belle Glade for away games. "We opened our arms to this study," City Commissioner Harma Miller later recalled of Whiteside and MacLeod's research, "and they bashed us with it."[6]

But the attention also brought in money from federal agencies and private foundations, which set up shop to study the AIDS epidemic in Belle Glade and to come up with solutions. They disproved Whiteside and MacLeod's more alarming theories but added to researchers' knowledge about heterosexual transmission of HIV. The two researchers had been wrong about many things, but they were right about one: many more people would be affected by the disease.[7]

The AIDS outbreak in Belle Glade was a harbinger of the epidemic to come. The South has been the epicenter of HIV infection in the United States for some time, and African Americans have come to make up a near majority of those newly diagnosed with the virus each year. Black women are also at much greater risk for HIV than women from other groups—in 2017 they were nearly fifteen times more likely to be diagnosed with HIV than their white counterparts. But even though the relatively high rate of heterosexual transmission has distinguished the HIV epidemic in Black America, Black gay and bisexual men have been among the hardest hit: according to a 2016 estimate, one in two will contract HIV within their lifetime. For Black transgender women, solid numbers are hard to come by, but the Centers for Disease Control and Prevention estimates that 44 percent are living with HIV, compared to 14 percent for transgender women as a whole.[8]

In short, AIDS has devastated Black America and continues to do so. This book tells the story of how African Americans organized to fight back.

AIDS WAS FIRST IDENTIFIED in 1981, when gay men started showing up at hospitals in New York, San Francisco, and Los Angeles with rare infections that usually affected people with impaired immune systems. That summer, as rumors of a deadly new disease swirled through gay communities, the *New York Times* reported the possibility of an emerging epidemic under the headline "Rare Cancer Seen in 41 Homosexuals."[9]

As the death count rose, gay men organized the AIDS education and support networks that would be the first wave of activism against the new disease. But due to racism and segregation, "out" gay communities in U.S. cities were largely white or were seen as such, even when those same cities had large minority communities. The organizations that emerged from urban gay communities tended to be staffed by white volunteers, supported by funds from white donors, and geared toward white clients. Their prominence reinforced the idea that AIDS was a disease of white gay men, even as doctors began to see cases of the disease among hemophiliacs and injection drug users, as well as their heterosexual partners and children. As mostly white groups of people with AIDS and their allies cared for one another, gathered at candlelight vigils to honor the dead, and later staged dramatic protests against the lack of a significant federal response to AIDS, they formed the public face of the disease.[10]

Meanwhile, the epidemic was raging in America's Black communities. The year that the Belle Glade story broke, around 25 percent of people with AIDS in the United States were Black, even though African Americans represented only 12 percent of the total population. In contrast to the white gay men who put a face on the early epidemic, in Black communities heterosexual and mother-to-child transmission were much more common. Some African American men identified as straight but had sex with other men, and those who contracted the virus sometimes passed it on to their wives or girlfriends. Injection drug use also accounted for a significant number of HIV infections among African Americans, especially in poor communities. The epidemic of crack cocaine use that exploded in urban areas during the 1980s further fueled the spread of HIV in poor communities of color, particularly among women who exchanged sex for drugs and money. Women, whether infected by a sexual partner or a shared syringe, could in turn pass HIV to their children either in utero or through breastfeeding. But these realities were largely ignored by the news media and policy makers and were invisible to the majority of Americans.[11]

Despite the lack of media attention to AIDS in Black communities, by the middle 1980s a small but growing number of African Americans knew first-hand that AIDS was not just a white gay disease. African American medical professionals such as Rashidah Hassan, a nurse and infectious disease control specialist in Philadelphia, or Pernessa Seele, an immunologist at Harlem Hospital, had seen Black people with AIDS come through their hospital doors who did not fit media stereotypes. The members of Gay Men of African Descent (GMAD) lost the group's founder, Charles Angel, to AIDS in 1986. Reggie Williams, the African American executive director of the National Task Force on AIDS Prevention (NTFAP), received his own diagnosis of AIDS-related complex in 1986 as well. Others, such as Dázon Dixon Diallo in Atlanta, focused their energy on educating Black women about AIDS. Over time, a diverse constellation of activists, including Black writers, religious leaders, medical professionals, and recovering drug users, would pursue grassroots strategies for fighting the spread of HIV and AIDS among African Americans. Since AIDS continues to wreak havoc on Black communities in the United States, understanding the work of African American AIDS activists is now more important than ever. This book aims to tell their story.

Although African American AIDS activists implemented a wide variety of programs to fight the spread of HIV in their communities, three themes run through their collective work. The first is that activists insisted on approaches that were tailored to Black communities—those that were, in public health parlance, "culturally competent." The second is that they worked through the institutions, large and small, that mattered most in the lives of those they wanted to educate about HIV/AIDS. In some cases that meant forming partnerships with the largest Black church denominations, while in others it meant going to the bars where Black gay men went to drink and dance. Finally, African American AIDS activists took aim at what sociologist Celeste Watkins-Hayes terms "injuries of inequality," which are more commonly known (in academic circles, anyway) as social determinants of health. But these approaches raised thorny questions about what it meant to be Black in America in the age of AIDS.[12]

African American AIDS activists very often saw themselves as uniquely qualified to educate Black communities about reducing their risk for HIV and AIDS. Much like other AIDS activists, they warned about the dangers of needle sharing or unprotected sex. However, they argued that in Black communities the messenger mattered as much as the message itself. Only culturally competent messages—those produced with Black communities in mind by those who knew members' values, language, and everyday activities—would be effective in educating African Americans about AIDS. But if people in Black communities needed to see and hear messages about AIDS that resonated with their culture, then what was "Black culture" to begin with? Was it to be found in Black churches? In hip-hop? In Kwanzaa and kente cloth? What was to be done when messages about drug use and safer sex conflicted with the claims to respectability that had been central to earlier struggles for civil rights? What about those Black cultural frameworks, including a significant portion of Afrocentric thought, that disavowed homosexuality entirely?

In addition to developing messages about AIDS that would resonate with Black audiences, activists had to find effective ways to deliver such messages. Very often they turned to existing institutions and social networks, hoping to capitalize on the everyday authority of community leaders and trusted friends. In some respects, their approach looks quite similar to that of white gay groups, who worked through gay bars, bookstores, and bathhouses to distribute condoms and deliver messages about safer sex. However, African American AIDS activists needed to reach not only self-identified Black gay men but also straight women, "down low" men, and intravenous drug users, all of whom were also at risk for contracting HIV. At the same time, the very Black community institutions that captured the biggest audience were sometimes the most ambivalent about becoming involved in AIDS prevention. Black churches in particular discouraged open discussion of sexuality, even denying that some of their parishioners could be gay. How could activists make room for messages about AIDS in such unwelcoming spaces? And how would they make inroads with populations that were otherwise considered "hard to reach," such as drug users and the urban poor?[13]

African American AIDS activists also approached the epidemic through the injuries of inequality that were a feature of everyday life in many Black communities. They reasoned that as long as unemployment, incarceration, and physically deteriorating neighborhoods threatened Black communities, preventing HIV/AIDS would not be a priority for many African Americans. During the first decade of the epidemic, these problems were getting worse, not better, as the progress made in alleviating poverty since the 1960s was rolled back. President Ronald Reagan took office in 1981, just before doctors recognized the first cases of AIDS in the United States. Reagan made good on his campaign promise to slash federal spending on welfare and social services, with massive cuts to jobs training, housing, and child nutrition programs. As a result, working families were plunged deeper into poverty. These cuts were aimed squarely at Black communities; Reagan had touted his support for states' rights in the heart of Dixie and attacked the "welfare queens" who were supposedly getting rich on the government dole. As Manning Marable observed, "The 'ideological glue' of Reaganism was racism." But Reaganism, as a manifestation of the long tradition of American anti-Blackness, was not merely a distraction from the fight against AIDS; it was at the root of the epidemic. That made activists' work much, much harder. How could they stop—or even slow—an epidemic rooted in forms of oppression that are older than the country itself?[14]

African American AIDS activists answered these questions through a variety of programs that aimed to stop the spread of HIV in Black America. In doing so they pushed at the boundaries of African American identity and community in two ways. On the one hand, many worked to make room for queer identity within prevailing ideas about Blackness, such as those found in the theology of African American churches or within Afrocentric thought. Here I borrow from political scientist and activist Cathy Cohen in using "queer" to include not only expressions of same-sex desire but also a wider range of marginalized identities, including women in public housing, recovering drug users, and the formerly incarcerated.[15]

On the other hand, African American AIDS activists frequently addressed AIDS in Black America as part of the pandemic among Black people around the world. In doing so they mapped a wide range of affinities among themselves, the peoples of sub-Saharan Africa, and the rest of the African diaspora. Some looked to Africa for essential Black values to guide AIDS programs, while some saw the continent as a place to redeploy the prevention programs they had developed in the United States. Their work at times was complicated by Africa's role as the point of origin and epicenter of the pandemic. To some, scientific reports that HIV had originated from a simian virus that crossed over into the human population of sub-Saharan Africa smacked of scientific racism, which represented people of African descent as animalistic, immoral, and diseased. Still others framed the AIDS epidemic among African Americans as part of the larger pandemic among people in the global South, including sub-Saharan Africa, where endemic poverty and underdevelopment fueled the spread of HIV. Such claims challenged persistent racial inequality within the world's wealthiest country while also creating opportunities for solidarity with those suffering under similar conditions around the globe.

Thus the title of this book has multiple meanings. As African American activists confronted AIDS, they aimed to make whole communities that were divided by homophobia, sexism, and classism. At the same time, by putting their work in a diasporic context, they struggled to heal older wounds, ones that stretched back through centuries of oppression to the beginning of the Atlantic slave trade. And by confronting AIDS as a problem of global inequality, African American activists sought to make whole a world wounded by a history of plunder, from the European empires that grew rich off the labor of enslaved Africans to the multinational corporations that dominate global markets.[16]

African American AIDS activists sometimes shared their white counterparts' goals, such as drawing the attention of federal agencies to the epidemic, delivering frank messages about HIV prevention, or getting seats at the table where AIDS policy was made. But African American AIDS activists also sought to address the structural causes and consequences of poverty, marginalization, and disempowerment—the injuries of inequality—that they saw at the root of the spreading epidemic. The issues that occupied many white gay AIDS groups, such as how much of a role the state should have in managing the epidemic by keeping track of the infected, policing sexual activity, and funding health care for people with AIDS, were certainly crucial to activism around the epidemic, but they do not make up the whole story. Adding African American activists to the mix gives us a more complete picture of the grassroots politics around HIV and AIDS in the United States.

A focus on African American AIDS activists also exposes the funding problems that Black AIDS service organizations often faced. These challenges were not unique to African American groups; their predominantly white counterparts also struggled to raise money to fight a stigmatized disease, especially during the first decade of the epidemic. However, this problem appears to have been more acute for Black AIDS service organizations. These groups emerged from Black communities that were already struggling financially, which made grassroots fund-raising more difficult. Moreover, these groups did not—at least in the beginning—have the professional staff that they needed to manage large grants from the federal government and private philanthropies. At the same time, the stories in this book make clear that the response to AIDS in Black America was part and parcel of what Katie Batza has described as the "neoliberal off-loading" of health and social services onto the very communities that were harmed the most by the deliberate unraveling of the social safety net.[17]

Recognizing the history of African American AIDS activism is crucial to the fight against the epidemic going forward. Without such an understanding, Black communities appear as passive, powerless victims of the epidemic. That narrative in turn makes it all too easy to shift the blame for an epidemic connected to virtually every form of inequality in modern America back onto the people who are most affected by it. As this book makes clear, African Americans have been neither passive nor powerless in the face of AIDS.

MANY HISTORIANS and social critics of AIDS in the United States have treated the epidemic among African Americans as peripheral to larger stories about gender and sexuality, health and medicine, or activism. Others have sought to explain that which they find lacking in African American responses to AIDS.

In *The Boundaries of Blackness*, political scientist Cathy Cohen laments the reluctance of organizations such as the NAACP and the Urban League to take up AIDS as a political issue. She sees this as evidence of the "breakdown of Black politics," as such groups' unwillingness to address an epidemic disease linked to gay sex, drug use, and poverty fractured the apparent unity that had characterized earlier struggles. The stories in this book likewise document the "hidden differences, cleavages, [and] fault lines" that hampered responses to AIDS in Black America. But in bringing sustained focus to grassroots responses to the epidemic, I show that AIDS occasioned not only the breakdown of Black politics but their reimagining as well.[18]

Looking more narrowly at the politics of AIDS in North Carolina, historian Stephen Inrig argues that both Black and white activists' efforts to reach African Americans with information about AIDS foundered on racial tensions and racialized poverty. While Inrig's focus on state-level responses to AIDS is valuable, this focus also leads him to conclusions about the extent and scope of African American AIDS activism that are very different from my own. Many of the actors in the stories that follow grappled with racism and poverty on a daily basis. While these problems complicated the work of African American AIDS activists—again, many Black AIDS service organizations faced persistent funding problems—they also shaped the way that these activists viewed and responded to the epidemic.[19]

A more recent wave of scholarship has focused specifically on the work of Black gay artists and writers who confronted AIDS. In *The Calendar of Loss* Dagmawi Woubshet examines the work of Melvin Dixon and Assotto Saint within the tradition of Black mourning. Here Woubshet finds a "poetics of compounding loss," in which Dixon, Saint, and others drew on the myriad ways that African-descended peoples in North America have wrestled with the precariousness of life and imminence of death, stretching back to the "many thousands gone" of the Atlantic slave trade. In *Evidence of Being*, Darius Bost similarly examines the work of Black gay artists and writers of the 1970s, 1980s, and 1990s as a site for Black gay community-making and caretaking in the midst of various forms of violence, including AIDS. Rather than write about Black gay life as overdetermined by such trauma, he "reimagin[es] black gay personhood as a site of possibility, imbued with the potential of creating a more livable black gay social life."[20] I likewise pay attention to the ways that African American AIDS activism fostered new ways of understanding the place of queerness and diasporic identity in Black America.

Just as Bost highlights the influence of feminists of color such as Audre Lorde, Barbara Smith, and Cherríe Moraga on Black gay men's AIDS activism, in *Mobilizing New York* Tamar Carroll traces the connections between feminist antipoverty groups and AIDS activist organizations such as the AIDS Coalition to Unleash Power (ACT UP) and Women's Health Action Mobilization (WHAM!). In this way she situates stories of AIDS activism within the larger project of multiracial feminist organizing. The stories in this book similarly flesh out some of those connections while putting African American activists, and occasionally white allies, at the center of the story.[21]

The chapters that follow also extend our understanding of the history of AIDS activism into the twenty-first century. Some of the key work in the field, such as Steven Epstein's *Impure Science*, predates this later period of AIDS activism. Inrig and Jennifer Brier both conclude their studies in the late 1990s, although Brier includes an epilogue on South Africa and the Treatment Action Campaign in the late 1990s and early 2000s. Here she argues that the center of gravity for rights-based activism by people with AIDS has shifted to the global South, and particularly to South Africa, although the story of ACT UP Philadelphia presented in chapter 6 suggests a somewhat different interpretation.[22]

Yet another vein of scholarship has described AIDS as an epidemic of globalization, both in the way that HIV has spread and in the international response to the disease. Genetic analysis of different HIV strains links the emergence of the virus to the Belgian Congo in the early twentieth century. There the colonial regime pushed locals into the jungle in search of chimpanzee meat; a cut or bite very likely allowed a mutated form of the simian immunodeficiency virus to cross over into the human population. From there the virus spread through workers in the rubber and mining industries to Kinshasa, which underwent rapid urbanization in the 1960s. Key to each phase of this story is the social, economic, and political dislocation that brought people in the Congo River delta into closer contact with one another, fostered broader sexual networks among them, and tied central Africa ever more closely to global markets and international affairs. Globalization has also been a key feature of other narratives about the emergence and spread of AIDS, from Randy Shilts's reporting on French Canadian flight attendant Gaëtan Dugas as "Patient Zero" (which has since been debunked) to stories about long-distance truck drivers as vectors of HIV infection in Africa and India.[23]

The international response to AIDS likewise reflects the globalization of the late twentieth century. Here nongovernmental organizations took center stage in the global fight against the disease, with key actors working above and across national borders. As Dennis Altman points out, the fact that many of these NGOs were based in the United States and Europe engendered "the dominance of Western discourses around HIV/AIDS" and thus "the introduction of human rights as a major issue, often linked to the so-called 'new public health' based on ideas of empowerment and community control."[24] As we will see, African American AIDS activists participated in this process and used those same discourses to challenge global capitalism, which fueled the inequities that made the AIDS epidemic worse. As this book makes clear, African American AIDS activists self-consciously used the language of globalization and diaspora to bring attention to the fight against AIDS among people of African descent, both at home and abroad.

In addition to the subject of AIDS history, this book contributes to conversations about the fight for health justice within the Black freedom struggle. From clubwomen in the Progressive Era to the physicians who traveled to Mississippi during the Freedom Summer of 1964, for over a century Black activists have battled inequities in the health and medical care of African Americans. In doing so they framed ill health as embodied racism, calling attention to the ways that discrimination and poverty made Black communities more vulnerable to death and disease. These struggles resonate through the work of the African American AIDS activists who carried on what Alondra Nelson calls the "long medical civil rights movement" by connecting the spread of HIV to myriad forms of anti-Blackness both in the United States and around the world.[25]

This book also joins a rich literature on Black internationalism, which has examined African American engagements with global affairs, including those of Africa and the African diaspora. Throughout this long history the meaning of Africa for people of African descent living in the United States has changed significantly. Some have seen it as a backward and timeless place to be disavowed. Others have pointed to the civilizations of a glorious African past to argue for Black equality in the present. After World War II, liberation movements in Africa inspired Black activists in the United States, who borrowed protest tactics and slogans, as well as music and fashions, from across the Atlantic. Some, particularly those on the Black left, looked not only to Africa but to the broader decolonizing and nonaligned world to forge anti-colonial solidarities.[26]

In their own time, African American AIDS activists also confronted a problem that unfolded simultaneously in their own communities and around the world. AIDS as a global pandemic was tied to Africa and its diaspora from the very beginning—first to Haitians as a "risk group" and then to central Africa as a likely point of origin. To Black observers, it seemed as though white medical authorities were trying to pin the blame for a new and terrifying disease *on them*. As the extent of the AIDS epidemic throughout Africa and its diaspora became clear, denial gave way to interest among African American AIDS activists in fighting the disease in both Africa and the Caribbean. At the same time, some looked to African tradition for values and symbols that would anchor

AIDS prevention and outreach programs in the present. In doing so, they wrote a new chapter in the longer history of Black internationalism.

THIS BOOK PROCEEDS through seven stories, told in seven chapters. Each story illuminates a different facet of African American AIDS activism; together they form a composite portrait of a larger movement.

The organizations that formed early on to fight AIDS in Black communities were responding in part to the failure of predominantly white gay organizations to reach communities of color. Different Black AIDS groups came up with different ideas about how to best reach African Americans, and especially Black gay men, with information about how to protect themselves from the disease. Chapter 1 describes the work of Blacks Educating Blacks about Sexual Health Issues, one of the country's first Black AIDS organizations, under the leadership of Rashidah Hassan, a Black Muslim nurse. Hassan maintained that Black gay and bisexual men could be reached only by canvassing Black neighborhoods outside of the downtown core, which was home to the mostly white "gayborhood." This approach, she argued, additionally would help prevent AIDS among the straight Black men, women, and youth who were also shown to be at increased risk of the disease. But this approach also drew accusations of homophobia and hurt the group's credibility with the Black gay men who were among the most at risk.

Whereas Hassan subsumed gayness within Blackness in her understanding of Black gay men's lives, AIDS organizations that were led by Black gay men saw things differently. Chapters 2 and 3 describe some of their work. The National Task Force on AIDS Prevention (NTFAP) produced some of the earliest knowledge about Black gay men's sexual practices in the age of AIDS through a nationwide survey that it conducted under the auspices of a CDC grant. At the local level, in San Francisco, the NTFAP also forged a multicultural model of AIDS prevention and safer sex education, situating Black gay men within the broader category of "gay men of color." Gay Men of African Descent (GMAD) built on the NTFAP's research, arguing that Black gay men suffered from low self-esteem due to both racism and homophobia, which made them more likely to put themselves at risk for HIV through drugs and unprotected sex. As a remedy, GMAD offered up affirming images of Black gay men, often looking to the past to do so. Discussion topics frequently included homosexuality and queer identity in African and African American history, including Egyptian and Yoruba culture, the Harlem Renaissance, and the life of gay civil rights activist Bayard Rustin. The group also sought to claim a place for Black gay men within Afrocentric ideology, at one point collaborating with the Black Leadership Commission on AIDS to produce an AIDS education and prevention program based on Kwanzaa principles. GMAD leaders argued that these interventions helped equip members with the self-esteem necessary to protect themselves from HIV by practicing safer sex.

From the beginning of the epidemic, African American AIDS activists had to contend with a variety of conspiracy theories, from the idea that the international news media were trying to pin the blame for AIDS on Haiti and Africa, to the rumor that AIDS had been cooked up in a government lab to wipe Black people off the face of the earth. Sometimes AIDS activists themselves propagated these stories. Such was the case with the Nation of Islam (NOI), the subject of chapter 4. Beginning in the early 1990s, NOI leaders became heavily involved in the fight over Kemron, a treatment for AIDS allegedly discovered by researchers in Kenya. They organized trips to Kenya for African Americans with AIDS so that they could be treated with the drug. Once they acquired the stateside distribution rights to Kemron, the NOI also began to advocate for a National Institutes of Health-backed clinical trial to prove the drug's effectiveness. Leaders sent emissaries around the country to speak to local Black community groups about the drug, arguing that, because of its African origins, Kemron would be uniquely suited to treating AIDS among people of African descent. The NOI did finally win approval for a trial in 1992, but the point became largely moot the following year, when the results of another large-scale study found Kemron to be totally ineffective. Nevertheless, the Kemron story sheds light on the complex dynamics within Black communities that have shaped their response to AIDS.

The Nation of Islam was not the only group that looked to Africa in the fight against AIDS in Black America; chapters 5 through 7 describe organizations that likewise connected AIDS at home to the epidemic abroad. One such organization is The Balm in Gilead, which grew out of the efforts of Pernessa Seele, an immunologist at Harlem Hospital, to organize local Black faith leaders to address AIDS. As Seele trained African American clergy to incorporate AIDS education into their ministry, she also confronted entrenched homophobia in Black religious institutions. Accordingly, The Balm in Gilead designed programs that would help churches accept and include gay members. In 2001, Seele contracted with the Centers for Disease Control and Prevention to extend her work with Black churches to sub-Saharan Africa, setting up programs in Côte d'Ivoire, Kenya, Nigeria, Zimbabwe, and Tanzania. She argued that because of Black people's particular relationship with church and faith, the approach that The Balm in Gilead had developed in the United States would work in Africa as well. As a result of the partnership formed with faith leaders in Tanzania, the group now maintains a second headquarters in Dar es Salaam, the country's largest city.

At the same time that The Balm in Gilead was expanding its work to Africa, the Philadelphia chapter of the AIDS Coalition to Unleash Power was becoming increasingly involved in the fight against global AIDS. ACT UP had been the most visible and outspoken AIDS activist group during the late 1980s and early 1990s, winning important victories that helped streamline the process for clinical trials and approvals of new HIV drugs. By 1996, however, most chapters had disbanded. Meanwhile, both white and African American grassroots activists at ACT UP Philadelphia redirected the group's protest politics to address the structural inequalities driving AIDS rates in poor communities of color, both at home and abroad. Just as some civil rights and Black Power activists had linked their own political projects for African American rights to broader anti-colonial struggles, ACT UP Philadelphia members situated their local work in the larger international movement against globalization and free trade. In Philadelphia, they focused on issues of concern to poor people of color with HIV/AIDS, including Medicaid privatization, needle exchange, and access to highly effective but expensive HIV drugs. The campaigns they waged at the local level fed into work on a much broader scale, as members joined forces with anti-globalization groups to protest American free trade policies in Africa. Today, the group claims at least a partial victory in the President's Emergency Plan for AIDS Relief, a massive funding package to support HIV prevention and AIDS treatment in sub-Saharan Africa and other parts of the developing world that have been hit particularly hard by the epidemic.

SisterLove, an Atlanta-based organization that takes an avowedly intersectional approach to fighting AIDS among Black women, also turned its attention to AIDS in Africa during the 1990s. Dázon Dixon Diallo, the founder and CEO of SisterLove, got her start in women's health as a student at Spelman College, where she became involved in the abortion rights movement as well as in the Black women's health movement. Those early experiences would shape her approach to AIDS education through SisterLove, where she took care to include all kinds of Black women in the group's outreach, at times focusing specifically on rural women, recently incarcerated women, and women in public housing. Starting from the notion that AIDS programs for African American women needed to address the ways that their lives were shaped by the simultaneous interlocking oppressions of racism and sexism, Dixon Diallo and SisterLove also considered the ways that other axes of power, including those of class, region, and nation, shaped Black women's experiences with AIDS and thus should shape SisterLove's work as well.

These stories travel around the United States and the globe, from San Francisco to South Philadelphia to South Africa. They proceed roughly in chronological order, from the middle of the 1980s to 2008. Many of them overlap in time, and here and there actors who are at the center of one story pop up in others as well. In this way these stories not only demonstrate the diversity and creativity of African American AIDS activists but also show that their individual work contributed to a larger collective struggle against AIDS in Black America. They reveal that African Americans responded to AIDS at the grassroots level early on and in everyday places—in churches and bars and public housing—and involve some unexpected but nonetheless important actors, such as leaders of the Nation of Islam. They show that African Americans frequently linked the epidemic in their communities to the epidemic in sub-Saharan Africa and to problems of global inequality. If these chapters seem varied and wide-ranging, that is because the same is true of African American responses to AIDS. The work of African American AIDS activists simply has not been recognized, either in popular media or in historical writing about AIDS in Black America. I hope that in this book they receive at least some of their due.

At the same time, I have tried to read the work of African American AIDS activists, whom I admire very much, with a critical eye. Responses to AIDS were and are shot through with homophobia, sexism, classism, and the stigma of addiction; this has at times been true of African American responses to the disease as well. Responses to "global AIDS" have also reflected and reproduced a divide between the global North (wealthy countries such as the United States) and the global South (less wealthy or poor countries in Africa, South Asia, and Latin America).

This book is not exhaustive—it is meant to be *a* book about African American AIDS activism, not *the* book about African American AIDS activism. There are so many other stories about this work that remain to be documented, stories of the everyday activism performed in communities large and small across the country. Future studies might examine the fight against AIDS in Black communities in the Deep South or in the Rust Belt. Others might focus on local battles over needle exchange programs or on advocacy by the Congressional Black Caucus for minority AIDS funding. I hope that future scholars will be able to use this book as a starting point to tell those stories, along with many others.

## CHAPTER 1

## A Disease, Not a Lifestyle

Race, Sexuality, and AIDS in the City of Brotherly Love

R ASHIDAH HASSAN WAS NERVOUS as she waited to take the stage in Philadelphia's LOVE Park on a wet September night in 1986. She knew that the short speech she had turned over and over in her mind would anger some of the crowd gathered for the city's first candlelight AIDS walk. They marched that night to remember the friends, lovers, siblings, and children they had lost to AIDS. Hassan shared their grief. Nevertheless, she was resolute about her message. As board vice president of Philadelphia Community Health Alternatives (PCHA), the parent organization of the Philadelphia AIDS Task Force, Hassan had grown frustrated at her colleagues' response to the growing AIDS epidemic among African Americans and other people of color in the city. During her speech she would resign her board position and call for a new approach to AIDS in the city's Black community.[1]

Hassan[2] presents herself as a lifelong skeptic and iconoclast, although her work has also been driven by a deep sense of faith. She recalls being a "fairly concrete thinker" even as a child, when she earned trips to the pastor's office at her Baptist church for "disrupting Sunday school by asking these very complex questions that the teachers didn't know how to answer." Curiosity led her to explore other faiths—Judaism and then Islam, to which she converted. She found the religion attractive because it emphasized "service to humanity, which tied back to my nursing, which was service to humanity, . . . in ways of care and treatment . . . which after a bit expands itself into social care and public health. And so there I landed, exactly where I was supposed to be, and in the midst of all that up came the HIV epidemic."[3]

That "exactly where" turned out to be a hospital room at Einstein Medical Center in the Germantown neighborhood of Philadelphia, where during the early 1980s she worked as an infectious disease nurse. One of the first African Americans with AIDS she encountered was a young man who had dropped out of high school and was living in poverty. He most likely contracted HIV either from the older men who paid to have sex with him or by sharing needles when injecting the drugs that he bought with their money. Either way, he landed in Hassan's hospital when his kidneys stopped working; they were clogged with the cornstarch he used to cut his drugs with before shooting up. Hassan recalls that as she entered the young man's hospital room, she found a horde of doctors, residents, and medical students, all looking at him "as a specimen." "They literally said to him, 'Your kidneys are shot. We're going to put you on dialysis, you have AIDS, and," gesturing to Hassan on their way out, "she's going to tell you what you need to do next." Hassan asked the patient if he understood. He replied, "My kidneys don't work. I'm not sure about what dialysis is, and I don't know whatever else it was they said."[4]

In the young man's hospital room, Hassan glimpsed the future of AIDS in the United States. Her patient—impoverished, "functionally illiterate," infected with HIV through drugs or sex work, and disregarded by his doctors—embodied the myriad ways that social, economic, and medical inequities would fuel the AIDS epidemic in Black communities. At that moment, Hassan realized "that this would be more likely the kind of people that would develop AIDS and HIV, and they would die not understanding anything that happened to them." In fact, the disease had already begun to "settle" in Philadelphia among the city's Black and Latino residents, and especially among those who were already poor and disenfranchised.[5]

Unlike San Francisco or New York, each of which is the setting for one of the chapters to follow, Philadelphia is neither a gay mecca nor a global capital of finance and culture. However, Philadelphia *is* a major city, home to over 1.5 million people. Its response to the AIDS crisis in the 1980s illustrates the ways that the postwar fate of many American cities shaped a growing epidemic. Like other urban centers in the Northeast and Midwest, Philadelphia was scarred by segregation, white flight, deindustrialization, and disastrous urban renewal schemes, which left the city with an eroded tax base and dwindling coffers on the eve of the AIDS crisis. Cities like Philadelphia were epicenters of the early epidemic but, thanks to systematic abandonment and disinvestment, lacked the resources to mount an effective response.[6]

At the same time, a vibrant gay and lesbian scene flourished in Philadelphia during the decades following World War II. Downtown Philadelphia emerged in these years as the nexus of local gay life, where gay bars, cafés, and shops near Washington Square and along Spruce Street coalesced into an enclave known as the "Gayborhood." Here, during the 1960s and 1970s, gay men and lesbians in Philadelphia began to organize for sexual freedom. Some groups, such as the Philadelphia Gay Liberation Front, were quite racially diverse;

others less so. In 1974 a group of mostly white gay and lesbian activists tried—and failed—to pass a bill through the city council that would add sexual orientation as a protected category under Philadelphia's Fair Practices Ordinance. The bill was defeated in no small part due to the united opposition of the city's Black clergy, who thoroughly rejected the activists' argument that homophobia was akin to racism. By the early 1980s, leaders of the Philadelphia Lesbian and Gay Task Force came to recognize the importance of racial diversity to their organizing strategy and accordingly built bridges to local Black gay activists. When a second nondiscrimination bill came before the city council in 1982, it passed. Wilson Goode, the city manager of Philadelphia, testified in support of the bill. The following year, with backing from the city's gay and lesbian community, he became Philadelphia's first African American mayor.[7]

Nevertheless, the "city of brotherly and sisterly loves" remained divided by race. The downtown gay scene comprised mainly white men, while Black gay men and lesbians instead set up their own social clubs in West Philadelphia. When Black gay men went out drinking and dancing downtown, they faced discrimination at bars that catered to white gay men. A bouncer might ask them for multiple forms of identification while letting white gays who appeared to be underage enter freely. Black gay men who did get inside reported being served last by bartenders and ignored by white patrons. The problem was not limited to Philadelphia; Black gay men in other cities described similar experiences with racial discrimination.[8]

As a result, a handful of bars catering mostly to Black gay men had cropped up in Center City by the early 1980s, including Smart Place near Tenth and Arch, Pentony's near Thirteenth and Arch, and Allegro II at Twenty-First and Sansom. However, as Black gay activist Arnold Jackson noted, "If blacks think they are escaping oppression by going to these bars, they are truly mistaken." Black gay men decried the bars' white owners for their "apparent refusal to spend money on upkeep." Philadelphia's gay bars, it seems, were both separate and unequal.[9]

Moreover, the treatment that Black men received at the city's gay bars was emblematic of a racial tension that suffused the community as a whole. Black gay men in Philadelphia reported that their white counterparts viewed "blacks as being inferior or less intelligent or sex objects." Others reported being made simply to feel invisible. Joseph Beam, a Black gay writer who lived in Center City, described being ignored by his "mostly young, white, upwardly mobile" neighbors, except when they wanted to see "if I had any reefer."[10]

Black gay men and lesbians felt similarly marginalized in local gay politics. In a 1986 letter to the gay newspaper *Au Courant*, Don Ransom, a Black gay man, criticized the "plantation mentality" in Philadelphia's gay and lesbian community. He pointed to the lack of local Black gay speakers at a protest organized by the Philadelphia Lesbian and Gay Task Force in response to the Supreme Court's decision to uphold state anti-sodomy laws in *Bowers v. Hardwick*. The group had invited Gil Gerald of the Washington, D.C.-based National Coalition of Black Lesbians and Gays to speak at the event, but Ransom saw this as evidence that the Philadelphia Lesbian and Gay Task Force "had to go out of town and find someone who wouldn't know about their behavior or their exclusionary policies."[11]

Racial divisions in gay Philadelphia were exacerbated by the role that gay men played in gentrifying Center City and the surrounding neighborhoods beginning in the 1960s. As they moved into the area around Washington Square and along the South Street corridor, they drove out residents who were disproportionately Black and working-class. Gay men were not the sole participants in the "back-to-the cities" movement that brought young, upwardly mobile professionals to the urban core. However, newspaper coverage framed the new urban residents as bourgeois sissies, describing the "quiche-and-fern bars" that they brought to neighborhoods like Queen Village, which bordered Center City along the Delaware River.[12]

Through both discrimination and gentrification, white gay men marked their downtown enclave as a space for affluent and middle-class whites. For Black gay and bisexual men in particular, the whiteness of the Gayborhood's bars and clubs also extended to its political institutions. This would have significant consequences for the way those same men, along with other Black Philadelphians, understood their risk for AIDS. With a cash-strapped city and with state and federal officials largely unwilling to address an epidemic associated with gay men and drug users, groups rooted in the Gayborhood took on the work of responding to a growing public health crisis. The whiteness of early AIDS groups in Philadelphia also reinforced the idea within the city's Black community that AIDS was primarily a *white* gay disease. As the disproportionate impact of the new disease on African Americans became clear, activists challenged local AIDS groups to improve their minority outreach.[13]

In the ensuing debates over Philadelphia's AIDS response, issues of race, sexuality, and the division of urban space took center stage. The predominantly white gay AIDS groups that grew out of the Gayborhood argued that prevention efforts should be focused on the bars, bathhouses, and bookstores that anchored gay life downtown. After all, gay and bisexual men made up the overwhelming majority of people with AIDS in Philadelphia. But critics, including Rashidah Hassan, argued that these groups failed to reach *Black* gay and bisexual men, who appeared to be at greater risk. For Hassan it was race, not sexuality, that structured Black gay men's daily lives. She argued that

Black gay men would best be reached by canvassing the Black neighborhoods that lay to the north, west, and south of Center City, and in 1985 she founded Blacks Educating Blacks about Sexual Health Issues (BEBASHI) to do just that.

Hassan's approach represented a view of Black gay identity that emphasized racial solidarity over sexual difference, one that was shared by at least some Black gay activists in Philadelphia. Yet this represents just one of the ways that African American AIDS activists made room for queerness within prevailing ideas about Black community and identity. As we will see in later chapters, other groups took diverging approaches.

## One New Case per Week

As in other cities, Philadelphia's first response to the AIDS epidemic came from within the predominantly white gay community. In 1979, gay health activist and regional health commissioner Walter Lear founded Lavender Health, a gay and lesbian community health group, which was renamed Philadelphia Community Health Alternatives in 1981. The following year, as reports of a new and deadly "gay cancer" began to spread, PCHA members formed the Philadelphia AIDS Task Force, a volunteer group dedicated to fighting the disease. Task force members distributed educational materials outside gay bars, operated an informational hotline, and provided "buddy" services to those who had become sick and had trouble caring for themselves.[14]

The downtown gay enclave in which the PCHA and the AIDS Task Force were found was in many ways a segregated neighborhood and was perceived as a specifically white space, especially by the Black gay men who felt excluded from it. As a result, gay men in Philadelphia developed overlapping but distinct racial and sexual geographies. Black and white gay men tended to live, work, and play in different parts of the city, or at least in different clubs downtown.[15]

Even as public health reports began to show that a disproportionate number of African Americans in Philadelphia were succumbing to AIDS, the Gayborhood's reputation as a specifically white space shaped the way that Black gay and bisexual men understood their own risk for the disease. In July 1983, Don Ransom and Len Bost, both members of the local Black and White Men Together (BWMT) chapter, told the *Philadelphia Gay News* that even as statistics showed that half of the city's cases were among African Americans, other Black gay men regarded AIDS as "a white man's disease." Both men urged the AIDS Task Force to reach out to the city's Black and Latino communities.[16]

The following year, the AIDS Task Force launched its "One New Case per Week" campaign to inform the public that AIDS affected all racial groups. It produced posters with three different faces—one white, one Black, and one

Latino—along with a tagline about the rate of new AIDS diagnoses in the city. Perhaps in a deliberate attempt to push its message beyond Center City and transcend the city's neighborhood divisions, the group placed the posters on Philadelphia's subway system.[17] Tyrone Smith, a Black gay activist, remembers, "They used to have on the subway . . . these posters up, and it would be how many folks had become infected within that week or within that month. And I started seeing these white faces . . . and then I got appalled one day when I saw Black faces there. I thought it was the enemy, I thought it was a trick, I thought that . . . if anybody was to get AIDS, it would be the Black children who fucked with white men."[18]

As Smith's story suggests, in the early days of the epidemic some Black gay men saw themselves as being insulated from the new disease. Jose de Marco, a Black and Latino queer[19] Philadelphia native, similarly remembers that "gay black men . . . thought this only happened to nasty gay white boys because [they] do nasty, dirty things. But in reality, a lot of black men and white men were having sex." For Black gay men, deflecting the identification of AIDS as a gay disease onto gay white men may have been a way of showing their frustration with racism and segregation in the downtown gay community, as well as a way to counter the historical association of Blackness with hypersexuality and disease. In framing AIDS as a white gay disease, Black gay men flipped the script on both their own mistreatment in the Gayborhood and centuries-old racist stereotypes.[20]

The "One New Case per Week" campaign angered other Black Philadelphians for the same reason. Task force president Nick Ifft defended the campaign to the *Philadelphia Tribune*, the city's oldest and widest-circulating Black newspaper: "Many of the calls we received suggested that we are doing something which is not true, but our reason for using three different images (Black, white and Hispanic) is because all people can get AIDS." Those viewers who objected to the posters saw them not as evidence of the disease's morbid equanimity but as a white organization's attempt to demonize African Americans by associating them with the epidemic. Given their initial relief—in the words of local AIDS activist Linda Burnette—that "finally it's something that's not about Black people," to learn that African Americans were also at risk would seem to be a terrible reversal of fortune. As Smith suggests, some saw it as a "trick," possibly one masterminded by some powers that be, to pin the blame for the epidemic on Black people.[21]

The AIDS Task Force also worked with the Philadelphia chapter of Black and White Men Together, an interracial gay men's group, to produce "Respect Yourself!," an educational rap single about AIDS that was aimed at African Americans. The record was funded by a grant from the United States Conference of Mayors and released in 1985, with an initial run of five hundred copies to be distributed to radio stations and dance clubs frequented by Black gay men. The project would come to be viewed as a flop: commercial radio stations in Philadelphia never played "Respect Yourself!," and the AIDS Task Force ended up selling copies at cost out of its Center City office. Don Ransom thought that the record's lyrics had been too explicit, while others thought that "Respect Yourself!" had been too much like "a Sesame Street rap," with the lyrics

> Be you a butcher, a baker, a candlestick maker
> AIDS don't care about the color of your skin
> You gotta keep your body strong
> Respect yourself and you will live long.

PCHA executive director Thomas Livers would later be accused of sitting on money left over from the grant because the AIDS Task Force "never took the rap record project seriously."[22]

When the PCHA and the AIDS Task Force did reach out to minority communities, their efforts were often frustrated. When Len Bost tried to distribute the task force's AIDS education literature at downtown Black gay bars, he was rebuffed. Some turned him away outright, while others threw the materials away as soon as he left. Although Bost himself was Black, this was apparently not enough to overcome the AIDS Task Force's reputation for not being "integrated," as one Black gay bar patron asserted, or its association with discrimination in the Gayborhood as a whole.[23]

Detractors of PCHA and the AIDS Task Force also saw these efforts as insufficient: some posters and a song would hardly make a dent in the growing AIDS epidemic among Black Philadelphians. Critics called on the groups to improve their minority outreach efforts. Some worked within the organizations. These included activists like Tyrone Smith, who joined Interpreting Minority Perspectives for Action (IMPACT), a volunteer committee within the task force that aimed to expand AIDS education for communities of color in Philadelphia. They also included Rashidah Hassan, who joined the task force as a volunteer around 1984 and became vice president of the PCHA board in May 1986. Around the same time, she and Wesley Anderson, who had experience tracking sexually transmitted diseases as a public health adviser for the Centers for Disease Control, founded BEBASHI, one of the nation's first Black AIDS service organizations. Others remained outside the PCHA and the AIDS Task Force. They included David Fair, a white gay man and member of BWMT/ Philadelphia who worked as secretary-treasurer of District Local 1199C of the Healthcare and Hospital Workers Union. Members of the union, who were mostly Black, had encountered some of Philadelphia's first AIDS cases while working in the city's hospitals. Fair, a political firebrand, often found himself at odds with the city's gay community leaders over what he saw as their racism and classism.[24]

From within and without, critics of the PCHA and the AIDS Task Force demanded greater minority representation among the groups' clients, volunteers, and staff. They argued that the agencies, which were made up primarily of white gay men, should look more like the AIDS epidemic in Philadelphia, where more than half of all people who had been diagnosed with AIDS were nonwhite. However, critics sought more than token representation of African Americans within the PCHA and the AIDS Task Force. They felt that more minority volunteers, staff, and leaders at the agencies would yield more effective AIDS services for people of color. For example, if the AIDS Task Force recruited more Black operators to its AIDS hotline, African Americans would be more comfortable calling and more likely to believe the information they received. Black volunteers for the buddy program would likewise be more sensitive to the needs of Black people with AIDS. Tyrone Smith recalls,

> [Gay white men with AIDS] were the Center Citiers, the Main Liners, they were the affluent who were being stricken with this disease. And what was being said to them is, "We want you to live a normal life, as normal as your life has been." Well, going to brunch was common for them, but going to brunch wasn't something my boys did. They just wanted a couple of dollars to go to a movie and basic stuff like that. So it was us who had to say to institutions, "Okay, well, but this is what these guys need." He wants a hoagie! I mean, he doesn't want truffles and luffles and luffles. He wants a hoagie, and he wants it where he wants it from.[25]

Here Smith frames the difference between Black gay men with AIDS and their white counterparts in terms of space and class, while his comments about brunch and "truffles and luffles" recalls the gentrifying "quiche-and-fern" set. To be sure, not all gay white men with AIDS took home hefty paychecks or lived in upscale parts of the city. That Smith associates white gay men with the Main Line, a wealthy white suburb disconnected from Center City and not known for having a visible gay presence, reveals the overlapping geographies that shaped Black gay men's sense of where they did—and did not—belong in the city. These in turn shaped their relationship to the PCHA and the AIDS Task Force.

Indeed, the debate over whom the agencies served was linked to the question of where their efforts should be concentrated. Critics and allies alike framed this question in terms of how race, sexuality, and class mapped onto

Philadelphia's physical geography. David Fair saw this as part of the problem of a local gay "movement" concerned only with advancing the interests of those who already enjoyed proximity—literally and figuratively—to power: white, middle-class, and affluent gay men and lesbians in Center City. As Fair told Dan Daniel, host of the local radio show *Gaydreams*, in 1985,

> The fact is that in Center City if you are gay, you can get information on "safe sex" and you can get information on AIDS. . . . But if you're a black kid who lives up at Broad and Columbia, or if you're a white kid who lives in Roxborough or K&A [Kensington and Allegheny], you can't get that information. . . . People are dying as a result of our racism, people are dying as a result of our elitism, and they're dying as a result of our lack of courage in being able to develop real strategies and real commitment, to involve people outside of the barriers that have been set up for us so far.[26]

Fair criticized the city's gay political leadership for focusing on the needs of gay "yuppies" in Center City while ignoring working-class and minority neighborhoods to the south, north, and west. Whether minoritized gay people had been shut out of the downtown by historical segregation, high rents, or outright hostility, they remained outside the orbit of the PCHA and the AIDS Task Force. For Fair, the failure of local gay rights and AIDS groups to reach beyond the Gayborhood evinced a deadly lack of political will, rooted in bias. Like Smith and other AIDS activists, Fair challenged the PCHA and the AIDS Task Force over questions of whose interests they represented and how their resources should be distributed.

The AIDS activists who attended BEBASHI's meetings around this time reflected this sense of division between a mostly white downtown, including the Gayborhood, and the rest of the city. Two extant sign-in sheets from BEBASHI meetings show that only about one out of six of those in attendance lived in Center City, while most of the rest lived in West or North Philadelphia. The location of the meetings is unclear, but around this time BEBASHI was using office space in the headquarters of David Fair's Healthcare and Hospital Workers Union at 1319 Locust Street, in the heart of the Gayborhood. Thus, it seems reasonable to assume that the location of the meetings does not explain the relatively low number of attendees from Center City.[27]

As the number of AIDS cases in Philadelphia grew, pressure for change at the PCHA and the AIDS Task Force mounted. But even those who agreed that a problem existed did not necessarily agree on a solution. Cei Bell, a Black transgender journalist who reported on charges of racism within the AIDS Task Force for the *Philadelphia Gay News* in April 1986, suggested that Black gays organize within the gay and lesbian community. She noted that bringing

Black gay men into an organization like the AIDS Task Force would be challenging but stressed the importance of Black and white gays alike laying aside their differences to work toward common goals. "It is not as though," she warned, "there are so many of us (both black and white) or as though we are so invulnerable we can not be eliminated en masse." Bell saw AIDS as bringing a "bizarre equality to the gay world that has never existed," by striking down people regardless of class, education, or race. In this new context, she argued, "we can no longer afford the luxury of fighting with each other."[28]

Rashidah Hassan, quoted in Bell's piece on racism at the AIDS Task Force, took a different stance. She argued that the AIDS response in Philadelphia reflected and reinforced patterns of inequality. Nevertheless, she allowed that the exclusion of people of color from the task force "hadn't been intentional" but rather resulted from white gay men's blindness to those outside their downtown gay enclave. But Hassan also argued that becoming involved with a gay-identified organization could put Black men in a precarious position: "Once you step out you label yourself. If you separate yourself from the black community, where does that leave you? In the black community, what affects one of us affects all." She argues now, as she did then, "It's not like saying, 'Oh, we'll go to the Gayborhood.' There's no black Gayborhood, so I've got to do the whole community, to make sure the most at risk hear the message." According to Hassan, AIDS educators would have to canvass the entire African American community in order to reach not only Black gay and bisexual men but also those who had sex with men but did not identify as gay or bisexual, as well as their potential female partners, who were also at risk of contracting HIV.[29]

David Fair, who was also quoted in Bell's piece, insisted that Executive Director Tom Livers hire someone "with proven community organizing skills in Philadelphia's black and Hispanic communities." Anything less would amount to nothing more than "pious proclamations" falling far short of a genuine effort to address AIDS among people of color in the city and indicate that the AIDS Task Force failed to take seriously the needs of Philadelphia's minority communities. For this reason, Fair remained reluctant to cooperate with Ifft and Livers in recruiting Black volunteers to the AIDS Task Force. In March 1986, he announced at a meeting of Black and White Men Together for Education, an offshoot of the interracial social group, that he had met with thirty-five Black members of his union "who were angry at having lost . . . lovers, friends, or family members to AIDS." When asked why he "kept those people in his hip pocket" while calling for the AIDS Task Force to improve its minority relations Fair replied, "I don't believe that the structure of the gay and lesbian community works for black people, and I will not input them into that structure."[30]

Bell, Hassan, and Fair each presented a somewhat different diagnosis of the AIDS Task Force's minority outreach problem, along with a different so-lution. Bell saw racism in the gay community as a problem of interpersonal relations: some white gay men were certainly racist, but closeted Black gays should overcome their personal misgivings so that they could join the "out" gay community in addressing a terrible crisis. Hassan and Fair argued that by concentrating its efforts in the Center City gay community from which it emerged, the task force failed to reach gay men in the city's minority and working-class white neighborhoods. Hassan contended that Black gay men lacked their own autonomous spaces and thus would be best reached when entire Black communities were canvassed. Fair, on the other hand, sought a movement by and for those who fell outside the white middle-class model of organizing presented by the downtown gay community, even as he pressed Ifft and Livers to hire someone to coordinate the task force's minority outreach.

Critics of the AIDS Task Force also focused on the question of funding. They argued that because the agency received money from city contracts and block grants, it should serve people with AIDS across lines of race, gender, sexuality, and neighborhood. A week after running Bell's piece on racism within the AIDS Task Force, the *Philadelphia Gay News* reported that Fair's union was considering a lawsuit against the group under the 1964 Civil Rights Act, which prohibits discrimination by institutions receiving federal funding. Similarly, a leaflet produced by Fair titled *Don't We Die Too?*, accused the task force of not using $100,000 of received public funds (a number disputed by Nick Ifft) to "serve the needs of the majority of people with AIDS" in a city where over half of the AIDS caseload was nonwhite. At a public meeting hosted by 1199C to discuss the leaflet, Darlene Garner, who served with David Fair as cochair of BWMT for Education, proposed that concerned people of color could continue to press the AIDS Task Force on minority outreach while setting up parallel services through Black churches. To this Gwendolyn Johnson, the chair of the meeting and an 1199C member, responded, "We don't want to do that. The Task Force has money. We want to get our share." Johnson stressed that she was concerned with the AIDS Task Force's funding sources and client popula-tion because, she said, "it's our tax dollars, too."[31]

Some white gay men who volunteered with the AIDS Task Force took excep-tion to the criticism. In a letter to Nick Ifft published in *Au Courant*, David Wentroble, a Presbyterian minister in Devon, a township outside of Philadel-phia, criticized Fair's allegations of a "racist attitude" at the agency. He took these "as a personal insult and an affront." Wentroble, who identified himself as a "suburban white middle-class gay professional," wrote that he had become involved in the AIDS Task Force "to help my community." Wentroble had ini-tially been paired with a young Black man, who had passed away, then with a two-year-old Black boy and the boy's family. He wrote that he had been "apprehensive at first" but was "blessed" to "have had my eyes opened about how people much different from myself live." When Wentroble described wanting to help his community by volunteering with the AIDS Task Force, these had not been the people he originally had in mind. Although he found some sense of connection with the toddler and his family, Wentroble's comments reveal that they were decidedly not part of the community that he had set out to help.[32]

Wentroble's letter points to the source of complaints against the task force as well as to white gay men's anger at the criticism. His lack of familiarity with his clients' culture and lifestyle—by his lights, "much different" from his own—speaks to the lack of and need for specific services for people of color with AIDS. He framed his volunteer work as providing an opportunity for personal growth, but how did the people with whom he was paired experience the encounter? Perhaps they sensed his wariness at working with them. For critics, this would be evidence of racism at the task force, but for Wentroble, his own story belied charges of bias. For him, racism would have meant denying services to African Americans, which the task force clearly did not do. As a volunteer and part of the task force's "community," Wentroble took the charge of racism personally, and Fair's allegations in particular left him "infuriated."[33]

By the fall of 1986, the two sides in the fight over minority AIDS education in Philadelphia had reached an impasse. Although the AIDS Task Force planned to hire a minority outreach coordinator, Rashidah Hassan had grown tired of fighting for change within the organization, where she often felt like the agency's "colored poster child." Hassan decided that she would publicly resign from the PCHA board in September 1986, during her speech at a rally following the city's first candlelight AIDS walk. She thought about the text of her speech that day as she bought a huge candle for the event—black in contrast to everyone else's white and large enough to make a statement. That evening, she marched through rain showers with over two thousand others, many holding signs stenciled with numbers to represent those who had died. Together, they walked to LOVE Park, where the assembled crowd waited to hear from a slate of speakers, including a woman who had recently lost her son to AIDS. Hassan felt guilty; as the mother of two young boys, she felt she had some insight into the other woman's pain. Hassan recalls that she approached the woman near the podium and explained, "I had a very painful task that I was assigned, and . . . nothing that I was going to say should reflect negatively on her son, or her grief . . . but . . . there was a socio-political statement that I needed to make in order to save the lives of others." According to Hassan, the woman hugged her and replied, "We all have to do what we have to do."[34]

When her turn came, Hassan stepped behind the podium, placed the giant black candle in front of her, and laid into the city's AIDS services establishment. She directed her criticism at the AIDS Task Force and the white gay community it represented by insisting, "Our people . . . have the right to be educated, have the right to have resources committed, have the right to stand here with you and say that we are dying from this disease and you are making it our disease." Since the task force "didn't, couldn't, haven't, won't provide education for the minority community," she had founded her own group, BEBASHI, to do so. Hassan and her BEBASHI colleagues had worked with the AIDS Task Force to improve the older organization's minority outreach but to little effect. In her speech she warned, "If in your presentations . . . you don't remember the Hispanics and you don't remember the Blacks, I guarantee you—I guarantee you we will be there to haunt you for it." She knew that her criticism of the AIDS Task Force, which provided much of what few local services were available, would anger some but told the audience, "I want you to be upset, [and] turn that energy to committing yourselves to seeing that minority people obtain the same treatment, the same empowerment to suffer from this disease and get away from it, to have health care, as you have." She ended on a conciliatory note: "I want you to remember that while you're fighting, there are those who are different from you who need to have a voice in how things are done . . . because they do not recognize that it is not just a white gay disease, and I ask your help and your support in trying to provide that information to that community."[35]

Today Hassan remembers this as her "Malcolm X speech," an "intense" piece of oratory that "was a little graphic about bending black butts over and feeling free to bang them without giving them the information or the protection they needed." However, a video recording of the rally shows that Hassan's speech contained no such language. She appears forceful and resolute, but not bombastic, in her criticism of the city's AIDS establishment. In the video, at least some audience members appear to cheer her on, shouting, "Tell 'em about it!" and "That's right!" Michael Hinson, who as a young Black gay man attended the rally and became an early BEBASHI employee, recalls, "I just haven't heard that many speeches where people have been so purposeful, so thoughtful, so powerful, but at the same time, so passionate and embracing."[36]

Looking back on that moment through the turmoil that came afterward likely makes the speech seem much more contentious in retrospect and helps explain why Hassan now frames it as "the skirmish of the war" for minority AIDS education in Philadelphia. After she split from the PCHA and the AIDS Task Force to pursue her own work with BEBASHI, Hassan drew fire for "creating division within the community." But just a few years later, as a greater number of specialized AIDS groups came on the scene, she became the target of the same criticism that she had once leveled at others.[37]

Although the crowd at the vigil seems to have been vocally supportive, the negative reaction to Hassan and her speech was almost immediate. A week after the march, the *Philadelphia Gay News* ran an angry opinion piece by Bill Whiting, a white gay visual artist who had designed the AIDS Task Force's "One New Case per Week" posters. Whiting criticized the event as a whole, and Hassan in particular, for her "intolerable" speech. He questioned the route for the march, which began north of Center City outside the State Office Building at the intersection of Broad and Spring Garden Streets before heading south to Benjamin Franklin Parkway and City Hall and finally to LOVE Park for the candlelit rally. The starting and ending points for the march were meant to draw attention to the lack of city and state funding for AIDS services. However, the route also intentionally avoided Center City; women on the march planning committee objected to the idea of a route along Spruce and Pine Streets, which cut through the heart of the Gayborhood, because those streets were "too white gay male." With statistics showing the disproportionate impact of AIDS on Philadelphia's minority communities, including women of color, march organizers wanted to disentangle the disease from its close association with white gay men and to portray the epidemic as "a growing concern that would effect [*sic*] everyone, not just gays."[38]

In comments to a *Philadelphia Gay News* reporter, Whiting insisted that the Center City neighborhood the march organizers had avoided was, in fact, diverse, with residents who were "blacks, whites, men and women, gay and straight, and families of a variety of ethnic backgrounds." From his perspective, a Center City route would have reached people from different walks of life. Instead, the march had gone "past bombed-out building sites, industrial warehouses and vacant lots," where "few people worth reaching live." He saw this decision as yet another example of Philadelphia gays "trying to be all things to all people at all times," lamenting, "We couldn't even do this thing right and remember our own in the setting where they had lived most comfortably."[39]

By "we," Whiting meant the AIDS Task Force and Center City's largely white and middle-class gay community. Though he excoriated many of the rally speakers as "blathering, ill-prepared, and often destructive," he heaped special scorn on Hassan, who "proved to be no friend to either the gay or the black community by acting out her own therapy at everyone's expense." He painted her as an interloper at the PCHA and the AIDS Task Force of whom he had only recently become aware when she "appeared on the scene to unleash venom for an unclear purpose," despite his having worked with both organizations for four years. He compared her to David Fair, "Philadelphia's own version of the Reverend Jim Jones," and warned readers not to "accept Kool Aid from either of them."[40]

Although Hassan and Fair criticized the Philadelphia AIDS Task Force for not doing enough outreach to the city's African American community, Whiting insisted that the group used half of its time and money "to help blacks." He meant this point not as a defense of the group but as a criticism—another example of the downtown gay community trying to be "all things to all people." Given that most of the volunteers at the AIDS Task Force were white and that "middle class white gay men . . . carried the financial burden of AIDS in Philadelphia," he argued that the group had a greater claim to AIDS services. To drive home his point, he asked readers to consider, "When was the last time that half of the monies and efforts by any black organization were used to further the health and welfare of whites?"[41]

For Whiting, the AIDS epidemic in Philadelphia was synonymous with its Gayborhood and the decision to hold the walk and vigil elsewhere, along with Hassan's critical speech, betrayed the memory of friends already lost to AIDS. With this view, Whiting ignored the constellation of factors that produced the Gayborhood as a white space. Those same factors in turn marked AIDS as a white gay disease, which made it difficult for PCHA and the AIDS Task Force to reach Black gay and bisexual men, much less the rest of Philadelphia's Black community. Even if statistics showed that people of color were disproportionately dying of AIDS, many white gay men in Philadelphia *felt* the epidemic most strongly in the ways that it cut down friends and lovers in their prime and threatened their own lives. Meanwhile, the epidemic raged in the city's poor and Black neighborhoods outside of Center City.

Hassan departed PCHA just as the AIDS Task Force finally hired a minority outreach coordinator as part of the agency's full-time paid staff. Delays in hiring someone to fill the post had been a source of animosity between Livers, who thought the funds to pay the salary of the new position should come from city block grants, and Fair, who argued that public funding obligated the agency to provide more meaningful outreach to communities of color. In early October, District Local 1199C hosted a reception for Ted Johnson, with speeches by Hassan and Fair, as well as by Tyrone Smith and Curtis Wadlington, two IMPACT members who had helped to interview Johnson for the position. Smith would go on to start his own organization for Black gay men, Unity Incorporated, while Wadlington would become a key early member of BEBASHI. At the reception Wadlington struck a conciliatory note, affirming, "We are all committed to something—services to persons with AIDS." Others pointed to the enormity of Johnson's task. Leon Bacchues, a Black gay man who served as secretary of PCHA's board, admitted that he had no idea how to educate the city's Black community about AIDS but offered his "professional and personal commitment to be with [Johnson] because he can't do it by himself."[42]

Johnson would hardly get a chance. The following February, after six months on the job at the AIDS Task Force, he was dismissed from his position and replaced with Wesley Anderson, who had cofounded BEBASHI with Hassan in 1985 but had resigned from that group's board due to internal politics. Johnson had recently criticized the task force in an interview for continuing to do a "fantastic" job for its white clients while providing "unequal and uneven" services to the city's Black and Latino communities. Johnson claimed that he gave the interview out of frustration after "not getting any results" from his new boss, Francis Stoffa, who had replaced Tom Livers as executive director of the AIDS Task Force. Stoffa claimed that Johnson had simply reached the end of his probationary hiring period and declined to further "discuss personnel issues or respond to complaints from a disgruntled employee."[43]

In contrast, an anonymous "advocate" of Johnson explained to the *Philadelphia Tribune* that Johnson had "brought about his own demise . . . by being outspoken . . . about the lackluster support he charged the group gave to educating" minority communities. Fair, speaking on the record, accused the organization of hiring minority staff and creating Johnson's program only out of fear of losing some of the $400,000 they received annually from the city. According to Fair, Black employees held little to no power at the AIDS Task Force; Johnson complained that he "did not even have a say-so in budgetary matters," while IMPACT, a committee of volunteers, held greater decision-making power at the agency. As a result, Johnson's program suffered from a lack of funding: on top of his own $25,000 salary, the AIDS Task Force set aside only $10,000 for minority outreach out of its $519,000 budget.[44]

Anderson remembers the Task Force differently. Whereas Nick Ifft was "a real great guy," David Fair "would put you on the outs" if you disagreed with him. The PCHA and the AIDS Task Force "did all that they could," he recalls, because "not one agency could do everything." When he replaced Ted Johnson, Anderson says, "there was never . . . [a] reflection of bias or anything like that, because they told me, 'We really don't know how to reach the black community.'" Even though during this time his "heart was always with BEBASHI," he recalls, "it got really bad, politically, and at times it made me feel a little uncomfortable."[45]

Indeed, Hassan and her allies continued to sharply criticize the AIDS Task Force and saw Johnson's unceremonious departure as evidence of the agency's racism. BEBASHI's 1986 annual report, released not long before the firing, charged that PCHA and the task force had been unable to overcome their "inherent limitations" as organizations "centered in [an] openly gay community that is overwhelmingly white, educated, and employed." According to the report's authors—presumably Hassan and Curtis Wadlington, the IMPACT member who had become BEBASHI's program director that October—Black employees such as Johnson had been hired "only as a result of intense political and community pressure," and their presence reflected no real change in the groups' power structure, since "PCHA/PATF [Philadelphia AIDS Task Force] continues to allow no meaningful black involvement in its leadership or decision-making." Even IMPACT, the minority outreach committee within the AIDS Task Force, served primarily "to provide a token black presence in PCHA/PATF in order to silence critics within the organized gay community of historical racism at PCHA/PATF."[46]

Beyond criticism of any one program, Hassan and Wadlington laid out a view of AIDS in Philadelphia that overlaid race and sexuality with urban space. As before, they argued, "For the most part, black communities do not segregate themselves by lifestyles; instead, people of all types and conditions live together in one community." Historically, this had been the key to collective survival in the face of enormous adversity. But while groups like the AIDS Task Force had apparently convinced many white gay men to adopt safer sex practices by reaching out to the public and commercial spaces where they congregated, the absence of a "clearly defined 'black gay community'"—bars like Smart Place and Pentony's notwithstanding—meant that "the only way to stop the spread of AIDS among non-whites is to orient AIDS education efforts to the *entire* non-white community." Hassan and Wadlington argued that the problem lay not only in the different structure of communities of color but in the way that minority gay men and other men who have sex with men (MSM) thought of themselves, since "*the primary characteristic of the communities most at risk of AIDS in Philadelphia is that they are black and Latino,* and that their homosexual/bisexual preferences are secondary factors from a public health education perspective." If race superseded sexuality as the salient category of identity for many gay men and MSM of color, Hassan and Wadlington argued, those men would respond better to prevention and education efforts targeted to minority communities than they would to those aimed at gay or bisexual men.[47]

Here Hassan and Wadlington deployed a vision of same-sex male desire in African American communities that resists easy characterization through gay or bisexual men driven to life "on the down low" by Black homophobia. To be sure, they acknowledged homophobic attitudes in communities of color as a significant barrier to AIDS prevention and education, just as homophobic attitudes in American politics and society more generally forestalled an effective and deliberate response to the epidemic at all levels of government.[48] This view was based, at least in part, on the authors' personal experience. Curtis Wadlington remembers a flamboyantly gay man with AIDS, a beloved and important part of the neighborhood, whose longtime partners also had wives and steady girlfriends:

> When Tommy died from AIDS . . . I went to preach his funeral, and I was standing there looking out, and I mean the neighborhood was devastated. The girls who were going with these guys were devastated because he was the one that kept their men responsible to them and their kids. This gay man now, that they'd been screwing since they were little. All of this dynamic is going on, and I said, "Somehow I've got to let them know that this is nice, this is good, this is beautiful, but there's something else. Tommy got AIDS, y'all. And y'all got to think about that. He did half this audience, and y'all did all of them women."[49]

The story of a Black openly gay man with AIDS who was nevertheless valued by his community points to a more complicated lived experience than caricatures of vitriolic Black homophobia and "down low" men. For Wadlington, the tension between racial and sexual identity was reflected in his choice to live in a mostly Black neighborhood, which was a source of conflict with openly gay African Americans as well:

> I said, "I don't think that promoting my sexuality as a feature of who I am should be in the front. 'Hi, I'm Curtis. And it ain't none of your business who I fuck. Is there anything else you want to know?' Because I'm not politically gay, I don't live in a gay community, most of my friends are not gay. So according to you, I'm not." And when I got into the community and found out what was going on, oh damn no, I don't want to be. I don't want to even be Black and gay, because you all let this shit go on. I can't believe that you all ain't had no riot or protest, and this has been going on this long. And most of the guys that I grew up with never considered themselves gay. Some got married, and you know, they did, and then they stopped and they didn't. But what I always knew was, I would be judged for being an African American man before I would for being gay. And then I said to myself, "That's who I am."[50]

Tyrone Smith describes himself in a similar way: "My sexuality is cute, my ethnicity is *wonderful*. Because my culture gives me the sustaining forces that are in my genes, in my DNA, that brought my ancestors from the Middle Passage to here. . . . But I celebrate the fact that whoever that was in my lineage that made it to this soil, and seeded on this soil, I am of them. They are me. We are one. That gives me a deep sense of humbleness, gratitude, and pride . . . it's the essence of who I am."[51]

BEBASHI did not dismiss the toll that AIDS was taking on the city's minority gay men and MSM but subsumed sexual identity within a constellation of other factors driving the epidemic. While white gay men were learning to protect themselves from AIDS and incorporating lessons about safer sex into their daily lives, their Black and Latino counterparts were not. The reason for their continued risk stemmed not primarily from their sexuality, Hassan and Wadlington argued, but from a host of other social pressures and inequities. Hassan and Wadlington predicted—correctly—that "without an urgent shift in the direction of AIDS policy, funding, education and service efforts, AIDS will become a disease identified mostly with the poor, with the non-white, with the uninsured and under-insured, with the uneducated and illiterate, with the homeless and outcast." Although it had initially been framed as an epidemic among white gay men, they insisted, "AIDS is a disease, not a lifestyle."[52]

## Anybody Can Get AIDS

Through BEBASHI, Hassan and Wadlington set about implementing their vision of AIDS education for Philadelphia's Black community. That meant expanding the conversation to include women, youth, and residents outside the Center City Gayborhood. BEBASHI volunteers and outreach workers held AIDS Awareness Days, which "resemble[d] neighborhood block parties," at public housing communities around the city. By October 1989, the group reported that "tenant councils at virtually all PHA [Philadelphia Housing Authority] developments have acted as hosts to BEBASHI at sometime [sic] during the past year." BEBASHI workers also regularly attended health fairs at local schools to raise awareness of the epidemic and produced *Choices*, an educational play about teenage sexuality in the age of AIDS at Freedom Theatre in North Philadelphia, the oldest African American theater in Pennsylvania.[53]

BEBASHI additionally included Black gay and bisexual men in their AIDS prevention efforts through the Brother to Brother program, which offered the *Hot, Horny and Healthy!* "playshop"—a safer sex workshop designed to be sexy and fun as well as educational—at gay bars frequented by Black men. Brother to Brother outreach workers and volunteers also sought out men cruising for sex or drugs late at night in Center City and West Philadelphia, distributing "survival packets" that contained literature about AIDS, condoms, and bleach that injection drug users could use to sterilize their needles.[54]

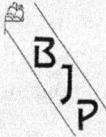

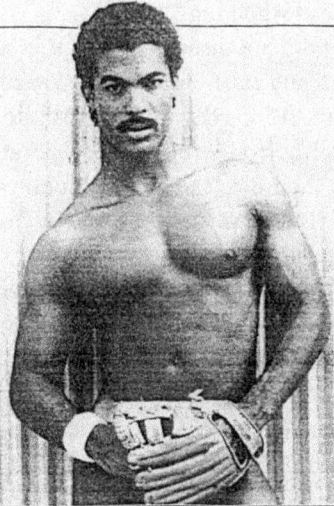

BWMT/PHILADELPHIA
will be hosting a
Hot, Horny and
Healthy Playshop on
Friday
November 9th
7 to 10 p.m.
at Bebashi
1528 Walnut Street
Suite 200
call
John Speer 692—6610
Hal Carter 546—4140

A SECOND HOT, HORNY & HEALTHY PLAYSHOP
WILL BE HELD ON
TUESDAY
NOVEMBER 13th
8 p.m.
AT Restaurant and Lounge
5300 Market Street
Philadelphia, PA 19139
BAR (215) 747-4953
Resturant (215) 747-4958
Disco (215) 748-5778

## Hot, Horny & Healthy!
### A Fun, Safer Sex Playshop
Come See How Great Safer Sex Can Be...
...In a Safe & Sexy Yet Non-Sexual Experience

FACILITATOR TRAINING SESSION
FOR THE HOT, HORNY & HEALTHY PLAYSHOPS
WILL BE HELD AT BEBASHI
10 to 4 p.m.
SATURDAY AND SUNDAY
NOVEMBER 10th &11th
You should also attend the Friday Playshop if you intend to be a facilitator.
All groups and organizations are encouraged to attend.
Please RSVP for the training session.

WE HAVE ARRANGED THESE EVENTS TO COINCIDE WITH THE PAINTED BRIDE'S
LIVING LEGACY PROGRAM
Some of us will attend the Bride's program at 8 p.m. Saturday evening.

Sponsored by: **bwmt** **BEBASHI**
Black and White Men Together—Philadelphia
1528 Walnut Street • Suite 1414
Philadelphia, PA 19102

National Task Force on AIDS Prevention
of the National Association,
Black and White Men Together

with funds from:
Phila. Department of Health and the Centers for Desease Control.

Flyer advertising the *Hot, Horny & Healthy!* playshop, sponsored by Black & White Men Together/Philadelphia, BEBASHI, and the National Task Force on AIDS Prevention, 1990. BEBASHI (Philadelphia, Pa.), Ephemera files, Ms. Coll. 35, John J. Wilcox Jr. Archives, William Way LGBT Community Center, Philadelphia, Pa.

Likewise, Hassan and her staff targeted the groups considered the most "hard to reach" for AIDS education: sex workers and drug users. In a 1992 radio interview Hassan insisted that the two groups were "not that difficult to talk to." By hanging out on street corners, BEBASHI outreach workers became a visible presence in the community and got to know the women plying the sex trade. Having established a rapport and some trust, they could offer condoms, answer questions, and teach the women how to negotiate safer sex with their customers. Personal relationships also mattered in getting access to the drug houses where needle sharing and HIV transmission took place. "We're familiar with people who do drugs in our community, we're familiar with people who run drug houses," Hassan told Terry Gross of NPR's *Fresh Air* radio program. BEBASHI staff and volunteers used that familiarity to gain entrée into places that other health workers could not in order to teach drug users how to steril-ize their syringes with bleach and to warn them about the danger of sharing needles.[55]

But these efforts to reach those who had been stigmatized and marginalized sometimes clashed with BEBASHI's own educational materials. In a training manual for BEBASHI volunteers compiled in July 1986, Hassan explained the disproportionate impact of AIDS on African Americans by arguing that "some within the African American community have adopted the social mores of the 'majority,' as indicated by the increases in cases of other sexually trans-mitted diseases and adolescent pregnancies." As a result, she continued, "the eventuality of AIDS entering the black population in even larger numbers is a real threat unless vigorous and aggressive educational action is taken." Here Hassan, like Tyrone Smith and Jose de Marco, flipped the script on stereotypes of Black sexual pathology. The problem, she suggested, was not Black sexuality but rather its white counterpart. But in doing so, she reinforced the dominant view of AIDS as a punishment for sexual immorality.[56]

The group's early brochures similarly played into the discourse of guilt and innocence that stigmatized those who had contracted HIV through sex or drug use. Several featured images of Black children, since at the time the major-ity of pediatric AIDS cases in the city were African American. One brochure paired the message "Anybody can get AIDS. Anybody," with a photograph of two Black children. The brochure itself was aimed at an adult audience; its message was that Black children were under threat. A similar brochure, emphasizing basic AIDS information and prevention techniques, paired the message "You don't have to be white or gay to get AIDS" with a drawing of a young Black boy. The brochure appeared to be aimed at heterosexual African Americans and emphasized basic AIDS information and prevention methods.

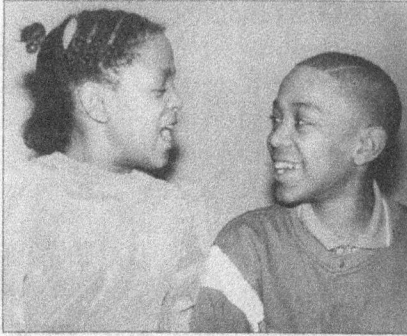

# Anybody can get AIDS.

## Anybody.

## Getting AIDS isn't easy.

And while the doctors and researchers study the virus that has been linked to AIDS, BEBASHI (Blacks Educating Blacks About Sexual Health Issues) knows there's another, equally important reason for why AIDS is reaching epidemic proportions — especially among Philadelphia's non-white communities.

Ignorance.

Because if you don't know how to protect yourself against AIDS, you're a lot more likely to get it. No matter how old you are.

## Getting AIDS isn't easy. Protecting yourself is.

It's so easy **not** to get AIDS, if you only know how. And BEBASHI tells that simple, life-saving message wherever it goes.

In churches. In community centers. In the schools. On the streets. Wherever the message that will save lives needs to be told, we'll tell it.

But we need your help.

Because even though most of the people in Philadelphia getting AIDS are non-white, education and service programs aimed at Blacks and Latinos have had to go begging.

We need your time, your energy, your money. We need you to care.

Please fill out and return the form on the reverse side to **BEBASHI, 1319 Locust Street, Philadelphia, PA 19107**. Or call 546-4140 for information or referrals.

TOMMOROW! SUPPORT THE WDAS 1480 AM AIDS RADIOTHON 581-2100 9 AM-9 PM

Promotional and educational flyer produced by BEBASHI, ca. 1987 Scott Wilds Papers, SPC MSS PP 061, box 4, folder "AIDS in Phila 1984–87," Temple University Manuscript and Special Collections, Philadelphia, Pa.

BEBASHI also used the same drawing of the boy's face on its reports and letterhead throughout the later 1980s and early 1990s, making childlike innocence the face of the organization. Another brochure produced slightly later used a different cover image, borrowed from a poster produced by Baltimore's Health Education Resource Organization. The image shows a Black woman cradling a toddler. Her blouse, pearl earrings, and hairstyle suggest gentility; given that BEBASHI sought to reach women in public housing projects, women's shelters, and on street corners, such a figure may have come across as more aspirational than relatable. In this way the image of Black respectability might have cut through denial about the epidemic among middle-class African Americans but also may have made it harder for poor and working-class Black women to recognize their own HIV risk.[57]

These brochures were not intended to educate children about AIDS. They were designed to capture the attention of Black adults by presenting the disease as a threat to children. Again, this was not without reason. The majority of pediatric AIDS cases in Philadelphia were Black, although the overall number (a total of five in the city as of April 1987) was still low. But by using images of children at risk to shock adults into awareness, BEBASHI reproduced the notion that some AIDS "victims" were innocent and others guilty. Children, as a powerful cultural symbol of innocence, had to be protected from those guilty others: the man "stepping out" on his wife and kids, the woman who contracted HIV through sex work or shared needles, or the predatory homosexual. That BEBASHI paired the image of a child with the message "You don't have to be white *or gay* to get AIDS" only reinforced the idea that gay men represented a guilty threat to "innocent" and "normal" people.[58]

After Hassan's break with PCHA, BEBASHI grew quickly, with support from disparate sources. Sponsorship from the Urban League resulted in a grant from the Philadelphia Foundation to cover the group's operating expenses, and District Local 1199C provided office space to the fledgling group. Meanwhile, a temporary position at the Philadelphia Department of Health kept Hassan afloat financially until she could draw a salary from BEBASHI. In its first two years the group held a jazz festival and birthday fund-raisers to bring in donations, but these paled in comparison to the amount of money that the AIDS Task Force could attract. While birthday parties for Don Ransom and Charlotte White, a Black community activist, brought in a combined total of around $2,000, a prom-themed fund-raiser for the task force housing program raised more than three times as much money and a benefit performance of *La Cage aux Folles* ten times as much. As Ransom told *Au Courant* in 1987, "BEBASHI doesn't have the resources or base of well-off supporters that other AIDS organizations have, so it's important that all of us do what we can individually to make sure that minority concerns around AIDS are addressed."[59]

That would soon change. In 1988 BEBASHI was awarded a five-year grant through the CDC's National AIDS Information and Education Program to help grassroots minority groups in Pennsylvania, New Jersey, Delaware, Maryland, and Virginia develop their own AIDS programs. The CDC grant, along with city contracts and private foundation funding, propelled BEBASHI through a

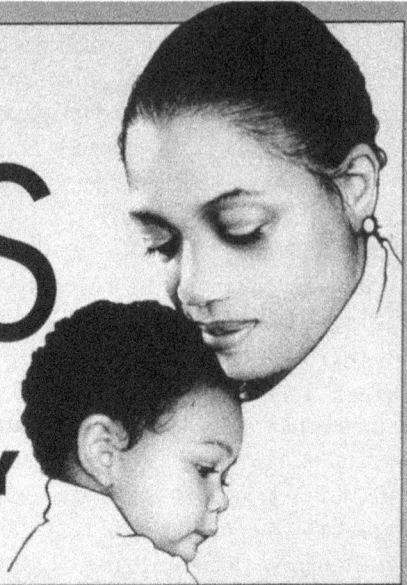

AIDS education poster produced by the Health Education Resource Organization (HERO) of Baltimore, Maryland, ca. 1987. BEBASHI used the same image of a Black woman and child for the cover of a pamphlet produced ca. 1988. U.S. National Library of Medicine Digital Collections.

growth spurt. By 1991 the group had a staff of thirty-five and an annual budget of over $1 million.[60]

BEBASHI drew international attention as well. Curtis Wadlington recalls that before long, "the Africans started calling us and saying, 'Can you teach us?' And we said, 'Nobody can do this in Africa!' And they said, 'You don't understand. The village is just like the hood.'" According to Wadlington, the framework of BEBASHI's approach would work elsewhere, so long as the programs were tailored to the language and culture of local communities: "We talked to [them] for hours about targeted, specific education, what things you add to the presentation, what things you highlight, and how to make them educational, and how you have to make the cultural connection first." BEBASHI's African contacts, according to Wadlington, "immediately understood that the message—they didn't know how to express it as 'targeted' or 'specific,' but they knew that this message couldn't be universal."[61]

Wadlington saw what AIDS programs developed for "the hood" looked like when they were translated to "the village" during a symposium on AIDS education in Yaoundé, Cameroon, in October 1989. "They did these little plays," he remembers, "because that's what was the culture of the village, they were used to that. But how they did them and who the characters were, and the language they used, all of that structure they got from us." According to Wadlington, the trip "made me understand how important preservation of culture was to them. So when I started to talk about AIDS, they immediately got it, that if we don't do this, all of this is gone, will disappear." He tells a story from his trip to Cameroon about an encounter that drove home the importance of culture to the fight against AIDS:

> There was one village in Cameroon I went to, and they took me to this giant stone. I mean, it was huge, it was maybe as big as two stories, and it had all these etchings on it. And the guy called this little boy who was three years old, and he said, "Watch this." And he said something to him and the little boy went up on the smaller rock on the side of this bigger one, and started putting his hand there. And he said, every kid here knows where his family began, from the eleventh century to today. And I went, "Goddamn, that's some powerful shit."

BEBASHI, Wadlington realized, was "right on track" in paying attention to culture as "a vehicle for the communication of important information. . . . Because it worked with Black people everywhere. And then we found out it wasn't just Black people. It worked with any minority group. Any group that you worked with, targeted specific education was really the hallmark, and it still is."[62]

Indeed, BEBASHI became an important model for other minority AIDS organizations, both locally and around the country, driven in no small part by Hassan's personal magnetism and no-nonsense approach to AIDS education. Carmen Paris of Programa Esfuerzo, a Latino AIDS group based in North Philadelphia, modeled her agency's one-on-one education program after BEBASHI's, crediting Hassan as a personal and professional mentor. Some of Hassan's staff ventured out to start their own organizations, as Michael Hinson did in 1991 when he founded COLOURS, a community empowerment group for LGBT people of color.[63]

But Hassan was not without detractors, who saw her as "arrogant" and called her a "diva." Moreover, as BEBASHI grew quickly, the group could no longer claim outsider status among Philadelphia's AIDS service organizations. David Fair moved into a new post as head of the city's AIDS Activities Coordinating Office in late 1987, which gave Hassan a key ally in city government but invited charges of political patronage because of their close working relationship. Nine months into his tenure in that position, a *Philadelphia Gay News* editorial criticized Fair for funding BEBASHI, claiming that the group had an "atrocious" record on outreach to Black gay men and IV drug users. Newer AIDS groups also found themselves competing with the former upstart for funding, creating resentment that echoed the conflict between Hassan and the AIDS Task Force just a few years earlier. Critics charged that Hassan had become part of the very system she railed against, while from her perspective the new groups were redundant in an already crowded field of service providers.[64]

For critics, Hassan's decision in 1988 to move out of the cramped 1199C offices to a separate space at 1528 Walnut Street, a stone's throw from the tony condos overlooking Rittenhouse Square in Center City, epitomized BEBASHI's transition from ingenue to insider. Fair was among these, accusing his former ally of "basically decid[ing] her survival means doing the bidding of a white AIDS bureaucracy not particularly sensitive to the black community's needs." Hassan shrugged off such criticism: "Center City is the seat of power. You cannot interface with power from out there in North Philadelphia."[65]

Nevertheless, the work and the criticism took their toll. "I get overwhelmed sometimes," she told the *Philadelphia Inquirer Magazine* in 1990, "like I'm rushing against the onslaught of a tidal wave." The problems that BEBASHI's outreach workers and Hassan herself encountered on any given day—teen pregnancies, a growing syphilis epidemic, crack cocaine, and a social safety net being deliberately unraveled at the highest levels of government—would be enough to disenchant even the happiest of warriors, and all pointed to a deepening AIDS epidemic in Black America.[66]

To cope, Hassan packed her days full of meetings, workshops, and conferences. The busy schedule kept her from dwelling on the bleak outlook for her community or on the number of dead and dying among the friends she had made through her work with BEBASHI. Long days and a busy travel schedule meant time away from home, her husband, Nimr, and her sons, Jameel and Bashir. During one conference presentation in 1990 she broke down crying, telling the audience, "I am a workaholic . . . I don't know how to say no." Still, the prospect of walking away seemed far worse. "I can't stop," she insisted, "because maybe I'm the finger in the dike."[67]

The CDC grant that BEBASHI received in 1988 also greatly expanded the scope of its work, from educating Philadelphia's communities of color about AIDS to helping grassroots organizations across a five-state area develop their own AIDS programs. That work meant more travel and an even greater burden on Hassan. Paula Michal-Johnson, a professor of communications who evaluated BEBASHI under a grant from the American Foundation for AIDS Research, found that Hassan and the agency were "given more than they could handle." It is easy to see why Hassan would want her organization to take on such an enormous task. The CDC grant brought needed funds to the fledgling agency, albeit with a vastly increased scope of work. Black communities across the country were being devastated by AIDS because, as Hassan saw it, they hadn't been given the information they needed to protect themselves from the disease. BEBASHI had made some headway in Philadelphia—shouldn't Hassan teach others how to do the same?[68]

Even as BEBASHI was hailed as "one of the most successful grassroots organization of its kind," cracks in the facade began to show. The agency had grown "far faster than most organizations do" and lacked the accounting expertise to keep track of the money coming in. The move to 1528 Walnut Street had plunged the group into debt almost immediately. Before long, BEBASHI was using grant money to cover what it owed. When the landlord at 1528 Walnut tapped the agency's bank account to pay back rent, BEBASHI shifted incoming funds to another nonprofit organization, the William J. Craig Foundation. Employees lost their health insurance when BEBASHI stopped paying the premiums. The chaos fueled low morale at the agency, which experienced high turnover among both the staff and members of the board, who accused the management of being "contentious, misleading, and generally inadequate." In the spring of 1993, BEBASHI filed for bankruptcy.[69]

Michael Hinson, who had left BEBASHI to form COLOURS, also criticized BEBASHI for being "less and less interested in the gay and bisexual community" as it grew. The Brother to Brother program had ended in 1991 with the resignation of Hal Carter, leaving BEBASHI without a program dedicated to men who have sex with men. In responding to this criticism, Hassan explained that Hal Carter had not been replaced due to BEBASHI's money troubles but allowed that as of late 1993 no "self-identified" gay men had worked at BEBASHI for over a year.[70]

BEBASHI's last-minute decision to cancel a conference in October 1993 on AIDS education for Black gay men fueled more accusations of homophobia. The conference, organized by Curtis Wadlington, was to bring together COLOURS, Adodi, and Unity Incorporated, three local groups serving Black gay men, for training with Gavin Morrow-Hall of the San Francisco-based National Task Force on AIDS Prevention. BEBASHI's image had been severely tarnished by this point; according to Morrow-Hall, "A lot of people had reservations working with BEBASHI." Financial difficulties were not the only reason for the group's bad reputation. Cliff Rawlins of Adodi remarked, "I don't know how [Wadlington] got appointed in charge. He doesn't have a good reputation with African-American gay and bisexual men."[71]

When it came to the office space at 1528 Walnut, "friends and critics agree[d] that the move into expensive Center City office space triggered the group's financial collapse." Hassan admitted that the move had been a mistake but defended her decision. "Why is it that minority groups can't be downtown?" she asked. "I still think we had to be at the crossroads of the city. Otherwise we would be just a North Philadelphia or West Philadelphia AIDS group."[72]

Reporting on the BEBASHI story trafficked in familiar anti-Black stereo-types. Echoing the "welfare queen" narrative that Ronald Reagan first popu-larized during his run for president in 1976, the *Philadelphia Inquirer* reported that "once BEBASHI got money, its tastes got expensive." The paper also noted that Hassan wore "stylish suits," suggesting that the executive director had used the agency's funds to expand her wardrobe. The fact that BEBASHI em-ployed Hassan's husband, mother, and older son didn't help matters, although the executive director insisted that she had neither personally hired nor di-rectly oversaw any of them. Indeed, Hassan's mother, Gwendolyn Jackson, was widely seen as "one of the most effective staff members."[73]

By all accounts neither Hassan nor anyone else on BEBASHI's staff had expe-rience running a major agency or managing multiple large grants. Perhaps no one at BEBASHI grasped the depth of the agency's dire straits until it was too late. Perhaps the professional plaudits and rapt audiences that greeted Hassan at AIDS conferences made it easy to ignore her own group's mounting prob-lems. Maybe the seventeen-hour days that distracted Hassan from the death and dying around her also kept her from thinking about the deepening fault lines within BEBASHI, which she had built from her kitchen table to one of the country's premier AIDS agencies in the space of less than a decade.

Hassan defends her actions as BEBASHI's executive, arguing that the choices she made brought a measure of financial security to her employees, who came from the community she so wanted to serve. In a 2012 oral history interview, she recalled, "I made a decision, with the understanding of my board, that if I have a staff of poor people who have jobs and families, and have been able to buy homes, am I going to make a choice between making sure their payroll is in, or paying the IRS?" She also insists that she didn't "run off with any dollars": "I didn't have a luxury home, I didn't have a big fabulous car, I rode the subway with everybody else."[74]

Curtis Wadlington similarly recalled being poor during his time at BEBASHI, when he was living off of food stamps and sleeping on a friend's couch. He also remembered the personal cost of AIDS work: "We were willing to give up anything. Rashidah broke up her damn marriage. I didn't have no damn relationships. You couldn't. It tore apart our families. She went through it. They wouldn't let her in the mosque to pray because she was 'messing with them faggots,' as they said. I went to preach and I remember the guy grabbing the back of my coat and said somebody had just told him that I did work with the sissies. In the middle of me preaching. I mean, we went through hell, but we wouldn't give up."[75]

Hassan resigned as BEBASHI's executive director in June 1994, and by the end of the year the organization had reached an agreement to pay off its debts. In the meantime, the group continued to provide HIV testing, counseling, and education. Gary Bell took over as executive director of the group in 1996 and remains in that position as of this writing.[76]

BY 1984 THE DISPROPORTIONATE impact of AIDS on Philadelphia's Black community was apparent. Some Black Philadelphians, mainly gay men or those working in medicine and public health, mobilized to draw attention to the growing epidemic and to demand resources for minority AIDS programs. Their efforts yielded BEBASHI, the nation's first Black AIDS service organization, which quickly became an important resource for others in the fight against AIDS. Half a decade later, minority prevention and education had become a key part of AIDS services in Philadelphia, with funding from the city's AIDS office. This was a testament to the difficult work of Hassan and her allies, if also to the growing AIDS epidemic in Philadelphia's communities of color. However, even though a general consensus within the city's AIDS service structure had been reached on the need for minority education and prevention programs, major disagreements remained about what such efforts should look like.

Such disputes stemmed largely from Black communities' complicated relationship to the new disease. In part, that relationship had been shaped by the initial identification of AIDS as a disease of white gay men, combined with homophobia in Black communities. However, that relationship was also shaped by the spatial disconnect between white gay community groups in the downtown core and more geographically marginal groups to the north, south, and west. Historical patterns of segregation and racism had produced different models of sexual identities and subcultures in Philadelphia's Black and white communities, with a mostly white gay enclave downtown, while Black gay men and women tended to live in neighborhoods defined by race rather than sexuality. In order to be credible to people of color, BEBASHI and its allies had argued, messages about AIDS would have to come from trusted sources within minority communities. However, as BEBASHI grew in size, moved downtown, and became integrated into the city's AIDS services structure, some critics contended that the organization could no longer claim the authority to do grassroots minority outreach. As before, communal identity, spatial politics, and the distribution of power and resources within the city shaped ideas about how to address the epidemic among Black Philadelphians.

In doing this work, BEBASHI argued that while Black gay men might be gay, they were primarily in and of Black communities. Others agreed. As Tyrone Smith put it, "My sexuality is cute, my ethnicity is *wonderful*." Certainly, many Black gay men in Philadelphia felt as though they didn't belong in the Gayborhood, although many also felt that they did not belong in the city's Black community, either. In this way BEBASHI claimed a space for Black gay men in Black communities while at times glossing over the homophobia that they experienced from other African Americans. Nevertheless, BEBASHI was part of a larger wave of Black gay organizing in Philadelphia. While Unity, Incorporated emerged from Tyrone Smith's work at IMPACT, COLOURS came out of Michael Hinson's work at BEBASHI. These were not the first or only Black gay groups in the city, but they made up a more visible, organized, politically powerful Black gay presence emerged in response to the AIDS crisis. As we will see, other groups articulated very different ways of linking Blackness and gayness to make the wounded whole. At the same time, BEBASHI's local efforts drew international attention, as Curtis Wadlington's trip to Cameroon makes clear. There he found that what worked in terms of AIDS education in "the hood" also worked in "the village"—a complicated claim to be sure, but one that prefigured the expansion of other African American groups into the fight against AIDS in Africa.

## CHAPTER 2

# Nurturing Growth in Those Empty Spaces

## Blackness and Multiculturalism in AIDS Education

R EGGIE WILLIAMS GREW UP in Cincinnati, the second oldest of nine children. His mother, Jean Carpenter Williams, "struggled long and hard to raise her nine kids by herself" in Washington Terrace, a public housing project that would later be torn down to make way for Interstate 71. Although Reggie Williams later recalled that in the project "there was a real sense of care and concern for your neighbor," it was also "an environment characterized by sub-standard housing, poor education, [and] lack of health care." The family was no stranger to tragedy: Reggie's older brother was murdered, and he lost another to prison. Jean Williams passed away in 1990, her "life cut short by cancer, which could have been treated if she had had proper access to health care." Reggie Williams knew what it was like to find community in the midst of hardship. He learned early on, as the saying goes, to make a way out of no way.[1]

Reggie Williams also knew from an early age that he was attracted to other boys. He "liked to do things that were very un-boy like," such as playing with his sister's dolls and combing his mother's hair. Tall, lanky, and dark-skinned with "nappy hair and big lips," he felt self-conscious about his appearance as an adolescent, and later found confidence in the Black Power rallying cry that "Black is beautiful." In the early 1970s he and a boyfriend moved to Los Angeles, where Williams hoped to become an actor or a model. He posed for *Playgirl* as a "guy next door" in 1979 and supported himself by working as an X-ray technician at Cedars-Sinai Medical Center. Around this time he met Tim Isbell, a white musician. Williams left his boyfriend to be with Isbell, and in 1981 the couple moved to San Francisco.[2]

In San Francisco Williams and Isbell joined the local chapter of the National Association of Black and White Men Together (NABWMT), the same group that later produced "Respect Yourself!" with the Philadelphia AIDS Task

Force. Black and White Men Together was a new organization at the time, having formed in San Francisco the year before Williams and Isbell arrived. Michael Smith, who was white, founded the group in part to meet other gay men interested in socializing and dating across the color line. For this reason, BWMT earned a reputation among some Black gay men as a haven for white "race fetishists." But the group also confronted racism in gay communities, such as the discrimination found in Philadelphia's Gayborhood. (Recall that BWMT for Education pressured the Philadelphia AIDS Task Force to expand its outreach to the city's Black community.) At the same time, San Francisco was more diverse than the name "Black and White Men Together" would suggest, with sizable Mexican, Chinese, and Filipino communities alongside whites and African Americans. Williams would become one of the country's most recognized AIDS activists, and San Francisco's multiracial environment would shape his activism in important ways.[3]

Williams began working in the radiology department at the University of California Medical Center. Part of his job was to administer X-rays, including the chest X-rays used to diagnose AIDS-related pneumonia. At that time, Williams and Isbell's friends were beginning to get sick and die from the new disease. In 1985, Williams helped found the AIDS Task Force of BWMT/San Francisco to "address the unmet needs of the non-white community in the present AIDS situation." Williams also became involved with other local minority AIDS efforts, including the Kapuna West Inner-City Child/Family AIDS Network, a group "committed to AIDS research education and prevention for black populations," and the Third World AIDS Advisory Task Force, which pushed for AIDS outreach to communities of color in San Francisco more generally.[4]

As Williams became more involved in AIDS activism, his own health began to fail. He felt tired all the time, and his already slender frame was shedding weight. Based on his symptoms, a doctor diagnosed Williams with AIDS-related complex in 1986. Williams took an HIV test to prove the doctor wrong, but the test came back positive. At first Williams "wanted to die, to let go." But soon, he later recalled, "my commitment to being involved in this epidemic deepened and I knew I had to do more. Now I had a different story to tell."[5]

Williams became outspoken as a Black gay man living with AIDS. He spoke to high school students about the disease and redoubled his efforts to educate other Black gay men on how to protect themselves from HIV. He shared this commitment with other members of the NABWMT national board, who wanted to integrate the work that Williams and other were doing in San Francisco around AIDS with similar activities by chapters in New York, Los Angeles, and Memphis. They saw the national organization's network of local groups as a way to scale up AIDS prevention programs to reach BWMT members across the country. In 1988 they applied for—and received—$200,000 in CDC funding through the National AIDS Information and Education Program. The grant, which was expected to be renewed annually over a period of five years for a total of just over a million dollars, established the National Task Force on AIDS Prevention as a project of the NABWMT.[6]

The NTFAP functioned as both a national training and advocacy group and a local AIDS service organization. It conducted a nationwide survey—the first of its kind—to find out how much Black gay and bisexual men knew about AIDS and what they were doing to protect themselves in the epidemic. NTFAP leaders also traveled the country to train BWMT members and other Black gay groups on how to facilitate *Hot, Horny and Healthy!*, a safer sex "playshop" targeted to Black gay and bisexual men, and developed other workshops focusing on Black gay men's self-esteem, HIV testing, and living with AIDS. Beginning in 1990 they organized the annual Gay Men of Color AIDS Institute, a conference where minority AIDS advocates from across the country could learn about strategies for fighting the epidemic in their own communities. Finally, the NTFAP partnered with other national organizations, such as the Black Gay and Lesbian Leadership Forum and the National Latino/a Lesbian and Gay Organization, to develop AIDS programs for their constituent communities.

Locally—that is, in the San Francisco Bay Area—the NTFAP also divided its efforts between programs specifically targeted to Black gay and bisexual men and those geared toward gay and bisexual men of color more broadly. Staff and volunteers targeted Black gay bars for condom "zaps" and designed an interactive video kiosk to teach Black gay men how to negotiate condom use with their sexual partners. Given San Francisco's racial and ethnic diversity, the task force pursued a multicultural model of local AIDS organizing as well. In 1989 the group joined several others, representing Latino, Asian American, and Native American gay and bisexual men, to form the Gay Men of Color Consortium (GMOCC). Out of "a shared sense of oppression" this larger group "developed cooperative strategies" to raise awareness about AIDS among gay men of color as a whole while finding "culturally sensitive and linguistically relevant" ways to educate members' respective communities about HIV/AIDS.[7]

This focus on Black gay men as a subset of gay men of color distinguished the NTFAP from other groups. In contrast, Blacks Educating Blacks about Sexual Health Issues located Black gay and bisexual men within the Black community as a whole and thus worked in Philadelphia's African American neighborhoods and institutions. Gay Men of African Descent, the subject of the next chapter, looked to Afrocentrism to "make the wounded whole" among Black gay men as well as to structure and guide AIDS prevention efforts, while the NTFAP framed the needs of Black gay and bisexual men in the AIDS epidemic

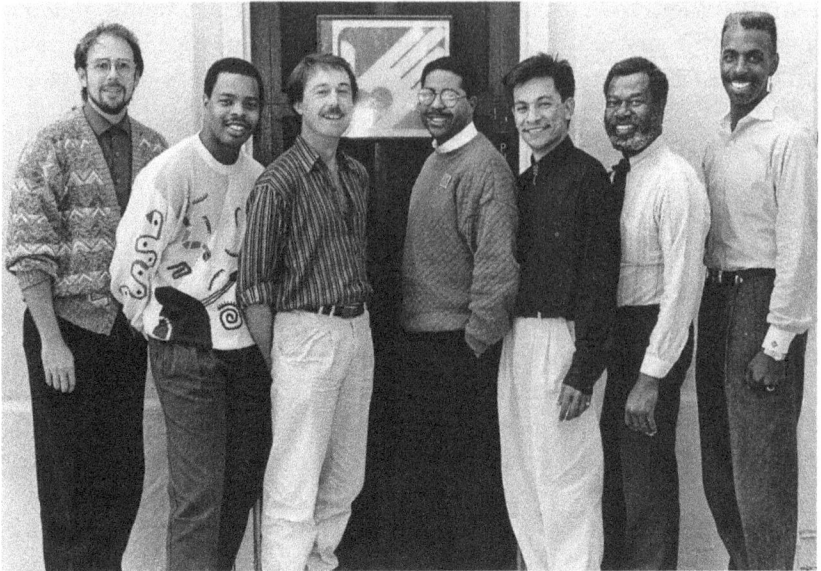

National Task Force on AIDS Prevention staff, 1991. *From left to right*: Alan McCord, Gavin Morrow Hall, Steve Feeback, Al Cunningham, Juan Rodriguez, James Fonduex, and Reggie Williams. Photo by Michael Emery. Courtesy of National Task Force on AIDS Prevention Records (2000-59), Gay, Lesbian, Bisexual, Transgender Historical Society.

as part of the needs of gay men of color more broadly. Of course, these strategies were not mutually exclusive. Rashidah Hassan saw her work as largely applicable to the needs of other communities of color and mentored Carmen Paris as the latter woman founded Programa Esfuerzo. George Bellinger also served as a Gay Men of African Descent board member while working as director of education and public information for the New York–based Minority Task Force on AIDS, which continues (as of this writing) to fight the epidemic across communities of color as FACES NY. For its part, the NTFAP sometimes framed its work in Afrocentric terms and named its technical assistance program for southern Black gay groups the Ujima Project after the Kwanzaa principle of "collective work and responsibility." Together, these groups point to the different ways that African American AIDS activists balanced interventions grounded in specific ideas about Blackness with collaborative approaches involving other communities of color.[8]

The NTFAP story also speaks to the changing politics of race in the 1980s and 1990s. As the United States underwent tremendous demographic change following the Immigration and Nationality Act of 1965, so too did Americans' vocabulary for talking about racial solidarity and difference. As discussion of the United States as a "multicultural" nation proliferated, so did confusion about the term's meaning and potential as a framework for community organizing. Activists and scholars alike asked themselves whether multiculturalism was "grounded in grassroots alliances," suggesting solidarity between different nonwhite groups in a push for substantive change, "or diversity management," which instead merely painted white institutions with a thin rainbow veneer. Indeed, minority or "multicultural" outreach (although perhaps well-intentioned) at predominantly white AIDS organizations such as the Philadelphia AIDS Task Force and the San Francisco AIDS Foundation (SFAF) often appeared to be tokenism at best and a cynical attempt to mollify critics at worst—recall that Rashidah Hassan felt like the "colored poster child" at Philadelphia Community Health Alternatives. In contrast, the NTFAP offers a useful example of multicultural AIDS activism from the bottom up, as the group worked with different communities of color to develop targeted interventions.[9]

At the same time, this story shows the struggles that even a large and well-funded minority AIDS organization faced. At its peak the group employed over sixty staff members and was supported by multiple large grants, but federal AIDS funding could be a double-edged sword. As the previous chapter also showed, running a large nonprofit and organizing a community to fight AIDS are both hard work and require very different sets of skills. Like many LGBTQ and AIDS groups, including Blacks Educating Blacks About Sexual Health Issues, the NTFAP struggled to balance the two. Federal funding made the NTFAP possible but also came with reporting requirements that could be onerous for a new organization. Reliance on federal money also opened the group to crippling political attacks that sapped staffers' time and attention and thus hindered their ability to fight AIDS.

The work of managing a large organization that included both local and national programs took its toll on those in charge, many of whom were also dealing with their own HIV-related illness. Reggie Williams stepped down as executive director of the NTFAP in early 1994 partly due to his own failing health. The personality conflicts and power struggles that ensued point to the weakness of organizations built on charismatic leadership, however capable and well-intentioned. After years of financial woes, high staff turnover, and leadership changes following Williams's departure, the group closed its doors for good in June 1998. But while the NTFAP would not survive the second decade of the AIDS epidemic, it paved the way for future organizing by gay men of color against the disease.

## Race and the San Francisco Model

As in Philadelphia, the first AIDS organizations in San Francisco were founded by white gay men to respond to the epidemic. Groups such as the San Francisco AIDS Foundation conducted outreach and education through institutions in the gay community, without recognizing just how segregated that community was. During the early years of the crisis the SFAF had few minority staff members, which fed the image of AIDS as a white gay disease. Tom Horan, reporting on "the mess at the AIDS Foundation" for the BWMT/San Francisco newsletter in May 1985, predicted, "The Foundation's basic effort to reach well-educated, 20 to 40 year old, Gay, White men will continue to succeed, but the word won't reach others except by spillover." In other words, the SFAF seemed unwilling or unable to reach gay men of color, much less communities of color more broadly, with the AIDS services they needed.[10]

For these reasons, AIDS service workers of color concluded that San Francisco's model of AIDS prevention and care, which was seen as perhaps the best in the country, was not working for minority communities. In response they formed their own organizations, such as the Third World AIDS Advisory Task Force, made up in part of frustrated SFAF staff and volunteers. Groups such as the San Francisco Black Coalition on AIDS formed to address the epidemic among African Americans, while existing Black community groups, such as the Bayview-Hunters Point Foundation, established their own AIDS education programs, although they often lacked experience in working with gay and bisexual men.[11]

At the same time, BWMT was working to address AIDS, both locally and nationally. Reggie Williams's AIDS Task Force of BWMT/San Francisco fought for better minority services in the city's programs for people with the disease. Following reports that the Shanti Project, a support center for people with AIDS, had treated minority clients and volunteers with everything from indifference to "outright discrimination," Williams and fellow BWMT member Larry Burnett met with Shanti's executive director and senior staff.[12]

Members of the task force also wrote to Dr. Paul Volberding of San Francisco General Hospital regarding racial discrimination in Ward 86, where AIDS services were concentrated. They charged that staff frequently failed to inform "Black and Latino people with AIDS ... about the nature of AIDS or about clinical, medical or alternative resources to aid in their treatment" and that "staffing at Ward 86 does not even approximately represent the racial/ethnic diversity of the city," especially in its lack of Spanish speakers. Moreover, the staff refused to "include others [aside from "White Gay males"] in the data gathering and research that represents much of the work of Ward 86."

This statistical erasure was used to further justify the facility's lack of minority AIDS education. To make matters worse, one doctor "felt free to 'humorously' speculate about AIDS being transmitted by African men having sexual intercourse with African green monkeys" and asked Black people with AIDS (PWAs) (but not whites) if they engaged in bestiality.[13]

In spite of this work, some questioned BWMT/San Francisco's commitment to fighting for racial equity. One African American member lamented that despite the group's name, "the membership is less than 1/3 black." He explained that he had joined the group "to meet new people and become more socially and politically involved," despite its "reputation as a club for race fetishists." Because "institutionalized racism is an everyday reality for black people," he was "more than a little dismayed" that the group "examines it only cursorily." Instead the chapter felt like "a little U.N." with observances of "Chinese New Year, Cinco de Mayo, [and] Jewish cultural activities." Such events, he suggested, represented a superficial multiculturalism that distracted from work on dismantling anti-Black racism.[14]

Some outside the group took issue with BWMT's "interracialism." At a forum on "Strategies for Survival of Black Gay Men," put on by the NTFAP in January 1990, longtime BWMT member Thom Bean opened the program by explaining that "Black males fall into two groups: Black-Black and Black-Interracialist. . . . Just like our oppressors, we are not too comfortable with differences and we need to get over with being judgmental with each other and on with supporting each [other]." Brandy Moore, a Black gay activist and assistant to Willie Brown, then speaker of the California Assembly, disagreed with Bean's call for understanding. In Moore's view, "White Gay men in the city don't give a damn . . . about Black people with AIDS and how they live or die because if they did, they would be down at the Black Coalition [on AIDS] making sure that they are volunteering efforts to save our lives." For this reason, he told Bean, "who you sleep with is my business, as an African American gay man. Because if you sleep with the wrong person, the action that you take . . . may constitute a political action against my existence and so who you sleep with is very well my business, darling." Here BWMT's reputation for "race fetishism" dovetailed with concerns about the white gay AIDS establishment; Brown suggested that both groups were made up of men who saw their Black counterparts as sexual objects and not as lives worth saving.[15]

Some likewise argued that because of BWMT's proximity to white gay men, the NTFAP could not effectively reach Black gay men with AIDS services. During a panel at the 1990 NABWMT convention in San Francisco, Cleo Manago, a Black gay activist and head of the AIDS Project of the East Bay, accused the group of "encouraging racism, attempting to position itself as the sole spokesperson for black gays and of undermining the work of black gay activists." In an article for the *Real Read*, a Black gay magazine that he coedited with Ron Grayson, Manago similarly accused BWMT of "riding on the apron strings of the white gay movement" and serving only "a small sub-culture of gay men of color who have a 'fetish' for white men." Moreover, he charged, "to avoid the Black community's disapproval ... BWMT has developed new organizations with new names to avoid possible scrutiny," a possible reference to the NTFAP, to Bay Area HIV Support and Education Services (BAHSES, a full-fledged AIDS service organization that had by then formed out of the BWMT/SF AIDS Task Force), or both. In contrast he offered his own group, Black Men's Xchange, as a means through which "Black Men Who Love Men" could access "comprehensive and sensitive AIDS education and other related services."[16]

Still, BWMT/San Francisco was not the only group within the NABWMT working to bring AIDS prevention programs to Black gay and bisexual men. In Philadelphia, BWMT for Education pressured the city's AIDS Task Force to expand its outreach to communities of color, while BWMT/Philadelphia co-produced "Respect Yourself!," a rap single that aimed to raise African Americans' awareness about AIDS, which Reggie Williams in turn promoted to Bay Area news outlets. In Shelby County, Tennessee, where the population was 54 percent African American, BWMT/Memphis was the only group to offer AIDS services to the local Black community—gay *and* straight. Phill Wilson of the Los Angeles chapter adapted *Hot, Horny and Healthy!* for Black gay and bisexual men. *Hot, Horny and Healthy!* would become a model for educational programs aimed at other groups of gay men of color, as well as a staple of the NTFAP's programming. But it would also become a source of controversy for the group, as conservative activists attacked the use of federal funding for such sexually explicit interventions.[17]

## "They Almost Couldn't Deny Us"

The National Task Force on AIDS Prevention grew out of a small cohort of BWMT members who formed an informal AIDS task force within the national association's board. The group included Reggie Williams along with James Credle, Tom Horan, John Teamer, and Steve Feeback. Building on the work of local chapters, in 1988 they put together an ambitious proposal for the Centers for Disease Control and Prevention that would lead to the creation of the NTFAP as the first federally funded group by and for gay men of color.

Williams, Credle, and the others did not expect to receive a CDC grant. Members of the Reagan administration and many in Congress were notoriously anti-gay, and the president himself all but ignored the epidemic. Feeback, a white gay anti-apartheid activist and former member of the group's New York chapter who put together the grant application in the spring of 1988, later recalled, "The grant was written in a way that they almost couldn't deny us, unless they wanted to use overt prejudice against a gay organization." The NABWMT lacked the name recognition of some other applicants, including well-established minority groups such as the Southern Christian Leadership Conference and National Council of La Raza. But whereas other applicants sought funds to *begin* work in AIDS education, the NTFAP was ready to hit the ground running, with an educational program and a national network of chapters through which to disseminate it already in place.[18]

The grant established the NTFAP under the auspices of the NABWMT. The new organization was to coordinate the AIDS education efforts of over twenty local chapters, train members nationwide to facilitate workshops on safer sex, and conduct a survey of Black gay and bisexual men's AIDS knowledge and sexual behaviors. The grant also allowed the NTFAP to hire paid staff, who were initially spread across the country. Reggie Williams, the NTFAP project director, set up an office in the Urban Life Center in San Francisco's Fillmore District. Steve Feeback worked as project administrator out of his home in Washington, D.C. (He later moved to San Francisco.) Phill Wilson, who had worked for the Stop AIDS Project in Los Angeles, served as health training coordinator. Meanwhile, Eric Perez worked for the group part-time from New York as a field outreach assistant on the East Coast.[19]

For those on the board who were committed to AIDS education, the grant was a giant step forward. However, the NABWMT was used to operating as a decentralized organization with almost no national budget, and Feeback later recalled that "many people didn't know how to deal with" the group's new status as a federal grantee. Even those who were supportive of the move had reason to be nervous. In August 1988 James Credle, a founding member of the NABWMT who had submitted the CDC grant application on his group's behalf, warned of "the dangers to our organizations and to our communities when we accept government grants without recognizing the potential negative consequences, especially when government funding sources are our primary ones."[20]

At the time it received the CDC grant, the NTFAP already had one major element of its programming in place: *Hot, Horny and Healthy!* The original version of *Hot, Horny and Healthy!* was developed in 1985 by Luis Palacios-Jimenez and Michael Shernoff, both of Gay Men's Health Crisis, to show that safer sex could stop the spread of HIV and still be pleasurable. Phill Wilson then adapted it to be "sensitive to the special needs of Black gay men." For

*Hot, Horny and Healthy!*, participants gathered in the back room of a gay bar or bathhouse, at a community center, or in someone's apartment. They started by sharing ways that AIDS had impacted their sex lives and talking about what they missed about sex before AIDS. They then discussed the good things about safer sex and made lists of "extremely erotic but safer ways of touching or being touched." Next, the playshop focused on eroticizing safer sex, with "condom races" to help participants learn to put on and remove a condom. Finally, participants used role-playing exercises to practice negotiating safer sex with their partners.[21]

NTFAP staff—first Phill Wilson and later Gavin Morrow-Hall, who succeeded Wilson as the group's coordinator of training and education—visited BWMT chapters to conduct *Hot, Horny and Healthy!* trainings. During these sessions, members completed the playshop before being trained as facilitators so that they could deliver it to others as well. In this way the NTFAP used a "train the trainer" approach, on top of the NABWMT's network, to amplify its AIDS education efforts. Participants offered the playshop in other spaces as well, such as Glide Memorial United Methodist Church in San Francisco's Tenderloin neighborhood and in bathhouses such as the Steamworks, which was located across the bay in Berkeley.[22]

*Hot, Horny and Healthy!* was meant to be sex positive. Rather than monogamy or abstinence, the playshop encouraged gay men to have "safer sex," defined as "on me, not in me, unless you're in me with a condom." This definition made no judgments about sexual relationships—as far as the NTFAP was concerned, it didn't matter if two men had been lovers for twenty years or had just cruised one another in a public park, so long as they used a condom and did so correctly.[23]

For the NTFAP the messenger and the context for learning about safer sex were just as important as the messages themselves. The group found that Black gay and bisexual men were "most likely to practice unsafe sex" and also were "the most likely to shun public sources of information" but would engage in "verbal, participatory methodologies" such as *Hot, Horny and Healthy!* Outreach workers would also have to earn the trust of their audience. That is, AIDS educators would have to be a "consistent presence" in gay bars and bathhouses that catered to Black gay men in order to gain the confidence of staff and patrons, and would need to show a "sincere and caring attitude" while delivering information about safer sex.[24]

*Hot, Horny and Healthy!* not only promoted safer sex but also untangled the knot of feelings surrounding the epidemic: the "great sense of loss, [the] overwhelming feeling of having had many things and people stolen away."

One source of grief was the "many men, wonderful men" who had passed away. Another was the discrimination faced by people with AIDS and those perceived to be at risk for the disease. Still another was the loss of what seemed, in retrospect, to be the carefree sex of the pre-AIDS era, the feeling "that man to man love is not as it was." But *Hot, Horny and Healthy!* also built a sense of community and identity by creating spaces specifically for gay men of color, and for Black gay men in particular, even if just in the temporary space of a gathering in the back room of a bar or a BWMT member's living room. In the midst of racism, homophobia, and the "compounding loss" of the AIDS epidemic, the NTFAP was "nurturing growth in those empty spaces."[25]

After receiving the CDC grant, the NTFAP wasted little time in seeking additional funding—not just to supplement its federal funding but to broaden its local operations in San Francisco. In 1989 the task force received support from Northern California Grantmakers, a regional philanthropic group, to "provide a multi-ethnic, risk reduction, train-the-trainer project" involving four different San Francisco communities. Using the version of *Hot, Horny and Healthy!* developed by Phill Wilson, participating organizations would produce "distinct culturally appropriate components for African Americans, Latinos, Asian & Pacific Islanders, and Native Americans." The participating organizations—Bay Area HIV Support and Education Services, which had grown out of the BWMT/SF AIDS Task Force; Community United in Response to AIDS/SIDA (CURAS); Gay Asian Pacific Alliance Community HIV Project; and the American Indian AIDS Institute—along with the NTFAP would together form the Gay Men of Color Consortium.

Under the initial GMOCC grant, each of the task force's four partner organizations hired a community representative to adapt the playshop curriculum for its constituency. For the Gay Asian Pacific Alliance Community HIV Project, this meant adding a discussion on "being Asian and gay" to the curriculum; for the American Indian AIDS Institute, it meant dealing with issues of tribal identification during the playshop. For Latino gay and bisexual men, the *Hot, Horny and Healthy!* had to be adapted in such a way as to offer "the chance to get clear and open information about AIDS in their own Lenguaje." In other words, the playshop needed to be translated not only into Spanish but also into the idiom of Spanish-speaking gay and bisexual men. Thus CURAS created *¡Caliente, con Ganas y Saludable!*, the Gay Asian Pacific Alliance Community HIV Project developed *Hot, Healthy and Keeping It Up*, and the American Indian AIDS Institute produced *Hot, Healthy and Snagging*, using a Native American slang term for sex.[26]

Working with GMOCC helped to "make NTFAP a multi-cultural HIV/AIDS

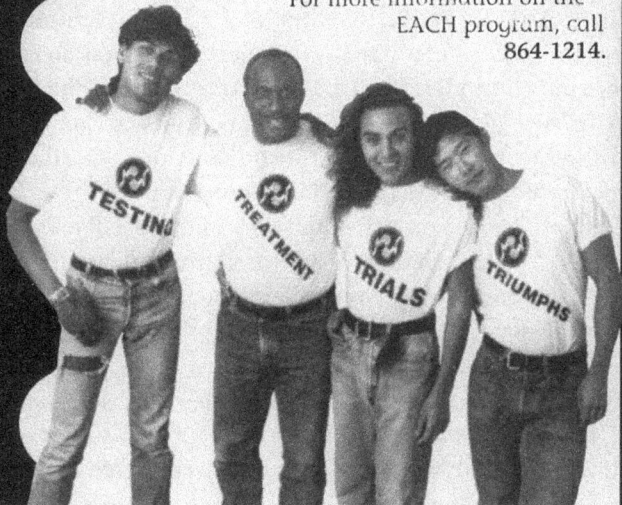

Flyer for the Early Advocacy and Care for HIV (EACH) program, ca. 1993. EACH was a program of the Gay Men of Color Consortium that focused on early HIV testing and treatment for gay and bisexual men of color. Courtesy National Task Force on AIDS Prevention, MSS 94–59, box 3, folder 16, UCSF Archives and Special Collections.

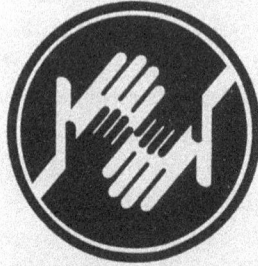

service organization" by extending the group's reach beyond a mostly Black and white national membership. Although each of the four communities of gay men of color represented in the larger group would be best reached through its own targeted, culturally competent programs, the groups also had experiences in common. Despite the disproportionate impact of AIDS on gay men of color, the groups "found themselves excluded from AIDS agencies and programs targeting gay white men or non-gay identified ethnic minorities." By collaborating through GMOCC, member organizations forged a model that they argued was "truly 'multi-cultural'" in that "programs are designed, implemented and administered by the communities themselves and not by dominant culture agencies attempting to expand or adapt their programs to communities they neglected in the past." Unlike the Shanti Project or the SFAF, which struggled to diversify, GMOCC offered a model for "multi-culturalism . . . carried into action." Here member groups worked together on grassroots AIDS programs that attended to their distinct cultures as well as to their common experiences.[27]

Gay men of color were excluded not only from white gay and minority AIDS agencies but from the communities they represented as well. That rejection was painful, and, according to activists, as a result many gay men of color subconsciously did not see themselves as worthy of the protection that safer sex afforded. For this reason, self-esteem was key to GMOCC's thinking about how to approach HIV education. Many similar campaigns targeting white gay men had "recognized the importance of promoting and strengthening self-esteem . . . in effect a resocialization that tackles head on the context of a homophobic society." That self-esteem was, in turn, "central to . . . self-efficacy, the perceived capacity to incorporate behavior change." But gay men of color endured living in a society that was homophobic *and* racist, making both self-esteem and the self-efficacy to consistently practice safer sex that much harder to cultivate. Hence GMOCC also drew on the work of Paulo Freire, the Brazilian postcolonial philosopher of education, in incorporating the social and historical context of its constituencies to "deliver a credible message, build skills, promote self-esteem and thus empower both the individual and the community to create a healthier set of behavioral and cultural norms."[28]

Working together as gay men of color also made financial sense: by presenting a united front to funders, member organizations avoided competing with one another and, by sharing resources and prevention models, could develop their programs more quickly and efficiently. And yet the partnerships were also based on a sense of solidarity, which was itself perhaps an outgrowth of the city's diversity and history of "Third World" organizing, as the agencies "understood that the health and empowerment of gay men in their community is based on the health and power of gay men in all communities of color."[29]

### "Being Informed Is Not Always Enough"

At the same time that the NTFAP was building intercultural partnerships through GMOCC, it was also creating new knowledge about Black gay and bisexual men. Under the terms of the CDC grant, the NTFAP needed to develop a research component. The task force elected to conduct a nationwide survey of Black gay and bisexual men's knowledge, attitudes, and behavior (KAB) surrounding safer sex and AIDS, using members as both survey takers and respondents. The effort was led by two NABWMT members: John Bush, a sociologist at Southeastern Massachusetts University, and Dan Minns, a political scientist at American University.[30]

The survey aimed to establish how much Black gay and bisexual men knew about HIV and its transmission and the extent to which they had changed their sexual practices in the context of the epidemic. Much had been written about gay men's adoption of safer sex practices, such as using condoms, but the studies that showed behavior change among gay men focused on *white* gay men. As the number of AIDS diagnoses among Black gay and bisexual men continued to rise, the NTFAP wanted to know what *they* knew about AIDS and what they were doing to protect themselves. The results, the task force argued, would help the organization target its AIDS prevention efforts.

The study also had larger implications beyond the NTFAP's programming. Studies about gay men's sexual behavior skewed toward white gay men because researchers considered gay men of color to be "hard to reach." By conducting a nationwide survey of Black gay and bisexual men, the NTFAP would show that they were not, in fact, "hard to reach"—at least not for those with the skills and the will to do so. And if one group of Black gay men could conduct such a study, then similar organizations could make claims on federal funding as well.[31]

Bush and Minns spent the fall of 1988 designing the survey and in the spring of the following year traveled to cities around the country, training chapter members to act as survey takers. They administered the questionnaire to 952 men, including both Black BWMT members and those who did not belong to the organization but could be found at bars and cruising sites such as gay bookstores and public parks. Interviewers were encouraged to target "Black men who are out of the 'information mainstream' about AIDS," meaning those who "are *not getting or are ignoring* [emphasis in original] the information available to the general public."[32]

The results of the survey, announced at a San Francisco press conference in June 1990, painted a troubling picture of Black gay men's sex lives and attitudes about AIDS. On the one hand, it showed that among respondents, "awareness of AIDS and its threat is practically universal" and the majority understood the risks associated with different sexual behaviors. On the other hand, the survey also revealed that "the commitment to safer sex behavior is weak in the Black gay and bisexual community"—the majority said they would be at least "a little likely" to "not worry about slipping and having unsafe sex once in a while." Black gay and bisexual men knew about AIDS, including the ways in which HIV was transmitted, but lacked either the tools or the will to practice safer sex consistently.[33]

Additionally, fewer than half of respondents had attended a safer sex workshop and just over half had attended an AIDS education program, even as the overwhelming majority believed that education was important for developing safer sex practices. For this reason, Williams argued, "there is an urgent need for more culturally specific education, risk reduction training and ongoing support, such as the programs the Task Force has pioneered and is continuing to develop." Put another way, "Being informed is not always enough"— Black gay and bisexual men would have to be taught how to negotiate safer sex through programs designed with them specifically in mind. For the NTFAP, this meant addressing the epidemic in ways that accounted for the daily trauma of living as a Black gay man in a racist and homophobic society.[34]

Williams also stressed that "Black gay and bisexual men do not segregate themselves into 'gay ghettoes,' as do whites." Instead, he reported, "they remain an active, involved part of the Black community, nurturing their immediate and extended families, and participating in every aspect of community life." A third of respondents also reported having at least occasional sex with women. The result, according to Phill Wilson, was a "chain of infection within our community" that included Black women and children. Williams concurred that the "Black community and its institutions must become more involved if we are to reduce the risk to women and children, as well as to Black men, regardless of their sexual orientation." He continued, "It's time to deal forthrightly with the issues of sexuality that the Black community has denied or ignored for far too long." Doing so, he argued, would "begin a community-wide healing process that will have far-reaching effects on the overall prognosis for African Americans' survival into the 21st century."[35]

In retrospect, these comments seem of a piece with the later controversy surrounding Black men "on the down low"—those who carried on sex with other men in secret and passed HIV on to their unsuspecting female partners.[36] However, in highlighting the implications of the NTFAP study for Black women, Williams and Wilson aimed not to demonize or scapegoat bisexually active Black men. Instead they aimed to encourage straight Black women to practice safer sex and to spark honest discussions about same-sex desire within Black communities that were long overdue.

The announcement of the survey results was timed to coincide with the start of the Sixth International AIDS Conference, held in San Francisco in June 1990. The previous year's conference, held in Montreal, had been marked by interruptions from the AIDS Coalition to Unleash Power, which objected to the absence of people with AIDS in high-level conversations among doctors, researchers, and policy makers. San Francisco was different—there, activists and researchers shared the stage for the first time. The NTFAP also found a place at the conference, through a poster presentation of the results of the KAB survey.[37]

Nevertheless, around fifty AIDS organizations, including the Gay Men's Health Crisis (GMHC), boycotted the conference over the United States' travel and immigration ban on people with HIV and AIDS. (It would be the last such conference in the United States until the 2012 International AIDS Conference in Washington, D.C., organized after President Barack Obama lifted the travel ban in January 2010.) In San Francisco, protesters demonstrated outside the offices of the Immigration and Naturalization Service, which was responsible for enforcing the travel ban, as well as outside the convention center and at the Marriott Hotel. At the end of the conference, thousands of activists and researchers joined together for an AIDS unity march through the streets of San Francisco. The only major disruption came during the closing ceremony and a speech by Louis Sullivan, secretary of Health and Human Services and the highest-ranking African American in the administration of George H. W. Bush. During Sullivan's address, ACT UP members blew whistles and chanted "Shame!" Dean Lance of DIVA (Damned Interfering Video Activists) TV, an affinity group within ACT UP, later claimed that "most of the delegates—by their own admissions—were looking forward to the anticipated obfuscation." Copies of the speech had been distributed in advance, and according to Lance, "Delegates could have heard it through headphones, [but] the majority of them turned their backs to the stage . . . in an expression of their outrage over the Bush administration's discriminatory policies."[38]

If delegates did in fact listen to Sullivan through their headsets, they heard him highlight the NTFAP study as evidence of a need to "develop culturally relevant and sensitive programs to combat the disease." They also heard his call to the audience: "Let us not turn our frustration into theater, searching for protagonists and antagonists." After the disruption, however, Sullivan became "very angry" at his treatment during the reception. He denounced the protesters as "un-American" and vowed, "I will not in any way work with those individuals."[39]

Phill Wilson, who served as a delegate to the conference, responded to Sullivan in an emotional letter full of frustration and grief. Wilson unequivocally sided with ACT UP. "Desperate people do desperate things," he wrote. "That's what I think the demonstration on June 24th was all about, Dr. Sullivan. Desperate people resorting to desperate means. Entire families are being wiped out and they want you to see their pain and have compassion." Wilson's own family had been ripped apart by AIDS; his longtime partner, Chris Brownlie, had passed away just seven months earlier in November 1989, and he had "lost nearly 200 friends and family members to the disease." He continued, "As a person living with this disease, it disturbs me that people are so quick to choose to play political football with my life."[40]

The day after the unity march that closed out the International AIDS Conference, the NTFAP held a meeting of its own. On Sunday, June 25, 1990, participants held a daylong Gay Men of Color AIDS Institute at San Francisco State University. The event brought together groups serving Latino, Asian American, and Native American gay and bisexual men to talk about the challenges they shared. As opposed to most AIDS conferences, which included only "brief sessions addressing the issues involved in working with the diverse communities effected [sic] by the AIDS pandemic," the Gay Men of Color AIDS Institute promised to "devote an entire day to discussing the unique needs of . . . gay and bisexual men of color and provide participants the opportunity to explore the impact of homophobia and racism in a safe environment." The Gay Men of Color AIDS Institute would become an annual event organized by the NTFAP and, along with its leadership in GMOCC, signaled that the group was committed to addressing AIDS among Black gay and bisexual men in the larger context of the epidemic among gay and bisexual men of color as a whole.[41]

## Too Hot and Horny for the CDC

When they received their initial grant from the CDC in 1988, NTFAP leaders were aware that their sexually explicit approach to HIV education might bring trouble in the future. In 1987, Senator Jesse Helms of North Carolina had made a political issue out of AIDS education when he held up *Safer Sex Comix*, published by the GMHC, on the floor of the United States Senate to denounce federal funding for such programs. He thus succeeded in passing the Helms Amendment, which prohibited the use of federal funds by the CDC to "provide AIDS education, information, or prevention materials and activities that promote, encourage, and condone homosexual sexual activities or the intravenous use of illegal drugs."[42]

In this context the NTFAP claimed some victory in having been awarded money from the CDC in the first place: "Helms's purpose was to prevent a group like ours from ever getting a Federal grant for AIDS prevention work.

His forces are not going to like it when they discover that one of the 31 successful applicants is an openly gay, multi-racial organization." However, the group's leaders knew that the Helms Amendment requirements could cause them trouble and thus pursued funding from the Robert Wood Johnson Foundation and the United States Conference of Mayors, because these groups were more insulated from political pressure than the CDC. (The group received some funding from the United States Conference of Mayors, but the Robert Wood Johnson Foundation grant, which totaled $223,000, never materialized.) Still, NTFAP leaders could not have predicted just how damaging it could be to run afoul of Helms and his political allies.[43]

Controversy over the use of federal funds for *Hot, Horny and Healthy!* erupted after the conservative syndicated columnist Cal Thomas attacked the NTFAP in newspapers nationwide. In a column published in early November 1990, Thomas lamented that in "tight budgetary times" the CDC had "found enough of our tax dollars to underwrite a program for a homosexual group called Black and White Men Together." He homed in on the playshop's condom races, which he argued were both an affront "to common sense and common decency" and prohibited under Helms's legislation. Thomas also groused that, because the NTFAP grant came out of funds earmarked for minority AIDS prevention, the program "bolster[ed] homosexual efforts to give their sexual behavior the same kind of legal approval that minority groups have under anti-discrimination statutes." Here he appealed to the notion that the gay rights movement had hijacked the agenda and language of the Black freedom struggle in order to promote a sinful lifestyle.[44]

At the same time, Thomas obliquely attacked the NTFAP for its focus on *Black* gay men. By referring to the group as Black and White Men Together rather than as the National Task Force on AIDS Prevention, he raised the specters of homosexuality and interracial sex while downplaying the group's public health mission. Thomas also contrasted the NTFAP grant with the situation of "poor old Lawrence Welk," who "has been getting a lot of flak for the $500,000 appropriated by Congress to restore his boyhood home in North Dakota." (Senator Quentin Burdick of North Dakota had attached the grant to a larger spending bill, sparking a public uproar; Congress later rescinded the bill.) By invoking the midwestern TV bandleader, Thomas appealed to readers' nostalgia for a bygone America that was both sexually *and* racially conservative.[45]

Thomas's readers wrote angry letters to their congressional representatives, who demanded that the CDC explain why it had funded such a program. The CDC, in turn, began to watch the NTFAP much more closely. Reggie Williams later testified to the Congressional Black Caucus that the oversight disrupted work at the task force, as repeated requests for information from the CDC meant that his organization, "already fighting with one Helms Amendment-tied hand behind its back, was forced to drop everything to respond to a litany of half-truths, whole fabrications and well-crafted innuendos." This, he insisted, was no accident. Instead, "the conservative forces in this country [had] made [the NTFAP] a target of their well-oiled 'disinformation' machine."[46]

In the meantime, the NTFAP learned that *Reader's Digest* was planning to reprint Thomas's column, which would both extend the controversy and publicize it to millions more readers. In a letter to the magazine's editorial desk, NTFAP media coordinator Al Cunningham rebutted Thomas's claims and stressed that the CDC grant represented "the *only* [emphasis in original] national funding for risk reduction programming specifically addressing gay and bisexual African American men," who made up more than twenty thousand HIV/AIDS cases in the United States by early 1991. In the bigger picture of AIDS funding, Cunningham argued, the money awarded to the NTFAP represented "a drop in the bucket." Besides, the condom races served an important function in encouraging safer sex by "address[ing] the oft-stated excuse that condoms take too much time to put on."[47]

Still, NTFAP leaders knew that they were unlikely to stop *Reader's Digest* from running the piece. Predicting that "Congress will get several thousands of letters complaining that tax dollars are being wasted on the likes of us," they encouraged local BWMT chapters to flex their political muscle by writing their own letters to their representatives in Congress. "But we pay taxes, too," they continued. "We have as much right as anyone else in this country to receive services, which are provided from the taxes taken out of every one of our paychecks." If conservative readers had been able to disrupt the NTFAP's operations through letter writing, then perhaps a similar campaign by gay men of color and their allies could help contain the damage.[48]

When *Reader's Digest* excerpted Thomas's column almost a year later, in September 1991, editors presented *Hot, Horny and Healthy!* even more pointedly as a waste of taxpayer dollars. They ran the story as part of "That's Outrageous!," a feature that carried the subtitle "Spotlighting absurdities in our society is the first step to eliminating them." Here editors juxtaposed Thomas's story with others, including one about a man who "made tanning booth appointments and honed his body in the gym" to prepare for the Mr. Massachusetts Male America Pageant, all while receiving worker's compensation payments from the state of Massachusetts.[49]

*Reader's Digest* invited readers to laugh at the man's queerness as a pageant contestant alongside the "absurdity" of the *Hot, Horny and Healthy!* condom races. But the magazine also positioned the news items as stories about the abuse of government largesse, which were embedded in a racially coded discourse used to justify deep cuts to public spending. Ten years after Ronald Reagan ascended to the White House in part by attacking "welfare queens," the idea that African Americans preferred living well on the dole to an honest day's work would have been firmly implanted in readers' minds. By placing Thomas's column alongside the Mr. Massachusetts story, *Reader's Digest* invited readers to consider *Hot, Horny and Healthy!* an "outrageous" abuse of public funds—not only by gay men seeking "legal approval" but specifically by *Black* gay men.[50]

After *Reader's Digest* ran Thomas's column more or less intact, the NTFAP struck back in a press release. It again argued that the CDC funds represented a relatively small grant and the only national funding for AIDS education aimed at Black gay and bisexual men. To the charge that federal funding for the NTFAP represented a waste of taxpayer dollars, it pointed out that "African American gay and bisexual men pay taxes too." It also asserted its leaders' credibility as AIDS educators—whereas Thomas and *Reader's Digest* suggested that the group lacked oversight or accountability, the NTFAP insisted that its programs were "professionally designed, repeatedly reviewed, and scrupulously evaluated."[51]

The fallout from the entire episode was devastating for the NTFAP. In September 1991 the CDC announced cuts to all of its national minority organization grantees for the following year. Although the agency described the cuts as "across the board," Reggie Williams and Steve Feeback later found that there were "wide differences in cuts" from organization to organization. For its part, the NTFAP lost the portion of the CDC grant that funded research and evaluation, which made up 43 percent of its funding under the program. As a result the group was forced to lay off two employees and to cut back time for those who remained. According to Williams, this made it difficult for the NTFAP "to do what we've set out to do and been funded to do, let along manage the day-to-day activities of an 'under attack,' underfunded national HIV/AIDS organization."[52]

For Williams, the difficulty was the result not only of political pressure on the CDC by conservative activists but also of "deliberate under-funding and deadly discrimination" by the agency toward the NTFAP. Likewise, Feeback later recalled that the group was investigated by the CDC more than other grantees, and the office was "constantly harassed by bureaucracy and piddling requirements." During this time, a CDC representative paid the office a visit to investigate its operations. Williams had recently blacked out due to the treatment he was undergoing for HIV, suffered a fall, and broken his jaw. Despite having his mouth wired shut, he told the representative "in no uncertain terms" that the group was doing everything right.[53]

Williams also soon found himself at odds with the NABWMT, which was still serving as the fiscal agent for the CDC grant. Some NABWMT board members questioned the task force's ability to manage multiple large grants at once and considered the group to be "out of control" under Williams's leadership. The CDC's decision to cut back funding exacerbated the tension. In November 1991, the NABWMT instructed that the task force should "operate within its means" and reduce expenditures in proportion to the CDC cuts. The national association also announced its intention to bill the task force for indirect costs and to require the NTFAP to submit future budgets to an oversight committee for approval.[54]

Williams resented the treatment. After months of negative press, pressure from the CDC, and budget cuts, being chastised by the board was yet another entry in a long list of indignities. He was recognized nationally as a preeminent AIDS educator and had testified before members of Congress; taking flak from his brothers at the NABWMT must have felt like an insult.[55]

Thus, the task force decided to formally separate from the NABWMT. It sought out certification as an independent nonprofit group, which it obtained with help from the office of Nancy Pelosi, the congresswoman from San Francisco. Now the task force could apply for—and manage—grants on its own. Gavin Morrow-Hall, who by then had replaced Phill Wilson as the group's coordinator of training and education, recalls that the separation from the NABWMT was "needed" and allowed the former group to push in new directions and to become more overtly political.[56]

## Campaigning for Fairness

Even before the CDC announced the funding cuts, the NTFAP had been looking to carve out a role for gay men of color in shaping AIDS policy. The *Hot, Horny and Healthy!* controversy gave the group new reason to do so, as well as some concrete demands to make in the policy arena. Its efforts would help change the way that decisions about AIDS funding were made across the United States.[57]

The Campaign for Fairness began in October 1991 at the second Gay Men of Color AIDS Institute in Los Angeles and called not only for the NTFAP's lost funding to be restored but for a dramatic increase in federal funds for HIV prevention among "gay and bisexual men of all colors." The campaign circulated a list of demands titled "A Campaign for Fairness! A Call to Action!" to AIDS organizations and elected officials across the country, drawing hundreds of signatures, and encouraged BWMT members to contact their elected officials about endorsing the statement as well. As a result, mayor of San Francisco Art

Agnos signed on to the "Call to Action," and San Francisco supervisor Carole Midgen wrote to CDC chief James Curran on the NTFAP's behalf. All twenty-six members of the Congressional Black Caucus signed on to a letter demanding restoration of the CDC's cuts to national minority organizations, the first time that the caucus had "been moved to action" as a body on the issue of HIV/AIDS. In June 1992 seventeen members of the House of Representatives also sent a letter to CDC director William Roper, urging him to restore NTFAP's funding to the full amount. One of these was Nancy Pelosi, whose legislation would help turn some of the NTFAP's demands into national policy.[58]

In March 1992 the campaign's national cochairs, Richard LaFortune (also known as Angukquac and Anguksuar), Steve Lew, H. Alexander Robinson, and Mario Solis-Marich, each of whom represented a different community of gay men of color, met with representatives from the Health Resources and Services Administration, who promised to include gay men of color in set-ting priorities for HIV funding. That July, Reggie Williams testified before a congressional subcommittee on AIDS prevention. He estimated that gay men of color made up 20 percent of people with AIDS nationwide but lamented that "gay men of color have been ignored and treated as if we don't have our own organizations, as if we don't have our own leaders, as if we don't have our unique health care needs, as if we are too hard to reach. At times we are treated like we don't even exist." Williams then quoted the CDC's own guide-lines, which directed that "communities or groups most disproportionately affected by this epidemic must be involved in the planning and implementa-tion of HIV prevention programs" to make his point: gay men of color should be at the AIDS policy table.[59]

Thanks in part to this pressure, in late 1993 the CDC directed that health departments in all fifty states, eight territories, and seven of the most affected cities in the United States would have to implement HIV prevention commu-nity planning. In other words, they would have to involve nongovernmental groups and individual community members in deciding how federal AIDS funds would be spent at the state and local level. This idea was not necessarily new, but pressure from the task force helped push it forward. Public health of-ficials credited Nancy Pelosi's proposed Comprehensive HIV Prevention Act of 1993, which would have tied federal HIV prevention funding to state and local planning councils, with driving the policy change. Earlier that year, Pelosi her-self had pointed to the Campaign for Fairness as "one of the primary reasons that my office is working on comprehensive reform of how HIV prevention services are delivered." The NTFAP also offered feedback on the CDC's planning guidance, which was incorporated into the final document.[60]

Task force leaders saw the advent of community planning as an opportunity to push directly for funding for gay men of color HIV programs. In a newsletter they opined that the CDC's guidance had "the immediate practical effect of opening up the process to input from all of you" and that "gay men of color will benefit a great deal from taking an active role." However, the process was not without its challenges. Bringing new voices into the conversation introduced conflict as well, and community members sometimes lacked the technical expertise of their colleagues in government. At the 1994 Gay Men of Color AIDS Institute, held about nine months after the CDC issued its guidance, H. Alexander Robinson and Mario Solis-Marich reported on "opportunities and dangers" in community planning as gay men of color (GMOC) "can be decisive in prioritizing local plans, and in establishing targeted prevention activities for GMOC." However, they continued, "The first year planning has already begun in several cities and states without adequate preparation of underserved and underrepresented groups such as GMOC. There are many more GMOC on the councils but these same GMOC are isolated and often lack support and skills to be effective."[61]

Nevertheless, the NTFAP's policy arm had helped democratize HIV planning nationwide. Campaign for Fairness cochairs Steve Lew and H. Alexander Robinson were also named to the Presidential Advisory Council on HIV/AIDS in June 1995. Gavin Morrow-Hall credits the group's policy efforts with changing the way the CDC treated AIDS in minority communities—specifically, with recognizing gay men of color as a group in need of targeted AIDS funding. Gay men of color had previously been invisible to federal agencies, which had treated gay men and racial minorities as separate categories of people, but would be invisible no more.[62]

## "This Place Needs to Burn"

Despite these successes, the work of the NTFAP was exhausting. Even before the CDC cut back its funding, the group was trying to accomplish a monumental task—educating gay men of color around the country about AIDS—with very little money. Tensions with the NABWMT and a hostile political climate only made things worse, and the group suffered other setbacks as well. By the end of 1993, two of the founding organizations in GMOCC—BAHSES and CURAS—were gone.

According to NTFAP records, BAHSES withdrew from GMOCC after some conflict over the nature of its mission. BAHSES was meant to be the consortium's African American agency and as such was responsible for a subcontract with the San Francisco AIDS Office to deliver culturally competent HIV prevention to Black gay and bisexual men. Instead, it "insisted on using a model that proved not appropriate to the target population," ironically enough, because it "felt that African American specific programming might compromise the 'multicultural' image of the agency." When BAHSES refused to make changes requested by the AIDS office, the NTFAP withdrew the subcontract and consolidated its local services for Black gay and bisexual men under the Brothers Network, a new initiative.[63]

Similarly, CURAS left GMOCC after a contract from the Office of Minority Health for a Latina lesbian health project was withdrawn. The group had undergone an audit by the San Francisco AIDS Office in the fall of 1992, which found a lack of oversight by the board of directors and major problems with the group's client files and case management procedures. As a result, the AIDS office recommended that the group's funding under the Ryan White CARE Act be terminated. The CURAS board of directors submitted a work plan for improvements at the organization, in which they argued that the problems outlined in the audit arose from "woefully inadequate administrative support," which was "not particular to CURAS but . . . indicative of a developing organizational infrastructure." The group had perhaps grown too quickly, as its annual budget had increased tenfold in less than two years. But that rapid growth, the board argued, was indicative of the fact that "the amount of funding given to Latino/a identified, governed and community based organizations is fully a decade behind the identified service need." In any case, the Office of Minority Health contract was withdrawn from CURAS and placed under Proyecto ContraSIDA por Vida, another project of the NTFAP.[64]

The notes from a focus group meeting of the GMOCC management team in late 1993 speak to the organization's successes and struggles. The departure of BAHSES had left a "vacuum," whereas the "CURAS Crisis" highlighted the "unevenness in development of member organizations." Tony Glover, who served as program director for the Brothers Network, noted that in places such as New York, "there seems to be more competition for the same pot of money," while in San Francisco "each individual community organization has become more powerful" through its involvement in GMOCC. But the group's structure also raised questions that were difficult to resolve: "How do you allow autonomy and empower a group such as GMOCC? How do you create a process in which people feel safe and can call on each other's shit?"[65]

Even apart from struggles with funding and conflict with other organizations, many NTFAP leaders, including Reggie Williams, were also fighting personal battles against HIV. Thus it was probably no surprise when, in late 1993, Williams announced that he was stepping down as head of the NTFAP. By this time he and Tim Isbell, the partner with whom he had moved to San Francisco, had split up. Williams had then met Wolfgang Schreiber at the 1992

International AIDS Conference in Amsterdam, and the two began a relationship. Schreiber had visited Williams in San Francisco, but the immigration ban on people with HIV meant that he could not move to the United States permanently.[66]

The task force threw a gala to give Williams a proper send-off. In his farewell address, Williams recalled that the "NTFAP spent the first five years of its life struggling to survive in a hostile political and economic climate that preferred to marginalize or ignore us as African Americans and as gay and bisexual men." Perhaps anxious about where the organization would go under new leadership, he continued, "But I am convinced that what we have painstakingly built in the past five years will not stand or fall on one person's presence or absence."[67]

Williams's nervousness about the NTFAP's future proved justified. The group was still in dire financial straits when he left, having received a $30,000 emergency loan from Northern California Grantmakers. The group did receive a second five-year grant from the CDC that same year but at a lower amount than requested and with a significant portion of the grant dedicated to a subcontract with Gay Asian Pacific Alliance Community HIV Project. Under the second five-year grant, the NTFAP would provide technical assistance and training to other groups around the country targeting gay men of color. In 1996 the NTFAP launched the Ujima Project in response to a CDC report that "HIV infection rates for gay and bisexual men of African descent were skyrocketing in the Southeastern United States." During this period the task force also helped other groups of gay men of color, such as the People of Color against AIDS Network in Seattle and Project Fire in New Jersey, to obtain their own federal funding.[68]

But the change in leadership led to problems at the NTFAP. Williams's successor was Randy Miller, who had served as program director for the San Francisco Black Coalition on AIDS's Rafiki Services Project before becoming director of local programs at the NTFAP. Steve Feeback, who had written the original CDC grant and been with the group since the beginning, left just a few days into Miller's tenure. Feeback later recalled that "things really fell apart" after Williams left and that Miller was "incapable of managing a complex organization." Miller stayed on as executive director until 1996 or 1997, when the group restructured. Mario Solis-Marich, who had been a cochair of the Campaign for Fairness, took over as the group's CEO, but some found him difficult to work with. Gavin Morrow-Hall remained with the NTFAP through this period but recalls that the group had "changed a great deal" and become "an unhealthy place." Around this time Williams came back to San Francisco for a visit. Seeing how much the group had declined, he remarked to Morrow-Hall,

"This place needs to burn." At the end of the second five-year CDC grant in June 1998, the NTFAP shut its doors for good. Reggie Williams passed away the following year, on February 7, 1999. He was forty-seven years old.[69]

THE NTFAP STORY POINTS TO some of the problems that have plagued minority AIDS groups. Supported as it was by a major CDC grant, the NTFAP was also vulnerable to political pressure, while being the only federally funded group for gay men of color made it a target for racist, homophobic harassment. White gay organizations suffered some of the same setbacks; the GMHC also found an enemy in Senator Jesse Helms. But the GMHC had gotten its start in the early days of the epidemic and had grown as the amount of available AIDS funding increased. By the time the NTFAP and others came on the scene, agencies such as the GMHC and the SFAF were established and well equipped to meet the expectations of public and private funders when it came to things like grant writing, budget reporting, and record keeping. The NTFAP did not have that advantage, but the group's funding and infrastructure problems had been forgiven up to a point because others respected and trusted Reggie Williams as the group's leader.

At the same time, the NTFAP example shows another way that African American AIDS activists thought about the place of Black gay identity. Whereas BEBASHI argued that Black gay men were primarily Black and secondarily gay, the NTFAP located Black gay men within the larger category of gay men of color. In this way it aimed to make the wounded whole through programs that emphasized the solidarity of nonwhite communities while attending to their cultural differences. Its effort to organize gay and bisexual men from different communities was unique as well as successful, at least in winning a seat for gay men of color, including Black gay men, at the policy making table. In the context of a racially diverse city and a country that was rapidly becoming more so, the NTFAP practiced multicultural organizing from the ground up by seeking input and leadership from different communities of color. Its model points to ways that multiculturalism can serve as a useful framework for grassroots groups from communities of color to work in powerful coalitions while maintaining their individual cultural identities.

## CHAPTER 3

# Black Men Loving Black Men
# Is a Revolutionary Act

## Gay Men of African Descent, the Black Gay Renaissance, and the Politics of Self-Esteem

N A MAY 1986 ESSAY FOR the *Philadelphia Gay News*, Black gay writer Joseph Beam took some of the nation's most prominent AIDS service organizations to task for failing to reach Black communities. "It comes as no surprise to me," he wrote, "that the Philadelphia AIDS Task Force has trouble getting AIDS information to North Philadelphia, that the New York City Gay Men's Health Crisis outreach doesn't quite make it to Harlem, or that the efforts of Washington, D.C.'s Whitman-Walker Clinic fail to extend east of the Anacostia River." Their failures, he argued, were part of a much larger problem: "The State (a euphemism for the ruling class)," which in his view included the white gay men running these organizations, "has never been concerned with the welfare of black people." Although themselves victims of homophobia, white gay professionals still had access to money and power that their Black counterparts did not and could not be counted upon to share those things with communities of color. "Our responsibility is twofold," Beam continued. "We should continue holding a gun to the heads of Philadelphia AIDS Task Force, Gay Men's Health Crisis, and the Whitman-Walker Clinic until minority outreach coordinators are hired and specific programs are implemented. But concurrently we must ensure our own safety and administer to our own sick." Beam summed up his cri de coeur: "Black men loving black men is the revolutionary act of the eighties."[1]

In nearby New York City, Beam's words became a rallying cry for the group Gay Men of African Descent. Through consciousness raising and discussion groups, members urged Black men to love Black men—to hold themselves in high esteem, to see themselves and each other as desirable, and to take care of one another in the midst of crisis. They did so in part by making Black gay men visible—to one another, to both Black and gay communities, and to the wider world.

Whereas Rashidah Hassan argued that Black gay men were primarily Black and secondarily gay, and the National Task Force on AIDS Prevention focused its energies on gay men of color more broadly, GMAD saw Blackness and gayness as more or less equally important parts of a holistic Black gay identity. Building on this notion, the group aimed to repair the psychological harm that Black gay men suffered from living in a racist, homophobic society. This, GMAD leaders argued, would be key to changing their brothers' sexual behavior in the age of AIDS and thus reducing their risk for HIV. Over time the epidemic came to make up a bigger and bigger piece of GMAD's work, as the grassroots consciousness-raising group morphed into a top-down nonprofit agency offering HIV prevention and care services to Black gay men.

GMAD emerged amid the Black gay renaissance, a larger artistic movement that aimed to make Black gay men and lesbians visible—to one another, to Black and gay communities more broadly, and to the wider world. The Black gay renaissance had its roots in the political and cultural ferment of the 1960s and 1970s, when Black Power and gay liberation (among many other movements) challenged the racism, patriarchy, and heterosexism that was baked into American society. But few of these movements made room for Black gay men and lesbians; Black Power groups and the Black Arts movement tended toward sexual chauvinism, while the growing gay rights movement was overwhelmingly white and, as the 1970s wore on, increasingly conservative. So Black gay men and lesbians forged their own path. They founded organizations such as Salsa Soul Sisters (which included Black and Latina lesbians) and the National Coalition of Black Gays and published newsletters and magazines for Black gay and lesbian readers, such as *Blacklight* and *Moja*.[2]

The devastating impact of AIDS in the 1980s gave these projects new impetus and urgency. According to Colin Robinson, who served as both a co-chair of GMAD's board of directors and as the group's executive director, the "creation of a culture and a consciousness and community" happened because "as people became ill," the "risk of coming out bec[ame] moot." As Darius Bost has observed, men in the Black gay renaissance wrote to fend off "the very real threat of historical erasure" by leaving behind a legacy that captured the fullness of their being as both Black and gay. Or, as Phill Wilson put it, "It was as if they were writing for their lives."[3]

At the same time, these writers complemented thinking among AIDS advocates as to why Black gay men seemed resistant to changing their sexual behavior. As Wilson wrote during this period, "High levels of denial and refusal to modify behavior in relation to the possibilities of HIV exposure and transmission is a further reflection of the cost being suffered by Blacks when we do not believe ourselves worthy of help or succor." "Black gay/bisexual men," he added, "are especially victimized by this phenomenon." In short, marginalization left Black gay men without the self-esteem they needed to protect themselves in the midst of a deadly epidemic. For this reason, Wilson wrote, "the center-piece of our approach" should be to endow Black gay men "with a sense of empowerment and personal efficacy." To this end, he continued, "it is essential that the Black community become educated about the critical roles Black gays and lesbians have played in the unfolding drama of gay life in America" and that "a *highly visible* gay and lesbian presence *within* the Black community" be developed. GMAD leaders likewise saw visibility for Black gay men as a means for individual and collective survival and cultivated a positive Black gay identity to help Black gay men see value in themselves. They also fostered a community that they hoped would help Black gay men feel less alienated and, later on, reinforce messages about safer sex and HIV prevention.[4]

Again, GMAD leaders built such programs on the visibility politics of the Black gay renaissance, a political and artistic movement with roots in Black lesbian feminism. That work included the excavation of a usable Black gay past, for which groups like GMAD looked to African American history and African tradition both to legitimate Black homosexuality in the present and to guide culturally competent HIV prevention programs for Black gay men. GMAD worked with the Black Leadership Commission on AIDS (BLCA) to develop one such program, based on the principles of Kwanzaa. That partnership ultimately fell apart but played an important role in GMAD's progression from a volunteer-run group into a nonprofit service agency with paid staff. As such, GMAD developed its own HIV prevention programs, including *Party*, a thirty-minute dramatic video that modeled safer sex through the stories of a diverse group of Black gay friends.

GMAD successfully courted both public and private funding of its HIV prevention efforts throughout the 1990s, but that growth came at a price. Professionalization and the pressures that came along with major grant funding weakened the group's grassroots base and narrowed its vision for social and political change. At the same time, the AIDS epidemic robbed GMAD—and the Black gay renaissance—of some of its most vital and challenging voices.[5]

## "Visibility Is Survival"

Growing up as a Black gay man, Joseph Beam felt invisible and alone. While attending graduate school in Iowa in the late 1970s, he later wrote, "I thought

I was the first Black gay man to have ever lived." After returning to his native Philadelphia and while working at Giovanni's Room, the city's gay bookstore, he "grew tired of reading literature by white gay men" in which "all the protagonists are blond; all the Blacks are criminal and negligible." At the same time, he felt that he could not "go home" to Black America, for there "I am most often rendered invisible, perceived as a threat to the family, or am tolerated if I am silent and inconspicuous." For Beam, invisibility meant annihilation, a fate worse than death. But, he wrote, "visibility is survival."[6]

Beam found comfort in art and writing by other Black gay men. He read James Baldwin's novel *Just above My Head*, one of the author's rare works depicting Black gay characters. He paged through newsletters and literary journals such as *Blackheart*, *Habari-Daftari*, and *Yemonja*, which featured essays and commentary by other Black gay writers. He danced to disco hits by Sylvester, the openly gay and femme Black singer, and corresponded with Blackberri, a stocky, dreadlocked singer-songwriter who toured West Coast coffee shops and galleries, performing original numbers like "Beautiful Black Man."[7]

Beam also found inspiration—and a model for his own work—in writings by Third World lesbian feminist writers such as Audre Lorde, Cherríe Moraga, Barbara Smith, and Cheryl Clarke. In anthologies such as *This Bridge Called My Back* and *Home Girls*, these women documented the ways that racial and gender oppression intersected in their own lives. In their writing Beam found both a framework for thinking about his experience as a Black gay man, living under the dual oppression of racism and homophobia, and a sense of revolutionary strength and resiliency. In the words of Jamaican American lesbian poet Michelle Cliff, these women claimed an identity they were taught to despise. As a writer and editor, Joseph Beam led the way in helping Black gay men do the same.[8]

Beam set out to produce his own anthology of work by Black gay men. He placed ads in gay newspapers soliciting essays, short stories, and poetry, which he published as *In the Life: A Black Gay Anthology* in 1986. The book was received with enthusiasm and acclaim for the mosaic of Black gay experiences it presented: a personal essay about fighting for citizenship as both "an openly gay person . . . [and] a foreign-born, Black individual," a manifesto on the need for a Black gay church, tales of erotic encounters, and an interview with the Black gay science fiction writer Samuel R. Delany. For Black gay readers who, like Beam, found themselves both missing from gay newsstands and exiled from Blackness, *In the Life* was a revelation.[9]

Work on *In the Life* eased Beam's loneliness by bringing him into contact with other Black gay writers around the country. One of these was Essex Hemphill, a poet and performance artist who lived in Washington, D.C. The two formed a close friendship, and after Beam's death in December 1988 (Beam was HIV positive, but as Darius Bost notes, his body was "found in such an advanced state of decomposition that the final cause of death could not be determined"), Hemphill took over responsibility for editing a second volume, *Brother to Brother*, released in 1991. At the same time that Hemphill was working in Philadelphia to complete *Brother to Brother*, the New York Black gay writers' collective Other Countries held a weekly writing workshop, along with regular performances and educational programs. The New York group would publish its own volumes of collected works, including *Other Countries: Black Gay Voices—A First Volume* in 1988 and *Sojourner: Black Gay Voices in the Age of AIDS* in 1993.[10]

Filmmakers in the Black gay renaissance also used their craft to explore identity on the margins of race and sexuality. In his 1989 film *Tongues Untied*, Marlon Riggs examined his own experience as an HIV-positive Black gay man. Isaac Julien's *Looking for Langston*, released the same year, explored the life of the iconic Black poet Langston Hughes, who was long rumored to have carried on affairs with other men. Two years later, in 1991, the lesbian filmmaker Jennie Livingston released *Paris Is Burning*, her documentary about New York City's underground drag ball scene. The film later became the subject of controversy, as many of the film's subjects, who were mostly Black and Latino, claimed they had been denied a share of the profits by Livingston, who is white. At the time of its release, however, it was warmly received by GMAD and the NTFAP, both of which hosted screenings.[11]

This artistic work overlapped with a growing wave of political activity by self-identified Black gay men and lesbians. National networks formed, such as the National Coalition of Black Gays (later the National Coalition of Black Lesbians and Gays, or NCBLG) in 1978 and the Black Gay and Lesbian Leadership Forum in 1987. Beam became editor in chief of *Black/Out*, the NCBLG's quarterly magazine, when it debuted in 1986. Black gay men and lesbians also organized at the local level, forming groups such as Philadelphia Black Gays, Salsa Soul Sisters in New York, and Black Gays/Lesbians United in Portland, Oregon.[12]

This movement sustained a liberationist model of gay politics—one that merged the fight against homophobia with struggles against racism, sexism, poverty, and imperialism. It also linked the struggle against oppression at home to the one abroad, evident in participants' use of the phrase "Third World" to describe nonwhite people in the United States.[13] Contributors to the National Coalition of Black Gays' newsletters *Habari-Habari* and *Habari-Daftari* criticized Reagan's "policy of military adventurism . . . in the Caribbean and Central America," which brought violence to people there and came "at the expense of child care programs, educational programs, aid for the elderly, aid to dependent children and an increase in poverty among women and Black people" at home. They likewise criticized leaders of the larger gay and lesbian movement for focusing narrowly on homophobia while ignoring other forms of oppression, including racism. At the same time, they encouraged support for those ensnared in the growing carceral system through their prison project and printed letters from inmates that testified to the abuse they faced on the inside.[14]

The intellectual and political projects of the Black gay renaissance were closely related, and both overlapped with Black gay men's AIDS activism. National groups like the NCBLG fostered networks of politically engaged Black gay men and lesbians who could be mobilized in the fight against AIDS, and activists used their meetings as an opportunity to conduct HIV and safer sex education workshops. Key figures also frequently crossed the line between movement politics and cultural politics. Gil Gerald helped to found the NCBLG and later served as the group's executive director; he also contributed to *In the Life*. Cary Alan Johnson joined the Committee of Black Gay Men in New York City in the late 1970s, contributed to *Black/Out* in the 1980s, and became executive director of GMAD during the middle 1990s. Colin Robinson helped to found Other Countries, worked as a field producer on *Tongues Untied*, and held a variety of leadership roles in GMAD during the group's first decade of existence. Artists and writers also engaged in direct action protest. Craig G. Harris, who contributed to *In the Life* and *Brother to Brother*, disrupted a session on AIDS at the 1986 meeting of the American Public Health Association in San Francisco. After seeing that there were no speakers of color included in the session, Harris stormed to the front of the room and snatched the microphone from San Francisco health director Mervyn Silverman, shouting, "I will be heard!"[15]

GMAD was born out of this political and cultural ferment. When Harold Robinson, Colin Robinson, and Charles Angel got together to write a statement of purpose for the new group in August 1986, they framed their project in expansive terms. GMAD would aim "to end any and all ills that interfere with the rights of all individuals to exist and co-exist in a free, democratic society," as well as "[to end] racism, sexism, class oppression, and all Lesbian and Gay oppression, wherever these may exist." They made no specific reference to AIDS, although a meeting later that month included discussion of the Minority Task Force on AIDS and the recently formed Minority Caucus of Gay Men's Health Crisis. By this point the disease was inescapable in Black gay circles, and GMAD members saw its impact in Angel's failing health. Within six months the GMAD founder would be dead of complications from AIDS, forcing the new group into a brief hiatus. Angel's death spoke to a looming reality, as the epidemic sapped the Black gay movement of some of its most vital and challenging voices. This would also become evident in the GMAD story writ large, as the group's world-making vision narrowed over time into a rearguard defense against a devastating epidemic.[16]

## Finding a Black Gay Past—and Present

By early 1988 GMAD had re-formed as "a support group of Black Gay Men dedicated to consciousness raising and the development of the Black Lesbian & Gay Community." Members gathered at the Lesbian and Gay Community Services Center in Greenwich Village or at someone's home for Friday Night Forum, a weekly event that included lectures, workshops, or discussion groups. Topics ranged from "Cruising and Coming On" and "Gay Parenting" to "Christianity and Homosexuality" and "Violence and Racism." The group also produced the GMAD *Calendar*, a monthly newsletter with events, announcements, classifieds, and artwork. GMAD took seriously Joseph Beam's call for Black men to love Black men, and both the Friday Night Forums and the GMAD *Calendar* explored the contours of that love. They portrayed Black gay men as desirable and diverse, with lives shaped by intersecting social differences, including race, gender, and sexuality. By seeing and sharing their own experiences in the larger group, GMAD members might come to love one another, and themselves, more fully.[17]

GMAD members also looked for a usable past to anchor their pride as Black gay men in the present. They found one in the Harlem Renaissance and the civil rights movement. Here, too, they built on the work of others in the Black gay renaissance. The April 1979 issue of *Moja*, a newsletter distributed by the Oscar Wilde Memorial Bookshop in New York City's Greenwich Village, reprinted an article from the feminist magazine *Sojourner* on J. R. Roberts's work to "document the biography, literature, music and other works—historical and contemporary—that speak to the lives of Black lesbians," which culminated in the publication of *Black Lesbians: An Annotated Bibliography* in 1981. The NCBLG's 1985 conference included a "well-received" workshop on "Black Lesbian and Gay Oral History" led by Mabel Hampton, who was also heavily involved with the development of the Lesbian Herstory Archives. In honor of Black History Month in 1986, Craig G. Harris, who would later that year disrupt the American Public Health Association meeting, wrote about the "seldom-told tale" of Black gay and lesbian history for *Au Courant*. Drawing connections between the Harlem Renaissance and the "black lesbian/gay movement of the '80s," he predicted that future generations would study the work of Beam, Hemphill, Audre Lorde, and a host of others. Harris lamented the need for "artist/historians telling both the joys and traumas of our lives," but his own work points to a self-conscious desire to both recover Black gay history and write the burgeoning Black gay renaissance into it.[18]

In the same vein, *In the Life* included a biographical profile of Black gay bohemian Bruce Nugent, who based the protagonist in his 1926 homoerotic short story "Smoke, Lilies, and Jade" in part on his contemporary Langston Hughes. Isaac Julien, a Black gay British filmmaker, also used Hughes's life as the basis for his 1989 film *Looking for Langston*, a "meditation" on "the role of the black [gay] artist in relationship to the black community" as well as on "the connections between black gay identities in the present and black gay identities in the past." George Bass, Hughes's former secretary and the executor of his estate, objected to the film and sought to block its U.S. release. Hemphill interviewed Julien for *Brother to Brother* and, in a separate essay in the same volume, criticized Bass and other "black academicians" for trying "to prevent black gays and lesbians from claiming historical affirmations and references for *our* desires."[19]

GMAD incorporated Black gay history into its weekly programs, arguing that this affirmed members' identity and would help them reduce their risk for HIV. At one Friday Night Forum in 1995, members learned about "the creativity and strategies of Black Gays and Lesbians during [the Harlem Renaissance] in creating or accessing social networks and spaces," concluding with a Black gay man in his seventies who shared "a candid personal history" about growing up in Jazz Age Harlem. According to a monthly report made to one of the group's funders, gay men's involvement in the storied Harlem Renaissance surprised many GMAD members, and most had never met a Black gay man so much older than themselves. The report's author asserted that such programming "support[ed] the development and maintenance of a healthy identity, a critical preventive measure to an array of risk behaviors."[20]

Bayard Rustin, the gay civil rights leader and "architect" of the 1963 March on Washington, also connected Black gay men in the present to a celebrated period in African American history. In a 1995 press conference in Harlem, GMAD board cochair George Bellinger pointed to Rustin as an example of the way that gay men had been made invisible in Black communities both past and present. "The Black community," he told the press, "believed that it would be better if the gay director of that momentous march took a backseat to a heterosexual spokesperson.... [Rustin's] contribution was rarely acknowledged and his silence was expected." He continued, "We have and will continue to defend you tooth and nail. We have been a part of every major activity and yet some of you dare not speak our names." Echoing the motto of the NCBLG, he

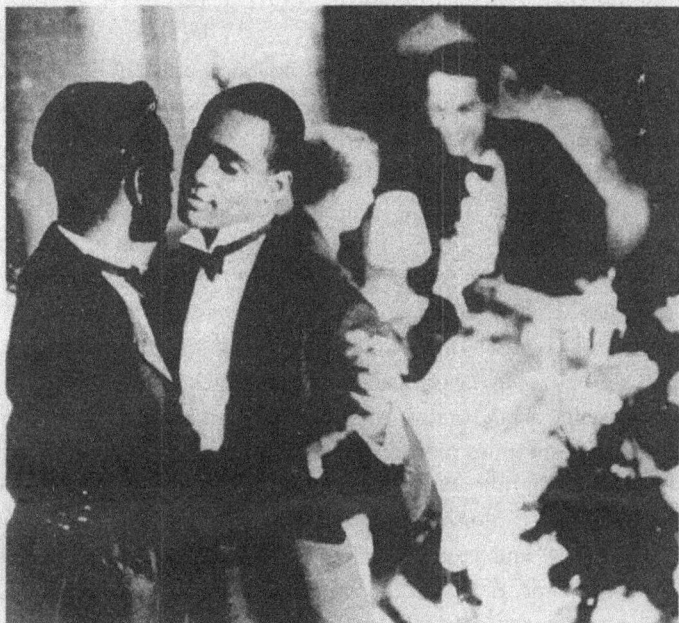

# GMAD
*Gay Men of African Descent*

FREE TO GMAD MEMBERS
Other friends, please send us $6 or more yearly, payable to Pilgrim Spikes/GMAD Treasurer.

# CALENDAR

**D E C E M B E R**

**1 9 8 9**

"Dancers in the timeless dance hall" from *Looking for Langston*
Photo: Sunil Gupta.  Courtesy Sankofa Film & Video

**GMAD is inclusive of African, Black, Caribbean and Hispanic/Latino men of color and welcomes your help in doing this better.**
GMAD meets weekly — generally Fridays at 8:00 p.m. at the Lesbian and Gay Community Services Center. *We encourage you to suggest other meeting spaces in the Black and Latino communities.* Meetings focus on different topics of relevance to the GMAD community. *(See pp. 2 & 3 inside for details of December and January meetings.)* Special events are also planned from time to time. Voter registration information and forms; safer sex information and rubbers; counseling and referrals are available at all meetings. Bring snacks and non-alcoholic beverages to share.

Help GMAD serve *your* needs by sharing your ideas for activities; or by helping to organize specific events. You can make suggestions by mail or phone *(see address and numbers below)*, or in person at any GMAD meeting.

Although you are welcome to attend most GMAD activities without becoming a member, we encourage you to support the organization by joining soon. Membership entitles you to voting privileges, notification of all meetings, plus this monthly calendar, and discounts on most fundraising events. Fees are $20 a year ($10 for six months). Membership forms are available at meetings, or you may write to the address below, or call Tito Malcolm Davis at (718) 498-3426 or Austin Pilgrim at (718) 464-0225 for membership information.

For more information, call (718) 802-0162 or (718) 756-1548; or write to the address below.

*Finding Community In Diversity*

P.O. BOX 2519, NEW YORK, NEW YORK 10185-0021

*GMAD Calendar*, December 1989, featuring a still from Isaac Julien's *Looking for Langston*. The text in bold specifies that "GMAD is inclusive of African, Black Caribbean and Hispanic/Latino men of color and welcomes your help in doing this better." Gay Men of African Descent Records, Sc MG 688, Schomburg Center, New York.

concluded, "We will no longer be rendered invisible, for we are as proud of our gayness as we are of our Blackness."[21]

GMAD also looked for a usable Black gay past in African history and tradition. Here members argued against Black Power icons like Eldridge Cleaver and Afrocentric thinkers like Frances Cress Welsing and Molefi Asante, who all saw homosexuality as a threat to the future of Black people. In his 1968 memoir, *Soul on Ice*, former Black Panther Cleaver declared it a "racial death-wish," while Welsing claimed it "was an almost non-existent behavioral phenomenon amongst indigenous Blacks in Africa" but had developed among African American men due to their emasculation by a racist society. Asante similarly claimed that homosexuality was not an "Afrocentric relationship" and thus was at odds with Black well-being. In one of his contributions to *Brother to Brother*, Marlon Riggs summed up their "pseudoacademic claims": "In precolonial Africa, men were truly men. And women—were women. Nobody was lesbian. Nobody was feminist. Nobody was gay."[22]

In contrast, GMAD highlighted same-sex desire on the continent, both in the premodern period and in the present, to validate Black gay identity. In this way the group presented an alternative Afrocentrism that made room for same-sex desire, even if it sometimes reproduced colonial tropes of Africa as a strange and timeless place. In July 1988 GMAD vice president Elbert Gates hosted two African gay men at his home for a Friday Night Forum. The event promised "exotic native foods" and asked attendees to "wear something traditional." At another forum, members learned about Black gay men in history, "from Africa to the present," positioning the continent as both spatially and temporally distant. Future GMAD programs and publications would also draw from African cultures that developed thousands of miles apart, flattening distinctions among them in a way that is common among Western observers.[23]

At other times GMAD looked more specifically to African history for inspiration. A May 1994 program, "Cross-Dressing in African Culture," asked, "Was the famous Hatshepsut a queen or a pharaoh? Or perhaps both? Did she rule wearing the drag of a king? Was Akhenaten an effeminate homosexual? What is the attitude of traditional Africa on cross-dressing and gender roles?" Such questions not only held open the possibility that queer embodiments such as female masculinity or male effeminacy might have been tolerated in "traditional Africa" but also attributed them to ancient Egyptian pharaohs, symbols of both political savvy and advanced civilization. Racist stereotypes, particularly in the United States and Europe, notably denied that African peoples could possess such qualities, and instead portrayed them as timelessly backward, primitive, even prehistorical.[24]

GMAD was not alone in this focus on Africa; the National Coalition of Black

Gays titled its early newsletters *Habari-Habari* and *Habari-Daftari*, Swahili phrases that mean "What's the news?" and "News register."[25] GMAD also supported and promoted the work of other groups that similarly called on queer African traditions. Adodi, a Black gay men's group founded in Philadelphia in 1986,[26] took its name from the plural of *ado*, a Yoruba word to describe "a man who 'loves' another man." "More than just a description of partners," the organization claimed, "in Africa, the ADODI of the tribe are thought to embody both male and female ways of being and were revered as shamans, sages, and leaders."[27] According to Michael Oatis, an Adodi member who profiled the group for *Black/Out* in 1987, the word itself "had a long spiritual heritage and tradition as well, being associated with the Santeria religion and the goddess Yemaya."[28] Here was evidence that Black gay men were not only accepted in at least one African society but awarded power and prestige as well.

Adodi members first met informally at the home of Clifford Rawlins, an art therapist in Philadelphia, to talk about everything from "the isolation they felt as Black gay men, to the alarming number of their brothers dying of AIDS, to the lack of institutions available to help them cope." Adodi organized an annual retreat in Pottstown, Pennsylvania, beginning in 1987. The theme of the first retreat, "Self-Esteem: Loving Ourselves through the 80's," echoed Joseph Beam's call for Black gay men to love one another, as well as Black gay AIDS activists' emphasis on self-esteem. According to a group member present at that retreat, Rawlins "felt the need to bring black men together to do some mourning rituals. We were all walking zombies, all of our friends and partners dying not knowing how to process. . . . It was a very sad time. . . . We all knew that we needed each other, we needed a space to be with each other." Adodi advertised its 1989 summer retreat, on the theme of "Self-Empowerment in the Age of AIDS," in the GMAD *Calendar*, which also periodically reported the deaths of Adodi members. In August 1991, GMAD hosted Adodi's New York chapter to talk about "exploring the spiritual side of our development . . . in the spirit of Umoja," the Swahili word for "unity" and one of the seven principles of Kwanzaa. The following month a Friday Night Forum titled "Older Black Gay Men Loving Each Other Is Seen as an Act of Survival" invited older members to take on the role of "ADODI, the wise men/healers of Yoruba society," and "enlighten us with their experience and instill in some of the younger GMAD members a sense of pride about their heritage."[29]

Over time, GMAD also increasingly used African language and symbols to describe its activities. Thus, "Can We Talk?," a series of "rap-style sessions with self-awareness and communication exercises," became "Can We . . . Ukwangela?," using a Nyakyusa word that the GMAD *Calendar* defined as "the enjoyment of good company and the mutual aid and sympathy which spring from personal relationships." This would offer members the "opportunity for us as Gay men of color to titter like sissies or palaver like princes in an unstructured, non-competitive setting," raising the possibility for members to embody both effeminate "sissies" and African royalty in the same evening.[30]

The cover of the first GMAD *Calendar* for 1992 urged readers to "Keep Kwanzaa Principles throughout the Year" with a list of the *nguzo saba*, the seven Kwanzaa principles defined by Maulana Karenga. A Friday Night Forum in late January promised to do just that, through a discussion of media representations of Black gay men. The program description asked readers, "How can we begin the process of defining ourselves in the mass media?" while urging them to "revisit the principle of Kujichagulia [self-determination] as we discuss and answer these questions tonight."[31]

As GMAD's programming became more explicitly Afrocentric in content, the GMAD *Calendar* communicated this shift with visual cues as well. The publication's pages frequently featured the outline or silhouette of the African continent or African iconography, such as the Yoruba door carving that adorned the cover of the June 1993 issue. Friday Night Forums covered topics related to Afrocentric or diasporic themes, such as the September 1993 workshop titled "Roots," which promised to "look at the roots of many of those things we inherit from the Motherland." Other events dealt with the status of Black gay men and lesbians abroad, as when GMAD hosted the well-known South African activist Simon Nkoli in October 1993 and representatives from Black gay and lesbian community groups from Africa, the Caribbean, and the United Kingdom in July 1994.[32]

Members of GMAD and Adodi looked for a usable Black gay past in order to challenge their own exclusion from contemporary ideas of Blackness, including the Afrocentric thought of the 1980s and 1990s. But they also looked to the past as a source of healing that could act as a balm for the psychological and spiritual wounds that Black gay men suffered at the intersection of racism and homophobia. In African tradition they found models of community in which to mourn friends and lovers lost to AIDS. In the long Black freedom struggle, they found examples of resistance and resilience to confront a devastating epidemic. For Black gay men facing an uncertain future, the past took on new importance.[33]

## Tongues Untied

The Black gay filmmaker Marlon Riggs framed history as a source of strength for Black gay men, and particularly for Black gay AIDS activists, in his 1989 film *Tongues Untied*. Riggs began work on the film in 1987 after testing positive for

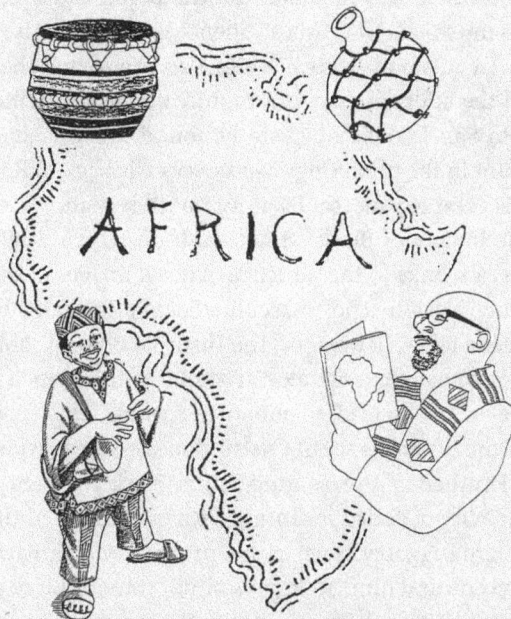

# GMAD
*Gay Men of African Descent*

A

SUPPORTIVE

ORGANIZATION

DEDICATED

TO

ADDRESSING

THE

NEEDS

OF

OUR

COMMUNITY,

FOCUSES

ON

ADVOCACY,

HEALTH,

EDUCATION,

AND

CONSCIOUSNESS

RAISING.

**CALENDAR**

*AFRICA*

*In The Spirit of Lesbian & Gay Unity...KWANZAA '94*

**DECEMBER 1994**

GMAD, Inc., 666 Broadway, Suite 520
New York, New York 10012-2317

Tel: (212) 420-0773  Fax: (212) 982-3321

GMAD *Calendar*, December 1994. The images of Africa, kente cloth, and a gourd rattle, along with the reference to Kwanzaa, mark GMAD's shift to a more Afrocentric style. Gay Men of African Descent Records, Sc MG 688, Schomburg Center, New York.

HIV and used it to connect the spread of HIV among Black gay men to the many ways that Black gay life was (and is) devalued.[34]

Riggs wove themes of silence and invisibility through *Tongues Untied*, exploring the experience of Black gay men in America through autobiography, poetry, and performance. Early on in the film, a conversation between two disembodied voices meditates on the perils and protections of silence: "Silence is my shield. (It crushes.) Silence is my cloak. (It smothers.) Silence is my sword. (It cuts both ways.)" Riggs also considered the meaning of his Blackness in the midst of a gay community defined by whiteness in recounting his move to San Francisco, where he found himself "immersed in vanilla." At one point in the film, Riggs' voiceover calls back to Ralph Ellison, lamenting, "In this great gay mecca, I was an invisible man," as exaggerated and pornographic images of Black "studs" flash on-screen. Riggs intended the film to serve as a rebuke to the "absence of black images in this new gay life," as well as to the "black macho" masculine ideal propagated by Welsing and Asante. One scene takes viewers to "The Institute of Snap!thology," where a group of Black gay men demonstrate variations of the snap, a flamboyant, nonverbal gesture meant "to read, to punctuate, to cut." The "snap divas" act out neither the macho performance of Castro clones nor the revolutionary bravado of the Black Panthers. By presenting actual Black gay men throwing snaps with a "multiplicity of coded meanings," Riggs challenged the contemporary vogue for "Negro Faggotry," seen in the "proliferating bit-part swish-and-dish divas" of television and film. To Riggs's mind, straight Black artists and intellectuals deployed the Negro Faggot in much the same way as blackface entertainers depicted shuffling Sambos: as the counterpoint Other, without interiority and authority, to construct a number of superior masculine images, including the tribal warrior, the fraternity brother of Spike Lee's *School Daze*, or the swaggering straight MC.[35]

In a poem that accompanies the film's closing sequence, Riggs turns to history to make sense of the loss of friends and his own imperiled health:

> I listen to the beat of my heart,
> let this primal pulse lead me,
> though lately I've lived with another rhythm.
> At first, I thought just time passing. But I discovered a time bomb
> ticking in my blood.
> Faces, friends disappear.
> I watch.
> I wait.

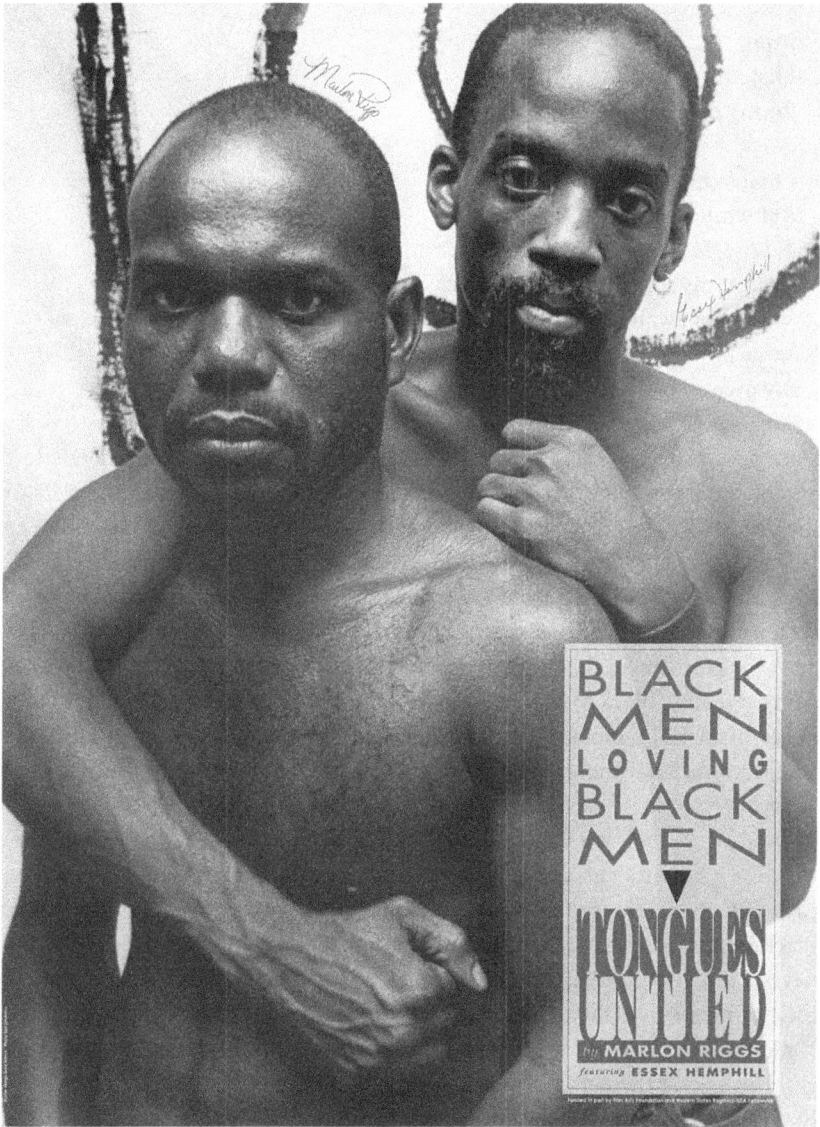

Poster for *Tongues Untied*, dir. Marlon Riggs, 1989. Collection of the Smithsonian National Museum of African American History and Culture, gift of Jack Vincent in memory of Marlon Riggs. Copyright Signifyin' Works.

I watch.
I wait.
I listen
for my own
quiet
implosion.
But while I wait,
older, stronger rhythms resonate within me,
sustain my spirit, silence the clock.
Whatever awaits me, this much I know:
I was blind to my brother's beauty, and now I see
my own.

Here Riggs struggles with a grief that defies representation—of friends lost and of the knowledge that his own name will soon be added to the rolls of the dead.[36] Yet he finds refuge in the past, drawing on ancestral tradition to "silence the clock" while writing himself and his brothers into historical time. Images of Black gay men lost to AIDS give way to photographs of past figures such as Sojourner Truth and Frederick Douglass, and footage of civil rights marches fades into a slow-motion shot of Black gay men marching with a banner that reads, "Black Men Loving Black Men Is a Revolutionary Act." With an eye to historical memory, Riggs wanted to make sure that future generations would know "that there was a vibrant Black gay community in these United States."[37]

*Tongues Untied* was well received by critics, but controversy surrounded the film when the PBS documentary film series *POV* decided to screen it in 1991. Due to the film's graphic nature, some local PBS stations refused to air it. Black leaders also criticized Riggs for promoting stereotypes of Black sexual deviance, although Riggs had produced such images precisely in order to show their oppressive quality. Congressional Republicans reacted by attacking the National Endowment for the Arts, which funded *POV*, for awarding Riggs a grant of $5,000 through the Western Regional Arts Fund. Like the attacks on the NTFAP and *Hot, Horny and Healthy!*, the censorship of Riggs's film were part of a larger set of struggles that ensnared work by Robert Mapplethorpe, Andres Serrano, and numerous others during the "culture wars" of the 1990s. At the same time, the story of *Tongues Untied* calls our attention to the ways that Black gay artists and activists in particular were vulnerable to conservative attacks during this period.[38]

Black gay leaders, including Reggie Williams from the NTFAP, Marc Loveless from the NCBLG, and Thom Bean from the Gay and Lesbian Alliance against

Defamation, were in Detroit in June 1991 for the annual meeting of the National Association of Black and White Men Together when they learned that the local PBS affiliate, WTVS, had decided not to air *Tongues Untied*. They met with the station's leadership to argue for the film's merit, but WTVS president Robert Larson refused to budge. In response, Bean insisted that by making the struggles of Black gay men visible to the viewing public, *Tongues Untied* would save lives. "That is why it is so important for Black gay men to see their common dilemmas in this society and recognize they are not alone," he said in a press release. "One less suicide, one less gay bashing would make airing 'Tongues Untied' worthwhile." Although Bean did not name risk for HIV as one of the threats to Black gay lives that the film might ameliorate, the NTFAP went on to develop a workshop for Black gay and bisexual men that combined a screening of the film with "discussions addressing issues of internalized racism, identity and self-esteem" that would make participants more open to protecting themselves from HIV through safer sex.[39]

Colin Robinson, then serving as co-chair of the GMAD board of directors, and Robert Reid-Pharr, who had been active in the NCBLG and contributed to *Brother to Brother*, also struck back in a trenchant open letter to the PBS affiliates who refused to air *Tongues Untied*. They claimed that the decision to block the film represented "not simply censorship, but a willful contribution to prejudice" and an abrogation of "public TV's fundamental mission ... to honestly represent Americans' rich diversity and complexity." Not only had "Black Gay Americans [missed] an opportunity to see our tax money spent in ways which directly seek to empower and affirm our lives," but the invocation of "chimeric 'community standards'" to block the film reinforced the exclusion of Black gay men from the national "community" whose standards PBS purported to enforce.[40]

The controversy over *Tongues Untied* went far beyond PBS affiliates' refusal to air the film. During the summer of 1991, just as NTFAP leaders were fending off attacks over *Hot, Horny and Healthy!*, Riggs was making the rounds on television talk shows to defend his work. Like Robinson and Reid-Pharr, he responded to critics who objected to the use of taxpayer dollars to fund and screen *Tongues Untied*, emphasizing that "we [Black gay men] are part of those Americans whose salaries are taxed to support the government." Meanwhile, conservatives used the controversy to strike at public institutions. Republican senators called for an end to the Corporation for Public Broadcasting, while Pat Buchanan used clips of Riggs's film in a presidential campaign ad that attacked George H. W. Bush from the right for "invest[ing] our tax dollars in pornographic and blasphemous art too shocking to show."[41]

Just as Craig Harris called for "artist/historians telling both the joys and traumas of our lives," Riggs delivered a film that was both deeply personal and political in the way that it wove Black gay AIDS activism into the longer trajectory of the Black freedom struggle in America. The decision by PBS affiliates nationwide not to air *Tongues Untied* illustrates the problem of Black gay men's representation that GMAD saw as crucial to its fight against HIV. At the same time, the controversy surrounding the film, especially when read alongside the backlash against the NTFAP over federal funding for *Hot, Horny and Healthy!*, highlights the ways that conservative activists used homophobia and anti-Blackness not only to attack Black gay men but to undermine the very notion of a public good.

## There Are No White People in the Room

While GMAD and NTFAP leaders agreed that self-esteem was key to stopping the spread of HIV among Black gay and bisexual men, they took different approaches when it came to deciding exactly who was welcome in their respective organizations. While the NTFAP explicitly embraced multiculturalism through the Gay Men of Color Consortium, GMAD moved toward an ethnocentric model. These ideas about Blackness did not represent the entire range of possibilities for Black gay identification. Instead, they point to the variety of ways in which Black gay men understood their identity in the context of an emerging epidemic.

GMAD members wrestled at times with the question of who exactly should be included in the group. From 1989 to 1992 the GMAD *Calendar* indicated that "African, Black, Caribbean, and Hispanic/Latino men of color" were welcome, and sometimes used "African American" instead of or alongside "Black," and added "Arab" for a few months in 1991. For a time, GMAD leaders tried to make the organization more inclusive of Latino gay men. For example, the theme for one Friday Night Forum in November 1989 was "Uniéndonos (Drawing Together)," with a program description printed in both Spanish and English that asked, "Are there issues of significance to Hispanic/Latino men that have not been attended to by GMAD? What can GMAD do to make our Hispanic/Latino brothers more welcome?" Whether they intended for the session to address the concerns of self-identified Afro-Latino gay men or of Latino gay men in general is unclear. Either way, beginning with the March 1992 *Calendar*, GMAD dropped specific ethnic labels and instead described the group as "committed to fighting racism, sexism and homophobia, while creating nurturing environments that affirm, celebrate and empower Gay Men of African Descent in all our diversity."[42]

In terms that echoed similar discussions within the Black gay community in the San Francisco Bay Area, GMAD also debated whether white men should be admitted to meetings and events. In May 1989 the group hosted a session titled "There Are No White People in the Room" to discuss a recent "controversial incident . . . where a White guest was asked to be silent." Two years later, in September 1991, the group hosted a similar session in which members discussed "Afrocentricity, security in self identity, and segregation," along with the question of whether "persons not of color" should "be allowed to participate" in GMAD.[43]

In March 1992 these questions came to the fore at a GMAD event, when member Bernard Jones asked "Anthony," a white gay man in attendance, to leave. The man left but wrote an angry letter to GMAD executive director Joe Pressley, decrying Jones's "hatred" and insisting both that other members had supported his attendance and that he should be allowed at GMAD events because he had a history of loving and dating Black men. Jones defended himself in a public response at a meeting later that month, claiming that "Anthony" had threatened him under his breath while getting up to leave and that the other man wanted only to "indulge [his] chocolate fantasies" anyway. Jones further argued that GMAD should be "a place of safety for those who desire and need it, removed from the everyday pressures of living in a white-dominated society." Drawing an explicit contrast between GMAD and groups like the NTFAP, he continued, "I am far less concerned about political correctness and the social fad of multiculturalism than I am about the clear work that we must first accomplish ourselves with a minimum of outside influence and participation."[44]

Pressley shared Jones's view. In 2013 the former executive director reflected on the incident and on the racial politics of the group's admissions policy: "I think identity politics are extremely important inasmuch as they provide an opportunity for people to enter into conversations. . . . I think that identity politics provide an avenue for getting people who may not even come in for any kind of discussion." Participation by white men, in his view, could prevent the kind of necessary healing dialogue that GMAD was trying to promote. He continued, "When there's a white person in the room, as liberal as that white person may be, it changes the conversation. So how do we have a conversation as only Black gay men?"[45]

Others disagreed. In the June 1992 GMAD *Calendar*, which contained the letter from "Anthony" and Jones's response, Pressley tendered his letter of resignation, citing frustrations with GMAD members and leaders who "kept/keep buying into the house negro and straight boy plans." He illustrated his point with statements made by fellow members, including two on the issue of allowing white people into GMAD meetings: "We just gotta allow white people in our meetings.

After all, it is *their* center," and, "It's wrong not to allow white folks into the meetings since many of y'all (GMAD members) attended *their* universities."[46]

Pressley defended the need to provide a space solely for Black men, asking, "Are we really so consumed by internalized racism and self-hatred that we've been brainwashed to believe that GMAD isn't legit unless white folks can enter and leave as they please?" He also castigated GMAD members for their disinterest in more explicitly political forms of activism, as the group could "sell out GMAD dances and fashion shows but [could not] get ten GMAD members to venture up to Albany . . . for AIDS Awareness Day or . . . to bring two hundred cans of food for clients of the Minority Task Force on AIDS Housing Project." In his view, GMAD members failed to fully realize the extent of their shared problems or their collective power. "AIDS Awareness Day," Pressley continued, "was structured to give disenfranchised people (*you know folks like us*) the opportunity to take our issues directly to our elected politicians." Alternatively, he raised the possibility of something like a Black gay general strike: "This city would come to a halt if every Gay/Bisexual Black man called in sick or took a vacation for just one day. Imagine if we joined forces with Black women. We have the power and we don't even know it."[47]

Pressley's frustration stemmed not only from GMAD's internal racial politics but from members' apparent reluctance to take up the tactics of movement politics. Around the same time, however, GMAD had begun to flex its power— not through lobbying or a general strike but by asserting its authority to shape the fight against HIV among its own.

## Lifestyles Genesis

Even as GMAD claimed inclusion in contemporary Blackness, it insisted that only Black gay men could design culturally competent HIV prevention programs to reach other Black gay men. The group clashed with the Black Leadership Commission on AIDS, a coalition of African American political, religious, and community leaders in New York City, over Lifestyles Genesis, an HIV prevention program based on the *nguzo saba*, or Kwanzaa principles, which GMAD had been contracted to deliver to its members. GMAD leaders found Lifestyles Genesis to be so poorly designed as to be ineffective, which they chalked up to the BLCA's failure to include input from gay and lesbian African American groups in designing the program's curriculum. Thereafter, GMAD created its own interventions, including a thirty-minute dramatic video intended to help Black gay men protect themselves from HIV.[48]

In 1990, GMAD contracted with the BLCA to present the latter group's Lifestyles Genesis Learning Series, an Afrocentric HIV education program based on the seven *nguzo saba*. In four meetings over the course of a month, groups of twenty-five Black gay men would meet with a licensed clinician, who would deliver the program's lessons on health, discrimination, sexual relationships, and identity management, all through the lens of the *nguzo saba*. While the BLCA administered Lifestyles Genesis through a contract with the New York State Department of Health AIDS Institute, GMAD and another group, People of Color in Crisis, would work on the ground as subcontracting agencies to deliver the program, conducting sessions and recruiting participants. Representatives from GMAD and People of Color in Crisis would also help craft the curriculum at a planning retreat with BLCA leaders, including Drs. Jerome Gibbs and Richard Dudley, the program's principal authors.[49]

The Lifestyles Genesis program meshed well with GMAD's emphasis on the psychosocial needs of Black gay men, not to mention with the group's increasingly Afrocentric orientation. Thanks to the NTFAP survey, which showed that Black gay men knew how HIV was transmitted but hadn't changed their sexual practices accordingly, GMAD leaders also saw the need for such a program. Lifestyles Genesis, with its emphasis on "identity management" and the *nguzo saba*, promised to strike a balance between healing individual Black gay men's sense of alienation and cultivating a sense of communal responsibility to reduce the spread of HIV through condom use.[50]

The contract with the BLCA to deliver Lifestyles Genesis to GMAD constituents also promised to help the latter organization grow into a professional organization with paid staff, but the collaboration did not go smoothly. Elbert Gates, GMAD's first executive director, negotiated the agreement with the BLCA much as he directed GMAD's other affairs—without consulting the board of directors. Unhappy with his single-minded leadership style, the board voted Gates out of office in April 1991, just months before the program was slated to begin. Colin Robinson, who helped found the group five years earlier and was elected to the board in the wake of Gates's departure, took the lead in dealing with the BLCA. When BLCA executive director Debra Fraser-Howze failed to fulfill Robinson's and the board's requests for a copy of the contract outlining GMAD's role in conducting Lifestyles Genesis, they grew anxious about the other group's level of investment in the program. As GMAD's first AIDS service contract, the Lifestyles Genesis program put the group in a precarious position. Although Fraser-Howze indicated that the point of contracting with GMAD to deliver Lifestyles Genesis had been to develop the group's infrastructure, Robinson and the rest of the board worried that, should the program fail, GMAD might not survive.[51]

Their fears about the BLCA's commitment to Lifestyles Genesis fed larger concerns about the program. The materials provided by the BLCA were "muddled and often incoherent," and one draft of the curriculum had misspelled most of the *nguzo saba*, suggesting the authors' ignorance of the program's supposed core principles. Although members of GMAD and People of Color in Crisis had attended the Lifestyles Genesis planning retreat and another group, Lesbian and Gay Voices of Color against AIDS and for Life, had offered input on the program at a special meeting arranged by Colin Robinson, none of their feedback was evident in the finished product. Robinson criticized the program's authors for their "faulty understanding of and scant respect for Black Gay community and culture." At times they seemed unable "to recognize the fundamental distinction between the terms 'self-identified Gay men' and 'men who have sex with other men.'" Even the program's title seemed "euphemistic and problematic," suggesting that Black gay men practiced a mutable sexual "lifestyle." For Robinson the program module on condom use typified the program's "heterosexist and patronizing" content. In one copy of the curriculum, where the authors instructed, "Latex condoms must be used at all times when having sex," Colin Robinson wrote, "What is sex?" and later, "Because sex = intercourse." By equating "sex" with penetrative intercourse, which made up only one part of gay men's sexual repertoire, the program ignored sexual acts far less likely to transmit HIV, such as mutual masturbation.[52]

The Lifestyles Genesis authors also failed to connect safer sex in theory to empowerment and safer sex in practice. While the curriculum advised, "Once one understands the consequences and is convinced of the necessity to practice safer sex, he becomes empowered and can better advocate for himself by actually practicing safer sex on an ongoing basis," Robinson doubted that information alone would lead Black gay men to modify their sexual behavior. He stressed the program's "need to MODEL" for participants how to negotiate safer sex with their partners, as well as the kind of positive identity that would empower Black gay men to protect themselves against HIV in the first place. Although he did not mention *Hot, Horny and Healthy!* in his comments, he would have been familiar with the playshop, which taught the very skills that were lacking in Lifestyles Genesis.[53] He showed his frustration at both the curriculum and the BLCA on the "Strategy for Achieving Empowerment Worksheet." Where asked to "identify four (4) means of becoming empowered for HIV positive persons," he answered

- zap[54] Debra [Fraser-Howze] and BLCA
- advocate for better spending of State $ for AIDS
- resign from BLCA Commission
- start an organization that really advocates for Black people w/HIV[55]

Robinson and the rest of the board believed that GMAD could be just such an organization. In late June, the board voted to form an HIV Program Initiatives Committee, composed of Robinson, GMAD executive director Joe Pressley, and George Bellinger, a longtime member of the group. Two months later, the committee met with representatives from the AIDS Institute to discuss expanding GMAD's role in revising the Lifestyles Genesis curriculum. As an alternative to the "learning series" format of four sessions, the committee proposed that the AIDS Institute support GMAD's effort to incorporate more gay- and sex-positive HIV programming into its ongoing activities. The revamped program would focus on building a system of social support for Black gay men to address problems of low self-esteem and alienation while establishing a community norm around condom use and safer sex. Unlike Lifestyles Genesis, which by design reached only twenty-five men at a time, the committee boasted that its own events regularly drew crowds of up to two hundred, ensuring a more efficient use of the state's AIDS dollars.[56]

Although the AIDS Institute at first seemed receptive to the idea of giving GMAD a larger cut of the Lifestyles Genesis grant, it later balked, and the BLCA worked with the department to have GMAD removed from the program. But while GMAD received only a small part of the $40,000 promised by the BLCA, the group leveraged its involvement in the program to win a $25,000 grant from the New York City AIDS Fund to hire staff and outside consultants and to increase distribution of the GMAD *Calendar*. This represented a turning point for GMAD, as it developed from an all-volunteer organization to one with paid staff supported by outside funding. Some would later wonder whether that shift "change[d] the soul of the organization." But for the time being, GMAD was occupied with developing its own AIDS education programs, including *Party*, a dramatic video that encapsulated much of the group's approach to HIV prevention among Black gay men.[57]

## Party

While working with the BLCA on Lifestyles Genesis, GMAD also began work on *Party*, a thirty-minute video that explored the challenges Black gay men faced in practicing safer sex. As with *Hot, Horny and Healthy!*, the goals of the video project were to make safer sex seem fun and erotic, to show viewers how to negotiate condom use, and to address the problem of safer sex "relapse" among Black gay men. GMAD collaborated on the project with AIDSFILMS, a nonprofit film production company that made educational films about AIDS. Alan Sharpe, a Black gay playwright from Washington, D.C., who himself had recently been diagnosed as HIV positive, wrote the script for *Party* with input from GMAD members. GMAD originally intended *Party* to serve as the core of an educational program, integrated with the group's alternative proposal for the Lifestyles Genesis grant, which would include a safer sex workshop and written guide to be distributed across the country. However, AIDSFILMS' executive director Donald Woods, who was also an Other Countries member and had contributed to *In the Life*, passed away from AIDS complications in 1992, and funding for the project from the New York State Department of Health AIDS Institute and a handful of other major grant-makers failed to materialize. GMAD nevertheless produced *Party*, distributed copies to Black gay and grassroots organizations free of charge, and used the tape in its own safer sex workshops.[58]

*Party* visualized diversity among Black men who have sex with men. Some characters in the film appear to be middle-class. Paul, the protagonist and host of the titular party, works as an airline ticket agent, while supporting characters Aaron, Curtis, and Vernon work as an office manager for a law firm, an advertising executive, and a nurse, respectively. Other guests at the party seem to be more working-class: Duane works in Curtis's office building as a security guard, and Kofi speaks in a street slang that marks him as different from the other characters. The video also presents visual markers of class status—when we see Paul's boyfriend Bryan in the opening shot, he's clad in "Calvin Klein sweats," and Antoine, "a sixty-ish grande diva from the old school" is accompanied by Steve, a well-muscled nineteen-year-old named Steve who carries two "designer shopping bags." Steve himself wears "overalls, workboots—and little else," but whether he's a construction worker or a hustler remains unclear.[59]

The characters also perform gender in different ways. Antoine frequently refers to herself as "Ms. Antoine" and speaks with a flamboyant affect; her blocking in the script likewise uses female pronouns (as I do here). Another character, Quiana, shares Ms. Antoine's diva affect. They call one another "miss thing" and "dear," although their exchanges have a sarcastic edge. Kofi, in contrast, appears more masculine, and insists that he's "not your typical brother 'in the life.'"

Each of the characters' subplots also offers a different lesson for sexually active Black gay men in the age of AIDS. The central conflict revolves around Paul and Bryan's relationship. They've been dating for a month but haven't had sex since their first date because Paul insists on using condoms, while Bryan wants to feel Paul "skin to skin." At the beginning of *Party* Bryan storms out of Paul's apartment over the condom issue and later gives Paul an ultimatum:

if he doesn't agree to give Bryan some "real loving," he'll find someone who will, even if that means leaving the party with another man.

Later on, the other characters in the film are busy negotiating safer sex for themselves. Ms. Antoine, who disappears into the bedroom with Steve immediately after arriving, later "sweeps into the kitchen" feeling "positively ravenous!" When the others ask about Steve she replies, "Ms. Antoine was just browsing, not looking to buy. Young men like that are too expensive ... one way or another. Too bad, though. They're so much safer at that age." Quiana presses her meaning. Antoine replies, "Don't be obtuse, darling. Ms. Antoine has no desire to become just another square-on-the-Quilt," but adds that she did not make Steve wear a condom. Vernon objects: "In the game of Russian Roulette, it doesn't matter whether the gun is old or new." Antoine continues, "My dear boys, one by one I've scrupulously relinquished all of my former ... diversions. I refuse to deny myself this final, remaining little pleasure. And I'm sorry, but it defeats the entire purpose to make someone wear a condom for oral sex ... besides which, it tastes terrible—like stale chewing gum." Vernon suggests, "Be creative, try some honey on it ... or strawberry preserves. Maybe dip it in brown sugar." When Antoine marvels at how "kinky" Vernon is, he replies, "Necessity is the mother of invention. Ever since Lonnie," his husband, "tested HIV positive, we've had to do some major adjusting." Still, he says, "in a lot of ways our sex life is more fulfilling and exciting than ever. Maybe since we know that whatever we do now is safe, we can relax and really enjoy ourselves."

In the next scene Curtis and Duane model another way that safer sex can be pleasurable. In the stairwell of Paul's apartment building Duane introduces Curtis to frottage, or "outercourse": erotic stimulation without penetration. He tells Curtis that he learned it in the army, where "a lot of guys are trying it cause it's safer." Curtis replies, "They must've been excellent teachers. It's like you found every erogenous zone in my body—including a few that I didn't even know I had." They leave together for Duane's place to continue their fun.

Not all of the characters are so successful in sticking with safer sex. At the beginning of the film, Paul's friend Aaron shows up at his apartment well before the party begins, utterly distraught. He's just been in the park, where he had unprotected sex with an anonymous stranger. The threat of AIDS had previously made him hypercautious in his sexual choices. He tells Paul, "I've been so careful for so long ... I wouldn't let *anybody* touch me. If I couldn't do it myself—it didn't get done." Now he's upset because it will be months until he can get a definitive HIV test result and because safer sex has become an important part of his social identity. He tells Paul, "The thing that really gets me is that I knew better. I'm the one who's always preaching to you guys about safer sex." Aaron represents the man who has "relapsed" into risky practices, suggesting that strict abstinence as a safer sex strategy can backfire. His example highlights pleasurable but safe sexual activity as an attractive middle ground between unprotected sex and absolute self-denial.[60]

Toward the end of the video, when Kofi returns to the kitchen after being gone from the party, the others ask where he's been. He replies that he's been "kicking it with Mr. Derrick Davenport in his 'Benz." Aghast, the others tell him that Derrick is nicknamed "the Human Torch" because he's "one of the biggest whores in town." When Kofi protests, "The brother is . . . very important in the community. He was featured in *Black Enterprise*," Vernon quips, "I don't care if he was featured in the New Testament, Mr. Respectable-Positive-Role-Model has burned more brothers than the Ku Klux Klan."[61] Even Antoine, who had been cavalier earlier about her own condom use, asks with concern, "You didn't do anything . . . reckless with him, did you?" Kofi asks why one of the others didn't warn him earlier. Vernon lays into Kofi, telling him that he's an "alright brother and all" but never wants to take responsibility for his own behavior. "Even with something like AIDS," he says, "you're the first one to argue that it's a white man's plot or the CIA scientists' latest conspiracy."

Kofi "storms out of the kitchen" and Paul catches up to him to say, "If it seems that everyone was coming down on you in there . . . it's just that we care about you and we want you to be safe." Kofi replies that he feels like he's on the outside of the group because he's not "your typical brother 'in the life,'" to which Paul comes back, "What is 'typical'? Each of us is different. But we're all in this together. Aren't you the one who's always preaching that black men should support each other, watch each other's back? That's all we're trying to do. We've got to help each other stay strong." Paul's speech reframes safer sex both as fun and pleasurable and as a necessary community enterprise. Here, safer sex becomes not only a means of protecting oneself against HIV but another way for Black men to show their love for other Black men.

## "I Cannot Go Home as Who I Am"

Over the next few years GMAD continued to grow, winning sizable grants, hiring additional staff, and expanding its slate of services. By 1993 the United States Conference of Mayors (USCM) recognized GMAD as "the most visible organization for African American gay and bisexual men in New York City today."[62]

Colin Robinson, perhaps more than any other person, shaped GMAD's development during this period. Robinson became the group's managing director in 1992 and left his job at the GMHC in 1994 to run GMAD's day-to-day operations full time as executive director. In funding proposals, he highlighted consciousness raising and community building as GMAD's unique contribution to the fight against AIDS among Black gay men, as the group worked to reduce not only risky behavior but "the *antecedents* of risk behavior—issues like identity, self-esteem, and social stability."[63]

To drive home this point with funders, Robinson used prose by Black gay renaissance authors to convey the shame and anger that he connected to unsafe sex and increased HIV risk. In one grant proposal to the USCM he quoted from Joseph Beam's essay "Brother to Brother," in which Beam invokes the panoply of Black institutions to which he could not truly belong as an openly gay man: "*I cannot go home as who I am.* When I speak of home I mean not only the familial constellation from which I grew, but the entire Black community, the Black press, the Black church, Black academicians, the Black literati, the Black left.... I cannot go home as who I am and that hurts me deeply." Robinson similarly quoted from Marlon Riggs on the suffering that Black gay men suffered at the hands of other African Americans: "The terrain Black Gay men navigate in the quest for self and social identity is, to say the least, hostile. What disturbs—no, enrages me—is not so much the obstacles set before my path by whites, which history conditions me to expect, but the traps and pitfalls planted by my so-called brothers, who because of the same history should know better."[64]

The USCM awarded the contract, and funding from the New York State Department of Health AIDS Institute, the Joyce Mertz-Gilmore Foundation, and the Henry van Ameringen Foundation followed, in no small part thanks to Robinson's fund-raising acumen. Nevertheless, Robinson remained at the head of GMAD for less than two years—conflict with the group's board of directors pushed him away from the organization. Some board members disagreed with Robinson's vision for GMAD as a professionally staffed service provider supported by external funding, and in August 1995 he returned to the GMHC to direct the agency's HIV prevention programs.[65]

After Robinson's departure, GMAD struggled through budget woes, staffing issues, and declining membership. Later that year, GMAD dismissed two staff members due to insufficient funding, and Robinson sued the group for back pay. In July 1996, the board of directors voted to expel a fellow board member for embezzling $7,500 from the organization. Just six months later, the executive director struggled through a bout of drug abuse, during which he missed appointments on the group's behalf. The board of directors, which was also concerned with his handling of GMAD's petty cash, voted to dismiss him immediately. These ongoing struggles damaged the group's reputation with members and funders alike. During an argument at a GMAD meeting in

February 1996, a member accused the group's leaders of being "petty robbers and shakedown artists." The following year, the AIDS Institute complained of not receiving progress reports on the GMAD programs it had funded for several years, again damaging the group's credibility with a major grant maker. By June 1997, the group's membership had fallen to 130 and the mailing list circulation to 800, from highs in 1991 of 300 and 1,200.[66]

GMAD recovered from these difficulties, in part thanks to the availability of new funding for the fight against AIDS in communities of color. In 1998 Black gay activists and their allies in the Congressional Black Caucus secured the creation of the Minority AIDS Initiative, which brought over $100 million to the fight against HIV/AIDS in communities of color in its first year. Kevin McGruder served as GMAD's executive director during this period, when the organization experienced another growth spurt. In a 2014 oral history, recorded while he was serving on the group's board of directors, McGruder recalled that the growth was "driven by the availability of funding" and focused tightly on HIV prevention and services at the expense of other parts of GMAD's mission. That money also came with strings—"program requirements, deliverables"—that limited what GMAD could do. As a result, he says, "We did more but in a narrower kind of range."[67]

For McGruder, the funding-driven emphasis on HIV prevention pulled GMAD away from the more expansive vision on which the group was founded. Efforts by GMAD and others to stop the spread of HIV among Black gay and bisexual men have failed, he says, "because the behaviors that are driving the infection rates are the result of something much broader than that. Education, family support, community support: all of those things are part of the solution." But subsisting on grant money leaves groups like GMAD in a precarious position. McGruder observes, "The challenge is for organizations trying to just exist, in a way." As a result, they have little room to push at the boundaries of conventional thinking around HIV prevention, which remains focused on individual behavior change rather than on ameliorating injuries of inequality.[68]

According to both McGruder and Joe Pressley, grant funding and the hiring of paid staff brought other negative changes as well. Pressley recalls, "HIV/AIDS funding was flowing then ... and I think it did change the soul of the organization." Before the group won its first grant for HIV/AIDS work, GMAD was "fantastic," "very organic," "very democratic," and "very grassroots"—an organization "that was really poised to really live up to its mission, which was about empowering Black gay men, both economically, socially, and politically." For both men, being an all-volunteer organization was one of GMAD's strengths, and so "there was a fair amount of loss with getting paid staff." According to McGruder, the sense of ownership among members that came with an all-volunteer structure went away: "GMAD in the late eighties, early nineties, I think people really felt it was their organization. And I know that's not how most Black gay men in New York feel now."[69]

Funding also complicated GMAD's relationship with its own constituents, which now included clients who relied on the group for services. McGruder presents this as another way in which the group has become alienated from the community it aims to serve: "There's a power dynamic, too, when somebody's a client—the bold ones may tell you what they really think. But the others might question, Is this going to mess me up here?" The transition from an all-volunteer organization to an agency with paid staff not only meant that members had less opportunity to push back against the leadership but also introduced a new group of stakeholders with good reason not to do so at all.[70]

Federal funding additionally brought its own problems, and the money that was available under President Bill Clinton seemed to dry up under his successor, George W. Bush. In March 2004, the CDC failed to renew two of GMAD's grants; as a result, executive director Tokes Osubu took a major pay cut and the organization eliminated a quarter of its staff. This points to some of the difficulties with grant-funded work in general: grants end, and the groups they support may not be able to stand on their own when they do. The universe of available funding can also change dramatically, as Joe Pressley makes clear: "HIV/AIDS dollars are not as plentiful as they once were and this has been a recipe for disaster for many of our organizations because ... their funding base isn't diverse and so if the HIV/AIDS dollars go, therefore those organizations go."[71]

Funding issues like these were by no means unique to GMAD. BEBASHI and the NTFAP struggled with their own financial woes, and, as we will see, so too did SisterLove. Each of these organizations fought to stay afloat while serving communities that are chronically underserved. They had to rely largely on grants from the federal government or from private philanthropies, which effectively limited the kind of work these groups could take on and left them vulnerable to public pressure and changes in the political environment. Nevertheless, groups like GMAD and NTFAP were groundbreaking in that they drew some of the first government funding to support the work of Black gay men. And as we will also see in the story of The Balm in Gilead, some groups successfully navigated the shifting political landscape and even turned such changes to their own advantage.[72]

Even so, as Pressley admits, it's easy to see why GMAD went after grant funding in the first place. The group was (and is) dealing with a community in crisis, and at the time other groups seemed ill-equipped to reach those who were the most vulnerable. In hindsight, alternatives can be difficult to discern:

"I get criticized because folks say, Well you're saying we shouldn't have gone for those dollars? How could you say that, Joe, given the fact that we were dying and continue to die?" McGruder suggests that GMAD could make up some of the difference by cultivating individual donors, but given that the group serves a community that is already short on resources, it's hard to see where those donors might come from.[73]

There are other ways to explain GMAD's "decline." The most obvious is also the most tragic: the AIDS epidemic robbed GMAD and the Black gay renaissance of their most vital and challenging voices. Charles Angel did not survive GMAD's first year. Donald Woods, who was involved in the production of *Party* and was also a member of Other Countries, passed away in 1992. So too did Craig Harris. Marlon Riggs died in 1994 of complications from AIDS, having finished a handful of other documentary films on intersections of race, gender, and sexuality; his final film, *Black Is . . . Black Ain't*, was completed after his death by his coproducers. Essex Hemphill passed away, also from AIDS complications, in 1995, around the time that Colin Robinson departed for the GMHC. These are just a few names, representing a tiny fraction of those who passed along the way. In the midst of such "compounding loss," maybe it's remarkable that GMAD survived at all.

GAY MEN OF AFRICAN DESCENT and the writers and artists of the Black gay renaissance articulated a holistic Black gay identity that built on earlier movements, including Black Power, gay liberation, and Third World feminism. They looked to Black history and African tradition, both to validate their place in Black America and to provide a framework for HIV prevention among Black gay men. Whereas AIDS activists in Cameroon had contacted BEBASHI to learn about how their American counterparts were tackling the epidemic, GMAD looked to Africa—or at least to mediated versions of it—for solutions. GMAD's use of Swahili phrases and Yoruba iconography speaks to a global community of Black gay men that was more imagined than material. Nevertheless, its work represents an attempt to suture the wounds of diaspora and create a sense of Black gay wholeness all at once.

## CHAPTER 4

We've Been Doing This for
a Few Thousand Years

The Nation of Islam's African AIDS Cure

O N DECEMBER 6, 1989, Dr. Davy Koech (pronounced "Koh-eech") made
an electrifying announcement: his lab at the Kenya Medical Research
Institute (KEMRI) in Nairobi had developed a medicine that, he told
Kenya's *Weekly Review* newspaper, "successfully reverses all signs and
symptoms of [AIDS] within a matter of days." The treatment, codenamed
KE089, was nontoxic and inexpensive, in contrast to AZT, which at that time
was the only drug approved for the clinical treatment of AIDS in the United
States. According to the *Weekly Review*, the announcement "generated an exciting ray of hope among local [AIDS] victims" and, if proven to be successful,
would "signal that African science has finally come of age."[1]

Over the months that followed, Koech's claims about the drug, now labeled
Kemron, grew still more fantastical. At a press conference in February 1990, he
announced that 10 percent of those treated with Kemron had later tested negative for HIV. The following month that number doubled, to nearly 20 percent of
the 101 patients treated with the drug. Although Koech was careful to say that
Kemron was not a cure for HIV infection, his announcements prompted people
with AIDS from other parts of the country, along with neighboring Tanzania
and Uganda, to come to Nairobi seeking the "Kenyan wonder drug."[2]

But even as the World Health Organization organized clinical trials in four
other African countries to confirm Koech's findings, the response from officials and news outlets in the United States and Europe was muted. The *New
York Times* reported that Koech's announcement inspired "hope and wariness" among AIDS researchers in the United States. According to one Kenyan
newspaper, a "war of words" over Kemron erupted in the capital as local journalists "accus[ed] Nairobi-based foreign correspondents of ignoring the discovery due to racist prejudice." For a time, within the United States only the

*New York Native*, a gay weekly newspaper, and AIDS treatment newsletters took the Kemron story seriously.[3]

Koech published his findings in the journal *Molecular Biotherapy* in June 1990 but, he complained, was met with "outright skepticism, disbelief, suspicion and rejection." Nevertheless, he was certain that history would vindicate him. At a ceremony to celebrate the beginning of a campaign to manufacture and market Kemron in July 1990, Koech compared himself to Galileo and Edward Jenner, both scientific visionaries who were misunderstood by their contemporaries.[4]

Kemron consisted of alpha interferon, a type of protein produced by the human body as part of normal immune function. By the time of Koech's announcement, doctors were using large injections of interferon to treat Kaposi's sarcoma, an opportunistic infection associated with AIDS. By contrast, Koech administered a low dose to his patients orally, in tablet form. If his claims were true, Kemron represented a tremendous leap forward.[5]

But skeptics had good reason to doubt Koech's findings. Previous reports of other "miracle" AIDS treatments later turned out to be dead ends, and ten years of research had uncovered little in the way of effective medicines, much less a vaccine or cure. Koech also conducted his trial without a control group, so it was possible that his patients' improved health was the result of a placebo effect. A significant number of Koech's subjects were also in the early stages of HIV disease and might have suffered from passing infections that happened to coincide with their Kemron treatment and would have resolved on their own. As for those who allegedly saw their HIV infections reversed, skeptics speculated that their initial tests had returned false positives that were later shown to be negative.[6]

While the *New York Times* and the *Washington Post* relayed Western scientists' skepticism, the African American press portrayed Kemron as a landmark Black achievement that was being ignored or deliberately suppressed. Here the conversation about Kemron among African American AIDS activists built on simmering resentment over the idea that AIDS had originated in Africa. Koech's story, and the unenthusiastic response from both scientists and major press outlets, also resonated with theories that HIV had been introduced as part of a genocidal plot targeting Black people worldwide. Even with mounting scientific evidence that Kemron and similar drugs showed little promise for treating HIV and AIDS, advocates continued to push for a full-scale clinical trial that might vindicate Koech and his Kenyan team.

The loudest voices in this chorus belonged to leaders of the Nation of Islam (NOI), who framed the debate over Kemron in terms of race pride and economic self-sufficiency. They argued that white American and European scientists discounted Koech because he was Black, that powerful pharmaceutical corporations wanted to keep Kemron off of the market because it would undercut the price of more expensive drugs, and that Western governments blocked Kemron because it would interfere with their plan to use AIDS to wipe out Black people around the world. At the same time, they promoted Kemron as a boon to Black economic power—or at least to their own organization, which held the rights to distribution of the drug in the United States.

The Kemron story has been told by historians only in limited ways. Cathy Cohen points out that the Kemron story allowed the *New York Amsterdam News* to cover AIDS within the boundaries of respectability politics, by emphasizing Black greatness rather than Black people dying of a virus they had contracted through sex or drug use. Journalist Elinor Burkett, in her 1995 book, *The Gravest Show on Earth*, is much more dismissive. She writes that the Kemron story showed how "Blacks with AIDS were betrayed by their own leaders—and by their own intractable paranoia." The belief that "whitey didn't want you to know about the cure," she continues, "was the best publicity the drug could get."[7]

But the Kemron story resonated for other reasons as well. Although NOI members made for unlikely AIDS activists, their messages about Black greatness, economic inequality, and medical genocide appealed to African American audiences. At the same time, their claims about Kemron addressed real concerns about the origins of HIV, the toxicity of the drugs approved to treat the virus, and racial inequities in AIDS treatment and care. Its leaders' inflated rhetoric make the NOI easy to dismiss from the history of AIDS treatment politics, but the Kemron story makes clear that its influence on the course of the epidemic in Black America has been significant.

### "What Are They Trying to Say We Did with That Monkey?"

For African Americans, theories about the origin of AIDS resurrected racist ideas of Black hypersexuality and barbarism, which have historically been used to marginalize people of color in the United States. Early on in the epidemic, most Western scientists had come to the consensus that the disease originated in Africa. Testing of old blood samples in Kinshasa and the discovery of a virus similar to HIV in green monkeys in the nearby jungle pointed to the Congo River delta as the epidemic's point of origin. The apparent eagerness of scientists to "blame" the epidemic on Africans and people of African descent aroused the ire of Black communities worldwide.[8]

In his 1989 essay "AIDS in Blackface," Harlon Dalton, a Yale law professor and member of the National Commission on AIDS, made clear that many

African Americans took the African origin theory as an affront: "Were I to go out tomorrow and speak about AIDS to a black audience anywhere in this country, I guarantee you that once the discussion got going, someone would ask about the disease's origins. The question 'Is it true that it started in Africa?' would quickly become 'Why do they keep trying to pin it on Africa?' 'Why do they keep trying to pin it on us?' and eventually I would be asked the clincher: 'What are they trying to say we did with that monkey?'"[9]

The belief that "they" conspired to pin the blame for AIDS on people of African descent dovetailed with a larger set of theories, widely believed within Black communities, that powerful interests were plotting to cover up some crucial truth about the epidemic. These conspiracy theories take many forms, including the idea that drug companies and government researchers erroneously promote HIV as the cause of AIDS (also known as HIV denialism), that a cure for AIDS exists but is available only to the wealthy, and that HIV was created by the U.S. government as a biological weapon to kill off "undesirables"— African Americans, drug users, and gay men.[10]

Belief in such conspiracies goes back almost to the beginning of the epidemic and has not faded with time. Survey after survey has found that many African Americans believe in some form of government conspiracy related to HIV/AIDS. Pernessa Seele, who founded The Balm in Gilead to help Black churches develop AIDS ministries, confirms, "Black people, all over the world, believe that HIV was created to kill them. We may not say it, we may . . . talk about it in private, but that is a fundamental myth that . . . wherever you find Black folks, behind closed doors we think that somebody created HIV to kill us."[11]

AIDS conspiracy theories are not unique to African Americans, and some of the most well-known HIV denialists and AIDS conspiracy theorists have been white. These include Peter Duesberg, a molecular biologist, Robert Strecker, a medical doctor, and Gary Null, a talk radio host and anti-vaccination activist. The success of such figures in sowing doubt about HIV and AIDS tracks larger, related trends in American society, such as the rise of alternative medicine and the advent of the internet and social media, where wild claims can circulate unchecked.[12] However, the prevalence of AIDS conspiracy theories in Black communities in the United States stems from particular histories of racial violence.

The Tuskegee Syphilis Study looms large in that set of histories. The study, officially named the "Tuskegee Study of Untreated Syphilis in the Negro Male," was conducted by the Public Health Service between 1932 and 1972 and examined the effects of syphilis on the bodies of 624 poor Black men in

Alabama. The men understood that they were being treated for their "bad blood," a folk name for the disease. But even after antibiotics revolutionized syphilis treatment in the 1940s, doctors in the study continued to administer ineffective mercury-based medicines so as not to compromise their results. Tuskegee showed the willingness of medical authorities, working under the aegis of the federal government, to put Black citizens at risk of death and disease. Moreover, in versions of the story that were later told and retold, the doctors infected the men with syphilis themselves. This was not the case, but as historian Susan Reverby discovered in recent years, patients who participated in a similar experiment in Guatemala *were* inoculated with syphilis, and by one of the very same doctors involved in the Alabama study.[13]

Around the same time that Tuskegee came to light, Americans learned about COINTELPRO, the FBI program that had worked for years to covertly disrupt "subversive groups," including civil rights and Black Power organizations. The report of the Senate committee tasked with investigating such abuses of federal power, released in April 1976, revealed that the FBI had harassed Dr. Martin Luther King Jr. and infiltrated the Black Panther Party in order to destroy the group from within. Clearly, the U.S. government was willing to go to great lengths to halt the struggle for Black freedom. Less than a decade after Americans learned about COINTELPRO, AIDS was ravaging Black communities across the United States. Might the two be related?[14]

African Americans also consumed news of Tuskegee and COINTELPRO alongside urban legends that highlighted the vulnerability of Black bodies. According to one set of rumors, the fast food chain Church's Chicken and makers of Tropical Fantasy soda put chemicals in their products to sterilize Black men. Other stories linked the kidnapping and murder of Black children in places like Baltimore and Atlanta to medical research facilities, namely Johns Hopkins University and the Centers for Disease Control. These tales bring to mind real-life examples, such as the "father of gynecology" J. Marion Sims's experimentation in the nineteenth century with surgical techniques to repair vaginal fistulae, which he practiced on enslaved women without the benefit of anesthesia. As anthropologist Patricia Turner argues, these rumors, along with conspiracy theories about AIDS, reflect individual and collective experiences of racial oppression and not just the "pathological preoccupations" of Black communities. In short, African Americans have good reason to be suspicious.[15]

Other stories point to the ways that Black bodies in the United States are made vulnerable by the denial of medical care. The legend of Dr. Charles Drew, a Black doctor who helped to pioneer blood banking techniques during the early days of World War II, has circulated widely within African American communities almost from the moment of his death in 1950. Drew was driving with several colleagues overnight from Washington, D.C., to a medical conference (incidentally) in Tuskegee when he lost control of the car in North Carolina's rural Alamance County. According to one version of the story, Drew died after being taken to a nearby hospital where white doctors refused to treat him on account of his race. In another version, the hospital declined to give him a transfusion of blood or plasma—as tellers of this story point out, Drew died after being denied the benefit of his own contribution to modern medicine. In reality, the doctors at Alamance General Hospital tried to treat Drew's injuries, but he passed away soon after he arrived. Many others were not so lucky; throughout the era of Jim Crow, countless Black southerners died because they were denied emergency medical treatment. In this sense, Spencie Love has argued, the myth about Charles Drew's death has been told and retold extensively in Black communities not because it is a "great story" but because "it is built on a many-layered foundation of Black beliefs, tales, and well-founded superstitions about the conditions of Black survival in white-dominated America."[16] The same could be said for conspiracy theories about the origin of AIDS.

Others have argued that such rumors serve a political purpose. Folklorist John Roberts takes a long view of HIV conspiracy theories in Black communities, framing them within the context of Black oral tradition, a "continuous process of creative cultural production" used to cement group bonds and warn one another about "potentially hidden dangers." Roberts's take on conspiracy tales resonates with Robin D. G. Kelley's work on rap narratives as both "a window into, and critique of, the criminalization of black youth." In a similar fashion, HIV conspiracy theories communicate and critique the exploitation of Black bodies in the United States, both past and present.[17]

However, when it comes to HIV, conspiracy theories take a toll on Black communities. Popular stories that deny a link between HIV and AIDS or insist that the virus was created by government scientists undermine efforts to educate vulnerable people about the disease. Researchers find that African Americans who believe in some form of AIDS conspiracy theory are less likely to protect themselves against HIV and are less willing or able to adhere to an HIV drug regimen. Those drugs are important for keeping a person living with HIV alive and healthy and for preventing the further spread of the virus. In some better-known cases, such as Fana Khaba, a popular South African DJ, or LeRoy Whitfield, a Black gay journalist in the United States, forgoing antiretrovirals in favor of alternative remedies or simply "better nutrition, good exercise and a low stress level" have meant early death. In the case of South Africa, where HIV denialists had the ear of South African president Thabo Mbeki, the consequences were disastrous. While the minister of health promoted the use of beets, lemon, and garlic to treat AIDS, the Mbeki government delayed the roll-out of antiretroviral drugs and AZT to prevent mother-to-child transmission of HIV, costing thousands of lives and leading to many more easily preventable HIV infections.[18]

In that case, as Nicoli Nattrass has pointed out, support for conspiracy theories at the highest levels of the governing African National Congress mattered a great deal for furthering their spread among Black South Africans. The agency of powerful political actors in promoting such theories, she argues, matters as much as the social and historical contexts that lend them credibility.[19] By the same token, the widespread belief in AIDS conspiracies among African Americans owes partly to their support from those with influence in the community. These include leaders of the Nation of Islam, who have promoted a wide range of AIDS conspiracy theories in the pages of the group's newspaper the *Final Call*.

## An Ideal Weapon

The Nation of Islam began covering AIDS in the *Final Call* years before the Kemron announcement. The newspaper primarily published a variety of conspiracy theories related to the new disease. Some of the coverage was surprisingly sympathetic to gays and lesbians, given the group's conservative gender and sexual politics. But for the most part, the paper stoked animosity toward gay and bisexual men, arguing that they were in one way or another responsible for the epidemic.[20]

The first article on AIDS in the *Final Call* appeared in 1984 as a letter from an anonymous inmate in Trenton State Prison. The man was anxious about the number of men in the facility who had become sick with AIDS but who, he claimed, didn't fall into one of the defined risk categories. The man worried that the disease might be spread in ways other than sex or injection drug use and proposed that the New Jersey Department of Corrections was covering up a "serious epidemic" within the prison's walls, where the majority of inmates were Black. Several features of this account—the ideas that a large number of Black men affected did not fall into any identified risk category and that authorities were covering up the truth of the disease—would be staples of the *Final Call*'s later AIDS coverage.[21]

Dr. Abdul Alim Muhammad, a spokesman for the NOI who would become the face of the Kemron campaign, also periodically weighed in on AIDS. He argued that the disease represented "the Judgment of the wicked by Almighty God" and that the influence of the "Gay Rights Lobby" kept authorities from telling the full truth about AIDS, including the possibility that the disease might be transmitted through casual contact or insect bites. This, he argued, would account for the large number of "ordinary men and women" who fell "outside the high risk group who are victims of AIDS." He theorized that AIDS might be linked to poor sanitation, which would "explain why Africans, who are not known for homosexuality and drug abuse, have gotten the disease in large numbers."[22]

Muhammad and leaders of the NOI also proposed that AIDS might be the product of a sinister conspiracy. AIDS, he argued, would be "the ideal weapon to 'depopulate'" Africa, thereby "giving the superpowers easy access to the mineral wealth of the land" and preventing the rise of politically and economically powerful African nations that might challenge the United States and the Soviet Union. Minister Louis Farrakhan similarly told the *Final Call*, "I suspect that [AIDS] is part of a long range plan to depopulate the earth of its Black inhabitants" due to predictions that the United States would soon become a majority minority nation. Another author, Hassan Omowale, repeated Robert Strecker's theory that HIV had been created by combining viruses found in cows and sheep, along with claims by Jacob Segal, an East German scientist, that AIDS had been created by American scientists as a weapon of war.[23]

Even as Muhammad railed against the "Gay Rights Lobby," the *Final Call*'s AIDS coverage was sometimes more sympathetic to sexual minorities. Omowale wrote that, as with "monkeys and 'niggers' in Africa," much blame had been "diverted to a small segment of the population (white homosexual males) who are victimized as scapegoats." Sovella X Perry went further in her coverage of the National Coalition of Black Lesbians and Gays' 1986 "AIDS in the Black Community" conference. She quoted NCBLG secretary Gwendolyn Rogers: "It is irresponsible not to address homophobia in the Black community. The hatred and fear of anything that has to do with homosexuality is allowing our brothers and sisters to die." Perry presented this perspective uncritically, even though NOI leaders, including Alim Muhammad, often espoused the very same homophobia. However, her article was the exception to the *Final Call*'s regular AIDS coverage. At best, the paper generally argued that homosexuality was rarely seen in Africa or among "normal" African Americans; at worst, that gays had brought AIDS on themselves and then engineered a government conspiracy to cover up the severity of the epidemic.[24]

These conspiracy theories were hardly limited to the pages of the *Final Call*. They found other outlets in Black media, and perhaps nowhere more than in the work of the journalist Tony Brown.

## Tony Brown's Truths

On his television talk show and in his syndicated newspaper column, which ran in Black newspapers nationwide, Tony Brown frequently gave HIV denialists and AIDS conspiracy theorists a platform to share their views. His show developed this approach over time, first questioning the African origin theory of AIDS and later giving airtime to rogue "scientists" and quack "doctors" peddling their own books, videotapes, and "miracle" remedies. Brown appeared to welcome these ideas in part because they challenged the notion that Africans and Haitians were to blame for the disease but also because playing host to such guests fit into Brown's view of himself as an unconventional thinker. At the same time, recordings of *Tony Brown's Journal* show that members of the host's studio audience brought their own ideas about AIDS and its origins to the discussion.

A 1985 episode of *Tony Brown's Journal*, which appears to be one of the first to deal with AIDS, featured Black gay author Craig Harris, Eddie King of the Baltimore-based Health Education Resource Organization, and Dr. Valiere Alcena, a Haitian internist working in New York. Brown asked Alcena about a pair of articles, just published in *Time* and *Newsweek*, that pointed to Africa as the point of origin for AIDS. Alcena offered a different explanation: that the disease had been brought by gay sex tourists from the United States. In Port-au-Prince, he said, "it became evident that you could go there as a gay man and for little or no money and have yourself a ball with your sexual habits." But when a new deadly sexually transmitted disease began to affect both white gay men in the United States and Haitian sex workers, Alcena argued, "white America . . . [found] some other way . . . of dumping [it] on the Blacks."[25]

But while Alcena questioned the idea that AIDS had originated in Africa and traveled to the United States through Haiti, he did not question the idea that AIDS was caused by a virus. When Brown pressed him on this issue, arguing (as would Alim Muhammad) that the disease might be caused instead by poor sanitation, Alcena pointed out that while the majority of Haitian AIDS cases were concentrated in the capital, sanitation in the countryside was actually worse. If AIDS were caused by poor sanitation, the reverse would be true.[26]

Alcena returned to *Tony Brown's Journal* in 1986, joined by Mark Whiteside of the Institute of Tropical Medicine and James Hebert of the American Health Foundation. While the panelists did not dispute that AIDS had a viral origin, they disagreed on its specific cause. Based on his research in Miami and Belle Glade, Whiteside proposed that in tropical areas AIDS was caused by repeated exposure to insect-borne viruses, although he had a harder time explaining why the disease also showed up in poor Black communities in New

York City. (Alcena also pointed out that if AIDS in tropical areas was caused by insect bites, many more people across the Caribbean would be affected.) Hebert disagreed, arguing that the viral cause of AIDS was probably related to African swine fever, likely spread through a Portuguese vaccination program, which meant that "although it's called African swine fever virus, [it] actually has a European link." Brown himself pointed out that the panelists disagreed with what "most of us have been told by the official government agencies," positioning his talk show as a forum for unorthodox ideas.[27]

In episodes of his show recorded in 1988 and 1989, Brown featured guests even further outside the mainstream of AIDS research. Gary Null, a radio host and promoter of alternative medicine, appeared on *Tony Brown's Journal* in 1988, claiming that HIV had been created through "genetic engineering" by crossing cattle and sheep viruses and then spread through a global smallpox vaccine program. He would appear on Brown's show several times over the next few years, arguing that HIV might not in fact be the cause of AIDS and touting the benefits of vitamins, juicing, ozone therapy, and a host of other "remedies" for the disease. Dr. Robert Strecker, producer and star of a ninety-minute video "exposé" on the origin of AIDS titled *The Strecker Memorandum*, also appeared on *Tony Brown's Journal* in 1989, similarly claiming that HIV had been created in a lab and spread through vaccine programs. Another guest, Dr. Alan Cantwell, argued that "AIDS was no accident of nature" and traced HIV to a hepatitis B vaccine trial.[28]

Other guests did not go quite so far. Peter Duesberg, a molecular biologist at the University of California, Berkeley, argued that HIV was not the cause of AIDS; he proposed instead that AIDS was caused by repeated exposure to toxic substances or infectious diseases. For gay men in the United States and Europe, this meant party drugs and repeated sexually transmitted infections. For Africans, the apparently new disease was the result of malnutrition, poor sanitation, and repeated parasitic infections. In short, gay men developed AIDS because of their libertine lifestyles (although Duesberg later distinguished between hard-partying gays and the "all-American homosexual from next door"), and heterosexual Africans developed AIDS because they were poor. In both cases, HIV was a harmless passenger virus wrongly identified as the cause of a pandemic. Duesberg would appear again on *Tony Brown's Journal* a handful of times during the late 1980s and 1990s and received sympathetic treatment from Brown, who portrayed him as a brave truth-teller ostracized from scientific circles for daring to challenge one of the "pet theories" of the medical establishment's "thought police."[29]

Some guests took more mainstream positions while still questioning "what comes down as official policy" on AIDS. Dr. Wilbert Jordan, an African

American doctor and infectious disease specialist in Los Angeles, complained that for "the first eight years [of the epidemic], Black people have had to sit and listen to every radio show, TV show, newspaper say that Africa was the source of AIDS. First it was Haiti, then it was Africa. And if there's nothing else to come out of this, I'm very happy to have someone from the US government finally say, 'It didn't begin in Africa. We don't know where it came from.'" Jordan's comment drew vigorous applause from the audience.[30]

Still other guests gave an Afrocentric twist to HIV denialism. On a 1989 episode, "Dr. Sebi" (also known as Alfredo Bowman) claimed that diseases like AIDS arose because people of African descent in the Americas had spent centuries eating food genetically unsuited to them. Sebi, who was Afro-Honduran, argued, "Our cells have been gradually breaking down, becoming weaker," to the point that "the whole Black race is sick." As a remedy not only for AIDS but also for "lupus, herpes, sickle cell, blindness and diabetes," Sebi offered a "substance" that was "consistent with that particular vibration" of Black people from the tropics. For making such claims, and for treating people at his Usha Herbal Research Institute in Brooklyn, the New York attorney general charged him with practicing medicine without a license. But in the face of legal challenges, Sebi argued that the "Black man has the right to use the substance that is genetically consistent with him."[31]

While some guests, such as Alcena and Jordan, criticized the African origin theory of AIDS, others, including Strecker, Cantwell, and Duesberg, offered alternative explanations for the emergence of the new disease. Still others, such as Null and Sebi, challenged the credibility of mainstream medicine itself. It is easy to see why these messages might have resonated with African American viewers. If Brown's guests were right, then prevailing theories about AIDS were either a projection of scientists' racist fantasies or the cover for a genocidal plot. Either way, they turned the old racist stereotypes about Black bodies as hypersexual and diseased on their heads. And if Null and Sebi were to be believed, then a cheap and accessible cure for AIDS was hiding in plain sight. All you had to do was believe.

Brown's guests made preposterous claims, and they often disagreed with one another. But giving a platform to those well outside the mainstream of scientific thought fit into Brown's idea of himself as an "equal opportunity ass-kicker." As he wrote in the introduction to his 1995 book, *Black Lies, White Lies*, "Most of all, I care about the truth. My journalism has been a search for that truth." Later in the book Brown once again endorsed many of Duesberg's views on AIDS, including that HIV was not the cause of the disease, and warned of "ethnic weapons" developed by the United States, along with other "potentially catastrophic biological threats . . . from medical research laboratories, where . . . the blind pursuit of scientific glory and financial gain overrides any sense of responsibility for human life."[32]

We would be mistaken to assume that Brown's readers and viewers uncritically accepted his messages about AIDS. At times it was his studio audience that pushed the envelope on ideas about the disease. During the 1986 episode that featured Alcena, Whiteside, and Hebert, a Black woman in the audience interjected in frustration to chide the panel for not asking why the disease was having such a disproportionate impact on Black people worldwide. On a 1987 episode featuring two Black health professionals, another member of the studio audience asked whether AIDS was the result of a "biological warfare plot bent on genocide." Brown himself seemed incredulous at the question, but before long he would be arguing the very same.[33] As the audience comments suggest, Brown was not the only influential Black voice to contradict the scientific mainstream or to suggest that powerful forces conspired to keep effective AIDS treatments out of the hands of those in the greatest need. Those claims would become central to grassroots support for a clinical trial of Kemron, which was just getting started.

## Out of Africa

In July 1990, a group of "doctors, teachers, nurses, social workers, and hundreds of curious citizens" gathered at Friendship Baptist Church in Brooklyn's Bedford-Stuyvesant neighborhood to hear about Kemron and discuss its significance. Speakers included members of a fact-finding delegation headed to Kenya to learn more about the drug: Gary Byrd of the local Black radio station WLIB, New York physician Dr. Barbara Justice, and Cedric Sandiford, an HIV-positive man who had been the victim of a brutal racist beating in the Queens neighborhood of Howard Beach four years earlier. Byrd told the *New York Amsterdam News* that even though "a cure is coming from the very place blamed for bringing the disease, skeptics say, 'Africa is too primitive to come up with this.'" Afrocentric historian John Henrik Clarke, "a longtime believer in the wonders of Africa," likewise encouraged the audience to feel a sense of racial pride in Kenyan president Daniel arap Moi's announcement: "I'm not at all surprised, this is old hat, we've been doing this for a few thousand years." Clarke received a standing ovation from the audience and, according to *Amsterdam News* reporter Vinette Pryce, "brought hope and inspiration to everyone who felt a part of this amazing discovery." While white scientists were eager to blame Africa for the AIDS epidemic, Byrd and Clarke were confident that the continent would instead produce a cure.[34]

For Black audiences like the one in Bed-Stuy, the mainstream media's silence on Kemron was bound up not only with the African origin theory of AIDS but with the way that members of the white press covered Black neighborhoods. An editorial in the *Amsterdam News* pointedly noted that it was "curious" for other news outlets to ignore the Kemron story "in view of the fact that the white press swarms Harlem whenever there is a rumor of a riot, or a shooting or a stabbing or a drug bust or of any white person who has contributed two dollars to support anything black." The Committee to Eliminate Media Offensive to African People also hit back at an article in the *New York Post* that described the delegation as a "Heartless AIDS Scam" and Kemron as "no effective cure for AIDS," threatening to sue the paper for libel. But in that committee's view, the dismissal of Kemron was part of a larger problem: the media's penchant for "savaging the image of Black folks with impunity." For Black New Yorkers, the way the *Times* or the *Post* reported on Kemron was not just an issue of what was happening *over there* in Nairobi but connected to the way that they themselves were misrepresented by the press as well.[35]

The *Post* was right about one thing, however: the delegation's trip to Kenya was expensive. Those who were going to KEMRI for treatment, including Cedric Sandiford, had to come up with thousands of dollars for the privilege. Sandiford called on friends and supporters to put together money for the trip, and on July 28, 1990, he traveled to Nairobi with Gary Byrd, Barbara Justice, and others. Sandiford reported that he regained some weight that he had lost due to illness and "became much improved" after starting Kemron but had his trip cut short after a few weeks so that he could return home to testify against his Howard Beach attackers.[36]

Sandiford's condition soon deteriorated. While attending the West Indian Day Parade in Brooklyn in early September he became "gravely ill" and spent the next three weeks in the hospital with pneumonia. Doctors put him on AZT, but he insisted on being treated with Kemron instead. He later told an audience at Abyssinian Baptist Church in Harlem, "I would rather die with Kemron than to take that AZT garbage." He also blamed the pharmaceutical industry for suppressing the Kenyan drug. "With its effectiveness, if Kemron hits the market in the U.S., AZT would be out," he told the audience at Abyssinian. "In my opinion that's where the problem lies."[37]

In fact, Kemron skeptics raised legitimate concerns about Koech's study, which had been conducted without a control group. (Koech countered that, given the drug's miraculous effects, it would have been unethical not to offer it to everyone.) Many of the patients in the study also had relatively high CD4 counts before taking Kemron, which undermined Koech's claim to extraordinary results; as the San Francisco-based treatment advocacy group Project Inform pointed out, they were "hardly people on their deathbed." Nevertheless, researchers investigated the Kenyan doctor's claims. A series of short clinical trials conducted in five African countries by the World Health Organization failed to replicate Koech's dramatic findings, but the group cautioned that it was "vital to await the outcome of controlled studies."[38]

Dr. Joseph Cummins, a Texas veterinarian, also challenged Koech's claim to a miraculous discovery. Cummins didn't question the effectiveness of oral alpha interferon for treating AIDS. Instead, he accused Koech of stealing credit for his idea. Three years earlier, Cummins had published a letter in the medical journal *The Lancet*, which recounted the dramatic recovery of a fellow veterinary surgeon from symptoms of AIDS after being treated with oral alpha interferon. In his telling, he then sought a clinical trial at KEMRI with human subjects, using samples of interferon provided by his company, Amarillo Cell Culture. In response to claims on Kemron as an African achievement, Cummins insisted, "This is an American invention—the Africans didn't invent this. They're certainly not honest about the story they're telling."[39]

Koech and Cummins had, in some way, collaborated. The two men were both listed as authors (Koech first and Cummins fifth) of an article in the June 1990 issue of *Molecular Biotherapy* that touted Kemron's beneficial effects. Cummins had also received a medal from Kenyan president Moi in July 1990, possibly as part of a ceremony celebrating KEMRI's success. But when Cummins, whose company also held the international patent rights for Kemron, learned that the institute had filed for its own patent, the Texas veterinarian threatened to take "appropriate legal action to defend my technology."[40]

Koech's other collaborator, Dr. Arthur Obel, also stirred up controversy. Obel was listed as the second author, behind Koech, on the *Molecular Biotherapy* article and coauthored a pair of articles with Koech for the *East African Medical Journal* as well. In December 1990 the *New York Native*, which gave the Kenyan researchers generally positive coverage, reported that Obel had turned around and sold both Kemron tablets and placebos from the KEMRI trial to a Ugandan doctor for the outrageous price of seventy-three dollars per pill. For some, the allegations cast a pall over the entire operation.[41]

But scientific skepticism, a brewing legal battle, and rumors of malfeasance did not discourage hundreds, if not thousands, of Americans with HIV and AIDS from seeking out Kemron substitutes. Different versions of oral alpha interferon became popular among buyers clubs, local networks of people with AIDS who imported prescription drugs not yet approved for sale in the United States and distributed them to members, with mixed results. Ron Woodroof, who would later be the subject of the feature film *Dallas Buyers Club*, claimed he and others were "getting clear benefit" from taking oral interferon. Lenny Kaplan, a treatment activist in Fort Lauderdale, likewise told Charles Ortleb of the *New York Native*, "It [oral interferon] really works." Members of the People with AIDS Health Group in New York City served the substance on Catholic communion wafers in an ironic jab at the church's stance on homosexuality but were disappointed with the results. Project Inform again took a dim view of Kemron, reporting in October 1990 that "two patients . . . were told they had experienced enormous CD4 rises while in Kenya, yet upon returning home found that the newfound CD4 cells mysteriously disappeared somewhere over the Atlantic, leaving them with the same low counts as when they began their journey." And at least one person with AIDS, a man in New York, died after stopping treatment for his Kaposi's sarcoma in favor of Kemron.[42]

In response to the craze surrounding Kemron and other "cures-of-the-week," Project Inform also published a guide to recognizing fraudulent claims about AIDS treatments. Authors Larry Tate and Martin Delaney may very well have had Kemron and Cummins in mind when they wrote, "A final common source of misinformation is reports of studies or proposed studies in developing countries. . . . All too often, so-called 'studies' there are just treatment observations done under totally uncontrolled conditions, with inferior laboratory facilities, sponsored by white middle-class entrepreneurs more concerned about promoting products than evaluating them."[43]

But for many of Kemron's African American supporters, the drug's supposed Kenyan origins were what made it attractive in the first place. Black news outlets around the country framed Kemron as a specifically African treatment for AIDS. The *Los Angeles Sentinel* informed readers that "a possible cure exists in Africa, called Kemron, that has been ignored by these American and European-based researchers simply because the discoverers of Kemron are Black" and urged scientists to "quit playing racist arrogance games and get to the business of finding a cure, no matter where the cure leads you." Writing for the *Michigan Citizen*, William Reed criticized "Blacks around the world who can't accept the proven success of the AIDS drug Kemron unless the white world says that it is O.K." Ron Sturrup of the *Atlanta Inquirer* opined that "the brightest ray of hope for people suffering from the debilitating ravages of AIDS comes from out of Africa, the continent alleged to be the birthplace of the dreaded, deadly disease."[44]

News of Kemron's effectiveness and the alleged effort to suppress it also spread through other channels. A photocopied packet of information about Koech and Obel's work at KEMRI and Gary Byrd's fact-finding mission to Kenya points to the ways that Black communities learned about the drug through rumor and gossip, as well as from the Black press. Echoing Sandiford's analysis, the packet's author(s) argued that mainstream news outlets wouldn't report on Kemron because it came out of "primitive/backward Africa" and "symbolize[d] financial disaster for those who have invested billions into the drug 'AZT' and other would-be-cures and treatment of HIV infection." The author(s) wed this argument to the conspiracy theories that found traction in the *Final Call* or on *Tony Brown's Journal*, writing that Kemron "may be the long sought after cure for that devastating virus that was created by the U.S. government" and had infected an "estimated . . . 80 million African people." According to the author(s), this man-made virus was being used to carry out a plan by "President Carter's World Commission to control population," which called for "2.7 billion non-white people [to] be eliminated from this planet by the year 2000, in order to ensure white survival." Finally, the packet included a pair of photocopied articles from a Kenyan newspaper touting the success of KEMRI and the instructions, "Please make 10 or more copies and pass it on."[45]

Some located the debate surrounding Kemron within popular Afrocentric ideas, claiming that African civilizations had accomplished far more than was previously recognized. For them, the fact that white scientists, the mainstream press, and even some African Americans continued to doubt the drug's effectiveness was yet another example of the ways that Black achievements had been ignored, forgotten, and covered up. But Kemron advocates found a host of other ways to explain the reaction to Kemron. Some saw criticism of the drug as evidence of a conspiracy to protect drug company profits or to eliminate Black people altogether. The Nation of Islam would bring all of these ideas to the fore in its campaign to promote Kemron.

## Selling Kemron

In many ways, the stories that Kemron proponents told about the drug mirrored the history of the Nation of Islam. The movement began in Detroit in the summer of 1930 with a man who called himself Wallace Fard. He claimed to come from the "Holy City of Mecca" and went door to door in the city's Black neighborhoods, peddling silks and a homegrown version of Islam. Customers who invited Fard into their homes learned that "black men in North America are not Negroes, but members of the lost tribe of Shabazz [who] must learn that they are the original people, noblest of the nations of the earth." Whites, on the other hand, were a devil race of "ice people" created thousands of years ago by an evil scientist named Yakub to divide and oppress the Black race using "tricknology." As word spread of Fard's teachings, his customers became followers of the newly formed Nation of Islam.[46]

Fard's appeal owed much to the dire situation that Black Detroiters found themselves in during the 1930s. Many had recently migrated from the South seeking jobs in the industrial North and respite from the horrors of Jim Crow.

As C. Eric Lincoln later observed, they found "hunger, confusion, disillusionment, despair, and discontent." African Americans in the North were confined by custom to derelict slums and the most menial jobs, and northern whites were no less racist or violent than their southern counterparts. Fard spoke to migrants' sense of alienation by spinning tales of Black greatness and white degradation. He also foretold a coming apocalyptic race war between white and Black, which his followers could hope to win only if they converted to their "natural religion," that being Islam.[47]

Fard mysteriously disappeared in 1933, never to be seen again. His successor, Elijah Muhammad, built the Nation of Islam into a truly national organization following World War II. Under Muhammad the Nation also pursued a program of Black capitalism, based on the idea that economic self-sufficiency was essential to the project of securing Black freedom. To this end the Nation operated a variety of small businesses and encouraged followers to start their own.[48]

During the 1960s, the NOI suffered greatly from the departure and subsequent assassination of Malcolm X, Muhammad's charismatic lieutenant; many believed the killing to be an act of retribution by Muhammad and his followers for Malcolm's apostasy. At the same time, the rise of new Black Nationalist groups drew off prospective members. Elijah Muhammad's death, with no named successor, in 1975 led to a schism between his son Wallace, who embraced mainstream Sunni Islam, and Minister Louis Farrakhan, who continued to lead the Nation more or less in the mold of his predecessor.[49]

Not unlike Fard in Depression-era Detroit, Farrakhan (re)built his flock by responding to the immiseration of Black communities under Reagan. Urban economies hollowed out by capital flight, a shrinking social safety net, the incarceration of an ever-growing number of young Black men, and the explosion of the crack epidemic (not to mention AIDS) left many faced again with "hunger, confusion, disillusionment, despair, and discontent." In this context, Farrakhan seemed like a vital and necessary voice in the wilderness, and the story that he and other NOI leaders told about Kemron both built on the group's mythology and spoke to struggling African Americans' desires and concerns.[50]

It made sense for the NOI to promote Kemron and to link its support for the drug to conspiracy theories about AIDS as a man-made disease. First, the narrative of AIDS as a man-made instrument of Black genocide resonated with the Yakub story. By the late 1980s, the NOI had blunted some of this rhetoric. According to religion scholar Anthony Pinn, in an effort to carve out a more mainstream image, "claims such as the demonic nature of whites were reconceived as a metaphorical attack on white supremacy." Nevertheless, NOI leaders talked about AIDS and Kemron in ways that reflected Wallace Fard's teachings. Perhaps, after all, some modern-day Yakub had manufactured AIDS to eliminate the Black race and used tricknology to keep them from learning about Kemron, the cure.[51]

The Kemron story also resonated with Fard's tales about the historic greatness of the Black race and with similar claims made by Afrocentric scholars in the 1980s. The Nation promoted such work through its newspaper the *Final Call*, which printed excerpts from books by Ivan Van Sertima, who argued that the scientific genius of ancient Africa had been lost to the horrors of European domination and the Atlantic slave trade. Like John Henrik Clarke at the Bedford-Stuyvesant meeting, Van Sertima and other Afrocentric scholars argued that African achievements had been ignored and suppressed by white historians, just as Kemron advocates argued that Dr. Koech's work at KEMRI was ignored by white scientists and the mainstream press.[52]

Kemron was also part of the revived business empire that Farrakhan built in the 1980s for the Nation of Islam. In 1985 he secured a $5 million interest-free loan from Libyan leader Muammar Gaddafi to develop a line of toiletries under the label POWER (People Organized and Working for Economic Rebirth). The program, according to the Nation, was "organized for the absolute purpose of restoring Black people in America to their original industrial and commercial greatness." POWER never really got off the ground—Gaddafi's loan and Farrakhan's frequent anti-Semitic remarks proved to be too much of a liability for producers—but foreshadowed the NOI's entry into the pharmaceutical industry with Kemron.[53]

Finally, the idea of Kemron as a natural and specifically African treatment for AIDS fit with the Nation of Islam's broader teachings about race and health, which stressed proper diet and purity of the body. Just as Dr. Sebi claimed that food unsuited for Black bodies was bound to make them ill, Fard told his followers that because "people in your own country . . . eat the right kind of food they have the best health all the time. If you would live just like the people in your home country, you would never be sick anymore." He instructed the NOI faithful not to eat pork because it was "created by God to attract the diseases and germs which the white man traditionally carries and wants to transmit to blacks with the aim of poisoning them, in order to weaken their race." Elijah Muhammad similarly emphasized the importance of healthy eating in accordance with religious prescriptions in his *How to Eat to Live* books, which were frequently excerpted in the pages of the *Final Call*. The idea that an "African" way of life was both key to Black well-being and a way to resist white oppression was part of the NOI worldview and would become part of the Kemron campaign as well.[54]

Around a year after the first delegation traveled to Kenya in July 1990, the NOI sent its own representatives to the country. In August 1991 Dr. Abdul Alim Muhammad, "the national spokesman for the Honorable Louis Farrakhan," and Abdul Wali Muhammad, the editor of the *Final Call*, visited KEMRI to investigate the "swirl of controversy" surrounding Kemron. There they met with another delegation that included Barbara Justice and over fifty of her own patients being treated for HIV infection.[55]

Upon their return to the United States, the front page of the *Final Call* declared "AIDS Treatment Found in Africa" in huge block letters alongside a photograph of Alim Muhammad and Justice meeting with Koech. Below the headline, two pill boxes—one of Kemron and one of Immunex, another form of oral alpha interferon—flanked the silhouette of the African continent, colored red, black, and green, the colors of the Black Nationalist flag. In eight pages of articles under the heading "Out of Africa: A Treatment for AIDS," readers learned about Koech's path to AIDS research, KEMRI's difficulties in securing distribution for Kemron, and frustration at the international scientific community's skepticism. Again, members of the delegation pointed to the drug's African origins in explaining the lack of news coverage in the United States. According to Justice, "If these reports (of Kemron's success) came from anywhere else, it would have caused a stampede."[56]

Koech similarly blamed those who questioned his findings for their own "racial bias," arguing that "those who know me as an individual and . . . know my academic background" knew he "must be telling the truth," while detractors took advantage of his irregular methodology to discount his results altogether. He explained that although he had set up his clinical trial of Kemron as a double-blind study, the clear difference between those taking a placebo and those taking the drug compelled him to break with scientific protocol and put all participants in the study on a Kemron regimen. Although this decision cast doubt on his findings, Koech insisted, "My responsibility is not to the WHO, it is not to the USFDA, it is to the Republic of Kenya and the people of Kenya. . . . Mainly posterity and the patients that we have will talk for us."[57]

The *Final Call* also included an interview with LaShaun Evans, who had accompanied the NOI delegation to seek treatment for her HIV infection in Nairobi. She suggested that a conspiracy of silence from the American "AIDS establishment" prevented information about Kemron from being circulated in the United States, speculating, "A lot of people will be out of jobs because Kemron is as effective as it is." Regarding the origins of the epidemic, she gestured more vaguely toward those responsible. Although she knew the man—a friend and former sexual partner—from whom she had contracted the virus and insisted that she bore him no ill will, Evans also told the paper, "I had to come back home [to Africa] to be treated for something they gave me over there, but that's another story."[58]

Like Cedric Sandiford, Evans had to raise money—$5,000—to cover the cost of her travel to Kenya. On a flyer for a fund-raiser benefiting her trip, Evans commented, "If somebody will help me finance my trip, I'll come back and say, it worked for me—or it didn't work." But Evans showed no symptoms of AIDS, so her case would offer little evidence of Kemron's efficacy. Nevertheless, upon returning to Washington, D.C., she became a vocal proponent of the drug.[59]

Cedric Sandiford made a second trip to Kenya around the same time. At this point his relationship with Justice had deteriorated, and some would later allege that she refused to treat him. When asked by the *New York Amsterdam News* about this rumor, she insisted that while others "wanted to use Sandiford for publicity and money," she had taken the "high ethical road" and refused. The thousands of dollars that Sandiford and others had paid notwithstanding, Justice asked, "How could we have charged poor people who are desperate and dying[?]" In any case, Sandiford stayed in Kenya for two months, again being treated with Kemron. He returned to the United States in mid-November even sicker—"a different person . . . like he was psychotic or something," according to his wife, Jean Griffith-Sandiford. Cedric Sandiford entered the hospital two days later, and four days after that he was dead. Kemron advocates seem to have paid his death little notice.[60]

Upon returning from Kenya, Alim Muhammad and other NOI representatives began promoting Kemron and another form of oral interferon called Immunex. In presentations around the country, they touted the drugs as natural, nontoxic, inexpensive, and remarkably effective treatments for AIDS that had been both suppressed by the powerful interests they threatened and ignored because of their African origins. In October 1991, at the NOI's University of Islam in Chicago, Alim Muhammad announced his plan to make the drug available by ending the media "whiteout," educating doctors about Kemron and Immunex, and staging a campaign to "bring the issue to the attention of the Federal Drug Administration and other federal agencies." Sylvia Taylor, an audience member who worked as a health educator at Cook County Jail, agreed with Muhammad's assessment, saying, "It's a political and racist reason that we haven't heard about these drugs." Representatives from Kupona Network, a group doing AIDS education on Chicago's predominantly Black South Side, expressed their enthusiasm about the "tremendous boost" the drug would be for their clients, some of whom were on complicated regimens of toxic drugs, and few of whom could afford the expensive medications imported by buying clubs.[61]

Kemron advocates liked to point out that the drug, unlike AZT, was made from a substance produced in the human body. In a presentation at the University of Cincinnati's African American Cultural and Resource Center, NOI representative Aaron X stressed that the drug had been "developed in Africa" using "interferon, a natural hormone produced in the body's immune system." In contrast, AZT was an *un*natural drug with "toxic side effects that speed up the process to death." Moreover, he told the audience in Cincinnati, "if a patient has been treated with AZT for AIDS, then the Kemron treatment will be ineffective." And at around $1,500 for a year's supply, Kemron was 80 to 90 percent cheaper than AZT, and thus much more accessible to those in the greatest need.[62]

Alim Muhammad and Justice also presented Kemron as part of a holistic approach to healing that was distinct from Western medicine. The Kenyan approach was different, they said, because it focused on "the holistic side of health when working with AIDS patients." This explained why an effective AIDS treatment had been discovered by African scientists rather than by their counterparts in Europe or the United States, since Western medical education teaches "that you can only treat the symptoms, but not the underlying cause." The doctors used a similarly holistic approach in their own clinics: Alim Muhammad stressed healthy eating and abstention from tobacco and alcohol with his patients and encouraged some to undertake periods of fasting, while Dr. Justice put her patients on a regimen of vitamins and herbs. This approach, they claimed, yielded a 90 percent success rate among patients treated with Kemron, although they were vague as to exactly what constituted "success."[63]

Kemron advocates and the Black press also stressed the drug's African origins. The *Call and Post*, Cincinnati's African American newspaper, covered Aaron X's presentation with the headline "African Treatment of AIDS Deliberately Overlooked." Regarding his trip to Kenya, Alim Muhammad reported that he had been "able to ascertain that active measures are being undertaken to ensure the production and world-wide distribution of both *African developed products* [Kemron and Immunex, emphasis added]." At a Philadelphia forum hosted by Blacks Educating Blacks about Sexual Health Issues, Alim Muhammad also reworked the Kemron origin story to amplify Koech's role, making the drug sound not just natural but primitive. He told the audience that after reading a journal article about the use of alpha interferon to cure viral infections in cattle, Koech had developed a "crude powder," which he then "administered to a Kenyan diplomat who was dying from full-blown AIDS." Miraculously, he recounted, the dying diplomat made a quick recovery.[64]

Despite his views on homosexuality, Muhammad's campaign also found some support from Black gay groups. In late 1991 the DC Coalition of Black

Lesbians and Gay Men offered a "Kemron Update" in its quarterly newsletter, which described an informational forum on the drug held by Drs. Muhammad and Justice along with LaShaun Evans upon their return from Kenya. The article hailed Muhammad for his efforts to "provide hope to all Black people living with HIV and to organize a local effort to make Kemron accessible" and celebrated the event for bringing together "Black nationalists, Black gays and lesbians, non-gays and transpersons" in "a growing movement of Black people willing and able to come together and take charge of their lives."[65]

Indeed, the NOI pitch for Kemron was a seductive one. Black gay journalist LeRoy Whitfield recalled his own reaction to a speech by Louis Farrakhan about the drug: "That word cure spoke directly to my soul. Thanks to the minister, I might not have to spend the rest of my life beholden for direction about AIDS to . . . insensitive doctors whom I deemed unreliable because of an alienating visit to one earlier that year. Nah, what Minister Farrakhan was offering, to my mind, wasn't just alternative medication but sorely needed liberation. To hell with trying to understand HIV or ever being a slave to oddball medical regimens, I thought: I am free." Others were more cautious. Rashidah Hassan of BEBASHI made clear, "We are not suggesting it is a cure. . . . We are not disclaiming its effectiveness." Above all she stressed that the public, and African Americans in particular, had "a right to demand this drug if it's appropriate, and to ask questions."[66]

As it turned out, those questions were not welcome if they suggested that Kemron was less effective than its proponents claimed. The day after the Kemron forum hosted by BEBASHI in October 1991, David Fair, recently hired as executive director of We the People, a local AIDS organization mainly serving poor people of color, wrote a letter to Barbara Justice. He began by enumerating the points on which they agreed, including "the genocidal nature of this epidemic worldwide and that the reaction of Western medicine to the Kenyan research is clearly consistent with a pattern of behavior . . . that will result in the decimation of whole populations of people of color." He also made clear that his group supported the establishment of a Kemron clinical trial in Philadelphia and would help educate others about the drug. But Fair took issue with the way Justice had treated a member of We the People's board during the BEBASHI forum.[67]

The board member, a white man with AIDS and "a strong advocate for many of the same objectives that you [Justice] articulated," had recounted his own experience taking Kemron. He felt that he had not benefited from the drug and told Justice that doctors advised him against taking it as a treatment for his illness. According to Fair, Justice responded by "attacking him for being white and attempting to isolate him from everyone else," to which the crowd reacted "by laughing at him and your [Justice's] pejorative comments." Fair concluded, "As an organization of people with HIV committed to protecting each other, we commend your efforts, but also must condemn your unfortunate and uncalled for attack on a person with AIDS whose only crime was to not fully agree with your perspective."[68]

While Kemron advocates framed the drug as a natural, holistic AIDS treatment "out of Africa," the reality was more complicated. On the one hand, there was where Kemron had actually come from, and who had developed it. On the other hand, there was the issue of whether or not Kemron was a "natural" treatment for AIDS.

When the *Final Call* reported the results of Muhammad's trip to Kenya, the paper described Kemron as the product of a collaboration among KEMRI, Joseph Cummins's Amarillo Cell Culture, and Hayashibara Biochemical Laboratories, a Japanese manufacturer. Kemron advocates would later shift the story over time to emphasize Koech's role in developing the drug and thus frame it as a specifically African treatment. But in November 1990 Joseph Oliech, Kenya's director of medical services, had "admitted that the drug was developed by Cummins and manufactured by Hayashibara in Japan and that KEMRI only conducted clinical trials."[69]

Advocates also touted Kemron as a "natural" AIDS treatment. While this was true inasmuch as clinical interferon was derived from proteins produced in animal cells, it was also one of a new class of drugs called "biologics": substances found in the human body but mass-produced through novel manufacturing techniques made possible by genetic engineering. Far from Alim Muhammad's story about a "crude powder," Kemron was produced in part through cutting-edge methods. Hayashibara, for example, used hamsters to cultivate human cells that had been exposed to a virus in order to stimulate organic interferon production. That interferon was then used to make Kemron.[70]

African American activists, Black newspapers, and especially the Nation of Islam touted Kemron as a natural, African remedy for a disease that was killing people of African descent worldwide. They told an appealing story. Black Americans were frustrated and insulted that blame for the new and terrifying epidemic was being pinned on Haitians and Africans. The Kemron story offered a much different narrative, with Africans not as victims or scapegoats but as heroes. At the same time, the apparent media "whiteout" to prevent news of Kemron from spreading fit a familiar script of conspiracy by the powers that be to discredit Black achievement. But the story behind the drug, including the way that it was initially reported in the pages of the *Final Call*, was more complicated. In the most generous reading, Kemron was not an African invention but the result of collaboration among doctors and scientists on three continents. It is also possible, as Larry Tate and Martin Delaney suggested, that Joseph Cummins chose Kenya as the site of a clinical trial that he hoped would make him rich. Either way, far from being a natural, African AIDS treatment, Kemron was the product of advanced biotechnology in a globalized world. In the United States, it would also soon become the subject of an ill-fated, controversial clinical trial.

## Clinical Trials and Tribulations

In February 1992 during a rally at Christ Universal Temple, a megachurch on Chicago's South Side, Louis Farrakhan delivered news sure to excite his followers: the Nation of Islam had acquired the exclusive right to distribute Immunex, a form of oral alpha interferon similar to Kemron, throughout the United States. He also announced that Alim Muhammad would take on the position of minister of health and human services for the Nation and be tasked with leading the group's efforts to combat AIDS. Taking the podium, Muhammad made clear that the Nation of Islam would seek FDA approval of Immunex. "However," he continued, "we can't wait. We will take any risk, bear any burden to free our people of a man-made disease designed to kill us all."[71]

For those who doubted the efficacy of oral alpha interferon in treating AIDS, this was an absurd turn in an already ridiculous story. Why would anyone trust what Farrakhan and Alim Muhammad had to say about Immunex when their organization had a financial stake in the drug's success? What made them any different from the pharmaceutical companies that they had accused of colluding to kill Kemron in the first place?

But selling Immunex fit within the Nation's goal of Black economic independence, which the *Final Call* promoted with headlines such as "We Must Depend on Allah and Ourselves," "Unity: The Key to Black Economic Success in the 90s," and "White Brutality Must Force Black Self-Determination." If Kemron and Immunex were found to be effective, profits would flow not to drug company executives and their wealthy shareholders but to Black communities—to Alim Muhammad's Abundant Life Clinic, which was located in Washington, D.C.'s Mayfair Mansions housing project, and to ordinary Kenyans through KEMRI.[72]

In April 1992, just two months after Farrakhan's announcement, the AIDS Research Advisory Committee of the National Institute of Allergy and Infectious Diseases dealt Kemron advocates a blow when it announced that "the original, exciting, positive results observed with this therapy [Kemron] have not been confirmed in preliminary results of subsequent well-designed controlled studies." The committee acknowledged that some ongoing studies had yet to be completed, but the report seemed to close the book on Kemron. Nevertheless, Muhammad was able to convince the National Medical Association, a Black physicians' group, of the drug's value. In August 1992 the group's legislative body voted to endorse clinical trials of Kemron in the United States. The following month, Boston's Multicultural AIDS Coalition also signed on to the effort to get a study underway. Barbara Gomes-Beach, the coalition's executive director, told the *Bay State Banner*, "This issue has become a political football. We would really like to know why. Is it because the drug comes from Africa and the positive studies done were done by an African[?]" In contrast to the Nation of Islam, she stressed her group's neutrality: "We are not marketeers but we are advocates for those who have tested HIV positive."[73]

The possibility of a new study was thus reopened. In October 1992 representatives from the National Medical Association and the National Institutes of Health met with Alim Muhammad, Barbara Justice, Wilbert Jordan, and Dr. Keith Crawford of the advocacy group Kemron Action Committee to discuss a clinical trial. Two days later, the NIH Office of AIDS Research and the National Institute of Allergy and Infectious Diseases announced that they would move forward with large-scale testing of oral alpha interferon, assisting advocates in designing a clinical trial. Although a panel of nongovernmental experts found "no benefit" to Kemron based on twelve existing studies of the drug, its underground use by buyers' clubs moved government scientists to conduct an official clinical trial in the interest of public safety. Jack Killen, a National Institute of Allergy and Infectious Diseases official who had previously criticized Koech's research, lamented to the *Washington Post* that people with AIDS "are opting to take low-dose interferon and declining to take therapy that, from our perspective, has been proved beneficial in good, sound clinical trials."[74]

Both sides acknowledged that the trial was also the result of political pressure. Malik Shabazz, reporting for the *Afro-American Red Star*, noted that the NIH was responding to "huge criticism from the African American community who felt that NIH was attempting to wrongfully discredit KEMRON." Not all of that criticism was directed at federal officials; Dr. Wayne Greaves of Howard University told the *Washington Post* that his and other Black institutions had come under fire from Black community leaders in the past for not backing a clinical trial. Victor Zonana, a spokesman for the Department of Health and Human Services, acknowledged the agency's desire to "build bridges" with African Americans who were "deeply suspicious of the research establishment" because of past abuses. He called the decision to undertake the trial "political, but good political."[75]

In response to pressure from Kemron advocates, federal officials also promised that Black physicians would be included in planning the trials. Dr.

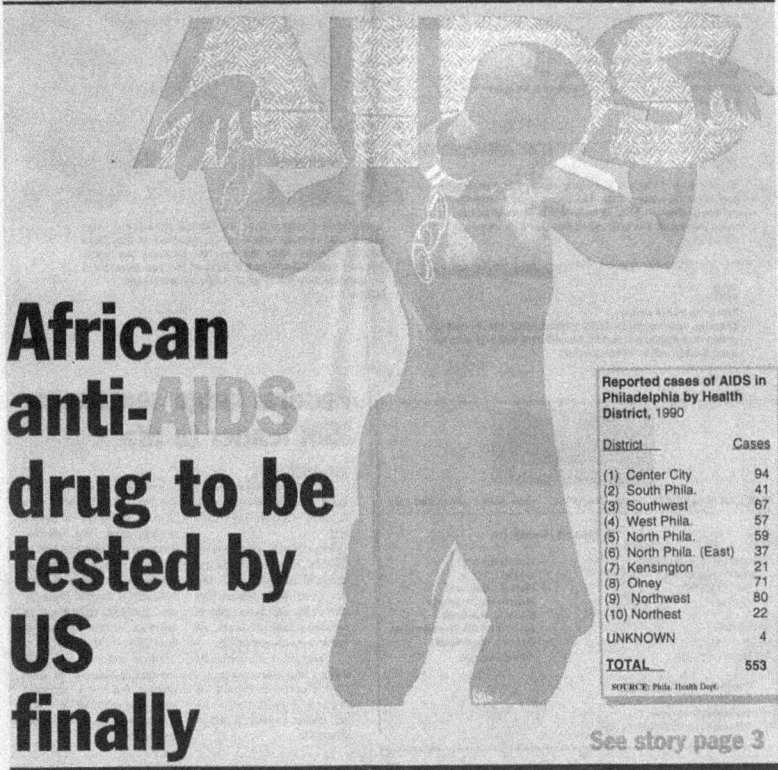

**THE PHILADELPHIA SUNDAY**

**SUN**

Volume 1, No. 6          October 18, 1992          75 cents

# African anti-AIDS drug to be tested by US finally

| Reported cases of AIDS in Philadelphia by Health District, 1990 | |
|---|---|
| District | Cases |
| (1) Center City | 94 |
| (2) South Phila. | 41 |
| (3) Southwest | 67 |
| (4) West Phila. | 57 |
| (5) North Phila. | 59 |
| (6) North Phila. (East) | 37 |
| (7) Kensington | 21 |
| (8) Olney | 71 |
| (9) Northwest | 80 |
| (10) Northest | 22 |
| UNKNOWN | 4 |
| TOTAL | 553 |

SOURCE: Phila. Health Dept.

See story page 3

*Philadelphia Sunday Sun* cover story on Kemron, October 18, 1992. Kiyoshi Kuromiya subject files on HIV/AIDS, 1990–2000, Ms. Coll. 18, John J. Wilcox Jr. Archives, William Way LGBT Community Center, Philadelphia, Pa.

Barbara Justice framed this as an issue of equity in the distribution of resources in the fight against AIDS: "We will be expanding that research to include researchers and physicians of color. . . . Those are tax dollars being used for research, we are 49 percent of the population of the United States that is so affected (by AIDS), yet our researchers, our scientists, our nation, our concerns have not been addressed to date." Alim Muhammad likewise told the *Philadelphia Tribune*, "There are billions spent on AIDS research each year, but institutions such as Meharry Medical School [a historically Black medical college in Tennessee] and Howard University get none of these funds." Additionally, he argued, putting Black researchers in charge of the trials would make their results more credible in the eyes of African Americans: "In order for these results to be verified for the Black community, trials must be done at Black institutions."[76]

Announcing further details about the upcoming trial the following spring, Muhammad once again touted the promise of "a product produced by Black people" and located the drug within the history of scientific genius in the African diaspora: "I think that historically Black physicians and scientists have always been in the forefront and have taken principled stands. This is just one further example in what I call the tradition of Imhotep, George Washington Carver, Ronald McNair and Charles Drew." He also moderated his earlier rhetoric, telling the *Philadelphia Tribune* that Western doctors had rejected the results of Koech's original Kemron study not out of explicit racism but because "it came from what was considered an unorthodox source, community-based people in Kenya."[77]

Meanwhile, the results of an African study of oral alpha interferon dealt a major blow to the U.S. clinical trial, showing "absolutely no differences" between the effects of the drug and a placebo on AIDS symptoms. Researchers reported their findings in June 1993 at the International AIDS Conference in Berlin. Project Inform called the results "the disappointment of this year's conference" and concluded that the study "seems to be the last word on Kemron and current trials will most likely be abandoned based on these findings."[78]

Yet even after the Berlin announcement, Muhammad pressed forward with his clinical trial. He maintained that oral alpha interferon had worked for his patients and that the controversy stemmed not from concerns about its effectiveness but from a conflict over funding for AIDS services. He criticized the local AIDS office for giving over a quarter of its $15 million budget to Whitman-Walker, D.C.'s gay health clinic, while the epidemic was "exploding" in Black and Latino communities. This advocacy, he insisted, was the real reason that interferon had been discredited.[79]

Muhammad had been successful, however, in securing over $200,000 in federal grants to provide a range of services for people with AIDS. An AIDS social worker with the Veterans Administration in Northwest Washington testified to the Abundant Life Clinic's appeal: "His holistic approach to care, his Afrocentric approach, is what my [clients] are looking for." But Muhammad's role as a minister of the Nation of Islam raised questions as to whether his clinic should receive public funds. Critics pointed to a record of anti-Semitic and homophobic remarks, although Muhammad insisted that over half of his AIDS patients at the Abundant Life Clinic were gay or bisexual. Even other interferon advocates disagreed with the clinic's religious messages. "He greets you in the name of Allah," Wilbert Jordan told the *Washington Post*. "You have the religious doctrine being pushed." But Muhammad's ambition went far beyond the walls of the clinic. In his quest to bring interferon to struggling communities of color everywhere, he told the paper, "I am literally out to save the world."[80]

Around the same time, Muhammad set his sights on winning a sizable contract from the District of Columbia. In 1993, for the first time since the beginning of the epidemic, the city invited bids for its $2 million contract to provide local AIDS services. In order to compete for the contract, the Abundant Life Clinic joined with a dozen other Black and Latino AIDS service organizations to form the Sankofa Community Coalition against AIDS. Its main competition would be the Whitman-Walker Clinic, which, like Philadelphia Community Health Alternatives, had started in the late 1970s as a health clinic serving primarily white gay men and had been among the first groups in the city to respond to the emerging AIDS epidemic.[81]

In arguing that Sankofa should win the contract over Whitman-Walker, Muhammad was quick to point out that the majority of people with HIV in the District were Black or Latino and "underserved" by the existing system. He also posited that the proportion of HIV-positive D.C. residents who were gay or bisexual men was "slipping" and that the growing number of HIV-positive heterosexuals would be uncomfortable being treated at a gay-identified clinic. Jim Graham, the executive director of Whitman-Walker, insisted that the majority of his clinic's patients were people of color. He also pointed out that the clinic's Max Robinson Center (named for the Black newscaster who died of AIDS complications in 1988) offered AIDS services in Southeast D.C., where the majority of residents were African American. Muhammad countered (quite improbably) that Graham had told him that he was interested only in serving "the *white* gay and lesbian community" and looked forward to the time when the Abundant Life Clinic "would relieve [Whitman-Walker] of the responsibility of having to be concerned about blacks and Latinos."[82]

But Muhammad also had to contend with the effect that his own public statements about homosexuality had on other members of the Sankofa coalition. During a "heated, three-hour exchange" just a month after the coalition formed, Black gay activists presented him with a list of demands, including that he add gay members to the Abundant Life Clinic board and publish an article in the *Final Call* on homosexuality in Africa. Muhammad told the *Washington Post* that he "essentially agreed to most of the requests" but that he had no authority over the content of the *Final Call*. H. Alexander Robinson, who served as president of the National Task Force on AIDS Prevention board and worked closely with some Sankofa members as president of the D.C. CARE Consortium, was unconvinced, saying, "I don't trust him to act in the best interest of gay and lesbian people." Others were more optimistic, if only a little. Greg Hutchings of Lifelink, a coalition member, allowed that working as a Black gay man with the Abundant Life Clinic was not "the best of alliances" but held out hope that "the coalition [could] ensure equitable funding for people of color with HIV in this city."[83]

That Black gay activists would choose to cast their lot with a man who had called for the government to deal with AIDS by enforcing "strong laws … against homosexuality" speaks to the persistent level of distrust they felt for the Whitman-Walker Clinic and other AIDS service organizations identified with white gay communities. Their choice also speaks to the desire among some to carve out a Black gay political agenda that was distinctly their own, apart from that of white gay activists.[84]

This dynamic was again on display in the months leading up to the Million Man March in October 1995, as Black gay and lesbian activists debated whether to be involved with the massive gathering. The National Black Gay and Lesbian Leadership Forum declined to endorse the event, out of objection to "its sexist and patriarchal tone and the homophobic comments made by some march organizers." Nevertheless, after deciding that participation in the march would "enable many black gays to abandon their masks of invisibility and assume or maintain their rightful place as citizens, mentors, and leaders," the forum encouraged "all black gay and lesbian people, and particularly men, to participate openly and visibly in the March." Moreover, it resolved, "we will no longer allow outsiders to dictate who is welcome at the black family table or to divide African Americans by sexual orientation or by gender."[85]

Muhammad also saw the Million Man March as an opportunity to promote Kemron and keep up pressure for a clinical trial. During the rally, which brought a crowd of hundreds of thousands—mostly Black men—to the National Mall, Farrakhan and Muhammad welcomed a man named Demetrius X

Haskins to the stage. Haskins claimed that he had tested positive for HIV in 1992 and, after being treated with Kemron at the Abundant Life Clinic, had been cured of the virus.[86]

With no hard evidence to back such claims, and a large number of scientific studies that showed otherwise, the interferon trial was slow to get off the ground. The arm of the study that would test the Nation of Islam's version of the drug, now marketed as Immulin, lacked FDA approval. Muhammad then blamed the NIH for the delay: "It's the same double standard. They make us jump over every hurdle and dot every *i* before we are heard." When the trial finally got underway in 1996, Muhammad told the *Afro-American Red Star*, "It can truly be said that it is the first clinical trial that is our very own." Barbara Justice framed the trial as a victory for race pride and social equity, telling the *New York Amsterdam News*, "This is the first time a treatment developed by an African has been placed for formal evaluation . . . and also the first time Africans worldwide have pressured whites into using our tax dollars for evaluation of a treatment we are interested in."[87]

The study, however, was short-lived. Soon after it began, Congressman Peter King of New York launched an investigation into Abundant Life, the same day that the IRS placed a tax lien on the clinic. A year later, in June 1997, the NIH terminated the clinical trial, pointing to low enrollment and retention. Dr. Beverly Austin, medical officer for the Opportunistic Infections Research arm of the agency, told the *Afro-American Red Star* that the end to the study did not preclude future research on oral alpha interferon but noted, "That will have to be determined by the (pharmaceutical) companies." Muhammad blamed the IRS for the poor outcome, telling the *Red Star*, "The day after the trials were open the IRS . . . attacked us . . . and the same with Dr. Barbara Justice in New York and Dr. [Wilbert] Jordan in [Los Angeles] whose funding was dried up and [enrollment] kept . . . low."[88]

For his part, Jordan blamed the NIH for assigning the study to the Division of AIDS Treatment Research Initiative, which was scheduled to shut down in 1998. Dr. Bill Duncan of the Therapeutic Research Programs at the NIH insisted that the future of the institute had no bearing on the demise of the Kemron study, but other treatment advocates disagreed. The Critical Path AIDS Project, hardly a supporter of Kemron or the Nation of Islam, reported that once Community Programs for Clinical Research on AIDS decided "that community interest in the drug had evaporated," Duncan "kicked the hot potato study" to the Division of AIDS Treatment Research Initiative, which was "nearly on the rocks." With Kemron's fate sealed, Jordan lamented, "They never really wanted to do the study in the first place." In a sense, he was right.[89]

MANY AFRICAN AMERICANS saw evidence of a genocidal conspiracy in the advent of a new and deadly disease, which seemed to come out of nowhere just as humankind had conquered so many epidemics of old. When scientists and journalists focused on Haiti and Africa as hot spots of infection, many more saw racist stereotypes being used to blame the latest global crisis on Black people. And when it seemed as though a miraculous treatment—even a cure—for AIDS had been discovered in Kenya, they saw the incredulity of those same scientists and journalists as evidence of their bigotry.

Skeptics were right to doubt Koech's results, especially as study after study failed to confirm his findings. But science does not exist in a vacuum, and that skepticism rankled Black activists and observers. Through political pressure, they won approval for a clinical trial of Kemron, which NIH officials saw as an opportunity to establish better relations with Black communities.

But the clinical trial did little to inspire trust of federal officials among Black communities. Alim Muhammad and other Kemron advocates thought that the NIH had not taken the trial seriously and said as much in the Black press. Even some of their detractors agreed. And for African American observers, Peter King's investigation and the tax lien against Abundant Life must have fit a familiar script of the abuse of Black leaders by powerful white political institutions.

At the same time, the fight over Kemron was about much more than the drug itself. For one, it built on African Americans' anger over the way that Haiti and Africa had been implicated in the origin and spread of AIDS. The drug offered a sharp rebuke to this "geography of blame," which African Americans felt affected them as well—"What are they trying to say we did with that monkey?" Kemron promised to flip this script on AIDS and global Blackness.

The economics of AIDS treatment and care also mattered to the Kemron story. Advocates insisted that the drug had been discredited because it threatened drug companies, which stood to make a lot of money from their own treatments. Kemron advocates were not alone in this criticism; other AIDS activist groups also made the pharmaceutical industry's greed a frequent theme in their campaigns, as the chapter on ACT UP Philadelphia will show. Alim Muhammad and Barbara Justice also pointed to real disparities in AIDS funding and resources, as the stories of BEBASHI and the NTFAP make clear.

Ultimately, the end of the oral alpha interferon clinical trial coincided with the advent of highly active antiretroviral therapies. The miraculous recoveries that Koech claimed to see in patients on Kemron *did* happen for some of those on protease inhibitors. This new class of drugs revolutionized the treatment of HIV and AIDS and turned the disease that had once been a death sentence into a chronic, manageable condition.

For those who could afford them, anyway.

Oral alpha interferon was different from AIDS drugs on the market because it was relatively cheap (the plane ticket to Kenya was another story). It nurtured the promise of a treatment that would be available to all, including the poor. Even if Kemron seemed too good to be true, advocates held out hope that it was not. And while protease inhibitors proved to be far more effective than AZT in treating HIV infection, their high price tag means that for many in poor communities of color, the revolution in AIDS treatment has yet to arrive.[90]

In contrast to other African American AIDS activists, Abdul Alim Muhammad and the leaders of the Nation of Islam did not try to create a space for queer sexuality within Black identity—not even close. To the contrary, they traded in a heterosexist idea of essential Black identity very close to the one that Gay Men of African Descent and others in the Black gay renaissance worked to overturn. But in Kemron the Nation of Islam and other advocates saw an opportunity to unravel the centuries-old racist stereotypes that contribute to the oppression of Black people worldwide. Kemron promised to validate claims to Black greatness, alleviate the suffering of millions of Black people across the globe, *and* provide for their economic uplift. Kemron's appeal, far from being a sideshow to the fight against AIDS, speaks to the close connection between AIDS in Black America and much older wounds that have yet to be made whole.

## CHAPTER 5

## There Is a Balm in Gilead

AIDS Activism in the Black Church

THREE DAYS into her new job, Pernessa Seele was already tired.

The thirty-four-year-old immunologist hadn't really wanted the job anyway. She was living in Brooklyn and working in a methadone clinic at Interfaith Medical Center when she noticed an ad in the *New York Amsterdam News* for a job as an administrator at Harlem Hospital. She recalls, "I knew that job was mine, but I did not want to work at Harlem Hospital. So I ignored it. Every weekend, every Friday, I'd look at the paper, saw the job. I knew it would never get filled because I knew it was my job." When the job ad kept reappearing week after week, she relented. "I went for the interview, and [Dr. Wafaa El-Sadr] hired me on the spot. And there I am, Harlem Hospital, because I knew that job was mine."[1]

Seele felt called to the job, but at first she wasn't sure why. The patients whom she saw in her administrative role "weren't really interested in the services I came to them about." Many were dying of AIDS; Harlem residents accounted for less than 1.5 percent of New York City's population but close to 8 percent of New Yorkers with the disease, and "they really wanted to talk. . . . No one was coming to see them. The family wasn't coming, the church wasn't coming. They wanted someone to sit by their bedside, hold their hand, and pray and be present with them." She realized why she had been called here: to bring the Black church into the fight against AIDS.[2]

Religion had been the center of Seele's life growing up during the 1950s and 1960s in Lincolnville, South Carolina, a small town founded by freed people after the Civil War. In Lincolnville, churches served as hubs for networks of mutual support, providing "whatever was needed, good or bad or indifferent," to the community and serving as "the first line of defense" when someone fell ill or died. Seele remembers that the church leveled differences in status among members and served as a refuge from life under Jim Crow. For African

Americans in the South, she says, "whether you were a doctor or a janitor, you had to sit in the back of the bus. But when you walked into church you were somebody."[3]

Historically, the Black church had been in the vanguard of struggles for social justice. But in the context of AIDS in Harlem, where over 90 percent of people with the disease were Black, churches had largely abdicated this role. Pastors seemed to have abandoned people with AIDS because the disease was associated with gay men and drug users, exposing fault lines of respectability within the church. And whereas churches had often taken the lead on a host of social and political issues in the past, now they seemed unwilling even to comfort people who lay dying from a disease of the abject.[4]

Seele saw the need to change things and had an idea of how to go about doing so. She would gather the neighborhood's faith leaders together for a week of prayer and education about AIDS. Their lack of action notwithstanding, Harlem's churches and mosques were already familiar with the disease. Pastors, with their intimate insight into personal issues of sickness and death, knew that they preached on Sundays to HIV-positive parishioners and at the funerals of young men and women who had died from AIDS, although ashamed families often listed cancer as the cause of death. Imams who ministered to former injection drug users, those who had kicked their habits in converting to Islam, also saw their congregations devastated by the growing epidemic. Seele believed that couching AIDS education in prayer would offer clergy and clerics a way to talk about a disease closely associated with homosexuality, sexual promiscuity, and drug use and so bring Black religious communities into the fight against AIDS.

As Seele tells it, she started by walking through the neighborhood herself, knocking on doors. "'Hi, I'm Pernessa Seele,'" she would say, "'and we are having a Harlem Week of Prayer.' And 'we' was me. And Thee. Me and the Lord was having a Harlem Week of Prayer for the Healing of AIDS." She tailored her message to Harlem's religious gatekeepers, emphasizing a program of prayer and healing with "education . . . in the backdrop." Seele believed that, through prayer, Harlem's ministers would find the resolve to "be bold and speak truth to power" with their congregations. They could then bring accurate information and an open mind back to their churches. "If we can get people praying for AIDS," she reasoned, "we can get them to do other things."[5]

The first Harlem Week of Prayer married elements of a church revival with more prosaic efforts to educate Black faith leaders, including workshops on HIV transmission, treatment, and pastoral care. On Sunday, September 10, 1989, nearly a hundred Black clergy, including Christian ministers, Muslim imams, Native American shamans, Yoruba priests, and Ethiopian Hebrew rabbis, gathered "to walk around Harlem Hospital like the folks walked around Jericho and blow the walls down." After an opening prayer, Seele recalls, "all of us African Americans with our different cultures and communities [were] walking around Harlem Hospital singing 'What a Friend We Have in Jesus,' saying our prayers in Arabic, saying our Yoruba prayers and messages." Outside the hospital, faith leaders addressed the community. Bishop Norman Quick of the Church of God in Christ told the crowd that he would have to leave the event early to conduct a funeral for a thirty-five-year-old man, the son of two members of Quick's church, who had died of AIDS. "The biggest thing we can do for our people is to get it out in the open," he continued. "It's all right to acknowledge that you have someone in your family who has contracted AIDS." Seele remembers Quick's address as a "revolutionary moment" because of his stature among Christians in Harlem and because he had previously rejected people with HIV and AIDS as sinners. Quick's willingness to talk openly about AIDS portended the sea change in community attitudes about the disease that Seele hoped to bring about. That change might in turn lead the neighborhood churches and mosques to offer more developed HIV prevention programs and advocate politically for people with the disease. As Wafaa El-Sadr, the hospital's chief of infectious diseases and Seele's boss, remarked, "The idea is to open up these churches for the word AIDS."[6]

Over the next few years the Harlem Week of Prayer for the Healing of AIDS grew, doubling the number of churches involved to two hundred by 1991. Seele began to hear from others around the country who wanted to replicate the model, and in 1992 incorporated a new nonprofit group, The Balm in Gilead, to do this work year-round. She drew the name for the new group from a verse in the book of Jeremiah, as well as an African American spiritual by the same name. The chorus of the spiritual goes,

There is a balm in Gilead
To make the wounded whole;
There is a balm in Gilead
To heal the sin-sick soul.

The call for both physical and spiritual healing fit the new group, which sought to mend rifts within the church around issues of sexuality and drug use in order to make headway against a deadly epidemic.[7]

With her professional expertise in immunology and her personal religious experience, Seele aimed to bring HIV prevention to churchgoing African Americans by bridging the worlds of science and faith. To combat stigma and silence surrounding AIDS, The Balm in Gilead encouraged Black churches to acknowledge the presence of sexuality, including homosexuality, in their

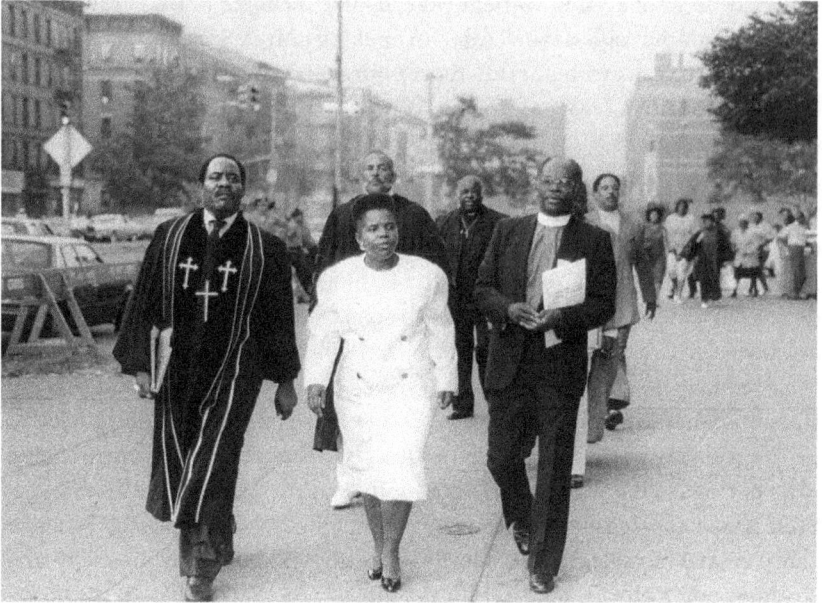

Pernessa Seele and clergy leading the first annual Harlem Week of Prayer for the Healing of AIDS, 1989. Courtesy of Pernessa Seele.

congregations. Seele also leveraged support from philanthropic donors and the federal government to expand The Balm in Gilead's model to churches throughout the United States, and then to the Caribbean and Africa. In the early 2000s, the organization set up programs in five African countries before establishing a permanent second headquarters in Tanzania. Throughout this process Pernessa Seele, as the leader and public face of The Balm in Gilead, argued that the church served as the focus of social life for disparate peoples throughout Africa and its diaspora, and thus her organization's approach to HIV prevention would work in Dar es Salaam as well as it had in Harlem. Working through Black churches, The Balm in Gilead tried to reshape the boundaries of Blackness by making churches more welcoming to gay parishioners and people with HIV and AIDS and by promoting a more open discussion of homosexuality. As the organization grew, The Balm in Gilead also sought to "bridge" the African diaspora in the context of a deadly pandemic that devastated Black communities around the world. But that meant forging partnerships with leaders—political and religious, at home and abroad—who threatened to undercut The Balm in Gilead's vision of a more inclusive Black church.[8]

## The Love That Dare Not Preach Its Name

In some ways, it made perfect sense for the Black church to take up the fight against AIDS. The Black church has a rich prophetic tradition, inspiring hope and envisioning deliverance during the darkest of times. The church has also functioned as a "nation within a nation," providing for worldly needs such as education and health care, not to mention the comfort of fellowship. Throughout a centuries-long history of dislocation, injustice, and murderous violence, the church has offered both spiritual and literal refuge to African Americans in need.[9]

At the same time, the Black church has a complicated legacy when it comes to issues of gender and sexuality. Women in the church have long resisted their subordinate place in an institution that relies heavily on their labor but valorizes male leadership. Some of those same women actively promoted the idea that African Americans would achieve political equality only through respectability, which meant conforming to middle-class standards of sexual propriety. Following the church's culture of silence on sexuality—and homosexuality in particular—many Black pastors avoided talking about AIDS; most of those who did condemned people with the disease as mortal sinners whose wicked behavior had brought a plague down from God himself. For the Black church, the association between the epidemic and homosexuality, which sat "among the worst of all sins," put AIDS activism from the pulpit beyond the pale.[10]

The roots of the modern Black church lie in the independent denominations founded by free African Americans tired of segregated worship, as well as in the "invisible institution" of slave churches. According to theologian Vincent Wimbush, for African Americans the Bible "came to function as a language-world," or the "storehouse of rhetorics, images, and stories" through which they could make sense of their shared experience. Stories of Hebrew bondage and exodus and of the trials and resurrection of Jesus Christ helped "an enslaved and otherwise dominated" people "imagine themselves as something other, in another world, different from what their immediate situation reflected or demanded."[11]

Even as the Bible helped African Americans to "imagine themselves as something other," the racist lies promulgated by whites were hard to shake. Slavery apologists used the myth of Black hypersexuality to uphold the peculiar institution and plunge the nation into Civil War. During and after Reconstruction white southerners pointed to the supposed threat of rapacious Black men who preyed on white women to justify the use of terroristic violence against the formerly enslaved. Elite and middle-class African Americans, including clergy and lay leaders in the Black church, countered this cruel fiction by cultivating for themselves an image of respectable sexual purity, in contrast to the image of the poor and working-class Blacks they sought to "uplift." As Evelyn Brooks Higginbotham observes, this approach "reflected and reinforced the hegemonic values of white America." The upshot, according to Black gay theologian Horace L. Griffin, is that the Black church has been haunted by "a large degree of sexual shame" ever since.[12]

Nevertheless, some found (or made) room for decidedly queer expressions of faith. During the social upheaval of the Great Migration, Black religious leaders such as "Sweet Daddy" Grace and Prophet James Jones gained large followings. Neither man conformed to the image of a respectable race man: Grace sported an ostentatious wardrobe, along with long hair and fingernails, while Jones's homosexuality was something of an open secret among both his followers and his detractors. According to Tim Retzloff, Jones's loyal working-class followers stuck with him, even after his arrest for soliciting sex from an undercover vice cop in 1956, "for he and they had common enemies: the middle and upper classes, orthodox religion, and law enforcement." The "messiah in mink," as Jones was known, appealed to those at the bottom of the social ladder because he, like them, bucked the conventions of middle-class morality.[13]

Nevertheless, it was the mainline Black Protestant churches, where the ethic of respectability prevailed, that stood at the center of the growing civil rights struggle in the years following World War II. Those who did not fit the mold found themselves marginalized by civil rights leaders or excluded from the movement altogether. Such was the case with Bayard Rustin, the Black Quaker and veteran activist who was imprisoned as a conscientious objector during World War II and who introduced Dr. Martin Luther King Jr. to Gandhian nonviolence during the Montgomery bus boycott. He was also gay and had been arrested in 1953 while having sex with another man in a parked car in Pasadena, California. Rustin's organizing acumen made him the target of petty jealousy within the movement, while his sexuality and arrest made him vulnerable to attack. Congressman Adam Clayton Powell, who also served as pastor of Abyssinian Baptist Church in Harlem, drove a wedge between King and Rustin in 1960 by threatening to charge the two with having an affair. Rustin resigned as King's assistant in response. Three years later, NAACP executive secretary Roy Wilkins prevented Rustin from becoming director of the March on Washington for Jobs and Freedom because, Wilkins said, "He's got too many scars."[14]

Some Black gay men and lesbians found refuge in the gay religious movement, which began when Reverend Troy Perry, a gay Pentecostal, founded Metropolitan Community Church in Los Angeles in 1968. Others found churches such as Perry's, which had predominantly white congregations, to be alienating. As James Tinney wrote in an essay for Joseph Beam's anthology *In the Life*, they longed "to hear the gospel in their own 'language of the Spirit,' respond to the gospel in their own ways, and reinterpret the gospel in their own cultural context—taking into account both race and sexual orientation at every step of the way." After he was excommunicated from Temple Church of God in Christ in 1982, Tinney founded Faith Temple Christian Church in Washington, D.C., where Black gays and lesbians could worship in a familiar style, without being judged for their sexual identity.[15]

Tinney started his church just as the AIDS crisis was beginning to explode in U.S. cities and at the same time that a generation of Black gay and lesbian clergy entered into the ministry. Many had been raised to see homosexuality as incompatible with Christianity. Archbishop Carl Bean attempted suicide and underwent shock treatment after being rejected by his church and family. He later moved to Los Angeles, where he founded Unity Fellowship Church, a Black gay congregation, and the Minority AIDS Project. As a "deeply, deeply spiritual" same-gender-loving young woman in the Church of God in Christ, Bishop Yvette Flunder lacked even the language to describe her desire for other women. Since "there were no words for it [her sexuality], not in our community," she married a man "who was struggling with the same kinds of issues . . . and I guess we figured that we would cancel each other out in some way." Her husband later died of complications from AIDS, and Flunder went on to found Ark of Refuge, a San Francisco ministry for people living with the disease. Darlene Garner, who would become one of the founders of the National Coalition of Black Lesbians and Gays, as well as cochair of BWMT for Education in Philadelphia and a reverend in the gay-affirming Metropolitan Community Church, left home for Washington, D.C., in her early twenties after coming out to her family as a lesbian. To explain Garner's departure, her great-aunt told friends at church that Garner was a prostitute who had skipped town after stealing money from her pimp, because "being a prostitute was, to her, far preferable than telling anyone I was a lesbian."[16]

Even though most Black churches approached homosexuality with an attitude somewhere between tacit disapproval and open hostility, many nevertheless relied on the work of gay men. As organists and choir directors, Black gay men in the church took an active role in producing a religious experience for the faithful every Sunday. Even as churches capitalized on their creative energies, Black gay men occupied an "open closet," trading their silence about sexual matters for membership in the flock. According to Reverend Renee McCoy of Metropolitan Community Church, "If Black lesbians and gay men are willing to check their sexuality at the door of the church, and come bearing gifts of talent, there are relatively few problems." However, as AIDS researchers Robert

Fullilove and Mindy Fullilove observed in a 1999 study of AIDS stigma in the Black church, "The homosexual man is cast out of the church, whether he stays or not." In an interview with Pernessa Seele, who ran focus groups for the Fullilovers' study, one participant recalled, "I used to hear ministers say they were going to find them a real sissy to play music in their church." The ministers' willingness to "forget the so-called theological issues in order to enhance their pocketbook" struck many Black gay men as cruel and hypocritical.[17]

The effect of religious homophobia on Black gay men in the age of AIDS also registers in the life and work of men in the Black gay renaissance. In Craig Harris's short story "Cut Off from among Their People," which appeared in Beam's anthology, the protagonist Jeff attends the funeral for his lover, who has passed away from an AIDS-related illness. The lover's family has cut him out of arrangements for the service, held in a Harlem mortuary because "a big church funeral would be both inappropriate and unnecessary." The African Methodist Episcopal minister who delivers the sermon, "simply dressed in a black suit, white shirt, and maroon necktie" rather than his vestments, tells the family and friends of the deceased that his death represents the "fulfillment of a prophecy." Citing Old Testament scripture, he continues, "There's no cause to wonder why medical science could not find a cure for this man's illness. How could medicine cure temptation? What drug can exorcise Satan from a young man's soul? The only cure is to be found in the Lord. The only cure is repentance, for Leviticus clearly tells us, ' . . . whoever shall commit any of these abominations, even the souls that commit them shall be cut off from among their people.'" Afterward, the undertaker tells Jeff that he has also recently lost a lover to AIDS and that he sees cases like their own all the time, with "tearless funerals, the widowed treated like non-entities, and these 'another faggot burns in hell' sermons."[18]

Similar scenes played out in real life. When Donald Woods, who had contributed to *In the Life* and as executive director of AIDSFILMS had worked with Gay Men of African Descent on *Party*, passed away from AIDS complications in 1992, his family cited cardiac arrest as the cause of death and erased any mention of Woods's sexuality from the funeral service. Furious, Woods's friend and fellow Black gay writer Assotto Saint "got up and began to shout at Donald's family about their hypocritical silence." Several years later, at the funeral of Black gay writer and spoken word artist Essex Hemphill, the minister "preached a sermon warning against the dangers of alternative lifestyles." Hemphill's mother, a devout Christian, claimed that her son had "given his life over to Christ" in the final month of his life. Meanwhile Hemphill—who had once promised,

When I die,
honey chil',
my angels
will be tall
Black drag queens

—had arranged for his papers to be donated to the New York Public Library. He passed away before the material could be transferred to the archive, and friends have since speculated that Hemphill's family destroyed the papers in an attempt to erase evidence of his sexuality.[19]

Black churches were not alone in condemning homosexuality or interpreting the advent of AIDS as God's punishment for sinful behavior. Conservative white priests and pastors did the same, as did Senator Jesse Helms, and their odious views shaped national AIDS policy. But for a variety of reasons, the Black church was uniquely positioned to make a difference in the fight against AIDS. For one, churches occupied a distinct place in African American life and had historically been part of struggles for racial justice. Moreover, AIDS educators struggled to reach not only Black gay men but also the large numbers of Black women and heterosexual men who needed to hear about the disease from a trusted source. Much like the Gay Men of Color Consortium and GMAD did, researchers and activists here argued that the shame Black gay men experienced as a result of the church's stance on homosexuality put them at increased risk for HIV. Theology notwithstanding, the church played a central role in the social and spiritual lives of many Black gays. Rejection from fellow churchgoers, combined with damning messages from the pulpit about homosexuality, left a "lasting and deep impact on the self-worth of [churchgoing] MSM [men who have sex with men]" and as a result made them less likely to protect themselves from HIV by using condoms and clean needles.[20]

Pernessa Seele realized that the church could shape the Black AIDS epidemic in powerful ways. Around the time that the Harlem Week of Prayer began, almost 70 percent of African Americans reported belonging to a church. This meant that ministers would be able to reach large numbers of Black men and women with messages about reducing their risk for HIV, especially if they were willing to bring frank discussions about sexuality into the church. By changing sexual norms among the laity, The Balm in Gilead could help churchgoers support one another in practicing safer sex. Campaigns targeted at both the pulpit and the pews could push Black churches to welcome people with HIV and AIDS as full members of the congregation. In turn, churchgoers would feel more comfortable getting tested for HIV and talking about the disease with their sexual partners. Church-based HIV education could also influence male congregants who had sex with other men but were not reached by other efforts because they either did not identify as gay or bisexual or did not frequent the gay spaces where a lot of AIDS outreach took place. Moreover, reducing homophobia by encouraging churches to embrace gay congregants would reduce the stigma associated with AIDS as a "gay disease." Finally, given the prevalence of mistrust among African Americans for the medical establishment, the church could serve as a trusted source for scientific information about the disease and its transmission. Aside from changing attitudes about HIV and AIDS, the church could offer infrastructure for education, testing, and counseling in communities where few such resources existed.

## To Heal the Sin-Sick Soul

As Pernessa Seele tells it, the name for her new organization came to her through divine revelation while riding her stationary bike one morning in her apartment:

> There was a book—I don't know where this book came from—there was a book on my bookshelf called *Balm in Gilead* by [Sarah Lawrence] Lightfoot, who was a nurse at Harlem Hospital. And I'm saying, "What am I going to call this organization?" And the Spirit said, "The Balm in Gilead." And I said, "That's a stupid name. How's anybody going to know what we do if we call it the Balm?" I'm just talking to myself in my apartment, "That don't make no sense." And I said, "Okay," I'm talking to the Spirit now, "If you think I should call it The Balm in Gilead, fine, but that sure don't make no sense to me."[21]

Here, as with the story about how she came to work at Harlem Hospital, Seele describes herself as a reluctant servant, someone divinely called to mobilize churches around AIDS but skeptical about doing so. By situating her work as a religious calling—as a vocation—she softens her challenge to church orthodoxy by laying claim to a higher power. She recalls that her lay status, her gender, and her gender presentation all might have undercut her credibility as she challenged religious orthodoxy on AIDS issues: "I was not clergy, I was a woman, I was bald-headed, I had nothing that looked like anything that I should be doing this work." By narrating her own reluctance to take up this calling, she adds to her authority; to those who might resist her message, she reveals that she too was skeptical.[22]

Seele also recalls being surprised to discover the origin of her new organization's name: "The truth of the matter is I really didn't get it until I was introduced and every time I was introduced, the organist or somebody sang, 'There is a balm in Gilead,' and it was the song and the name of the organization that came together . . . [and] I got it. Like, 'Wow, look at this, I didn't even know we had a song.' Because I was very young and crazy and stupid and just doing what I thought I was being called to do." As she later explained on The Balm in Gilead's website, the phrase comes from both biblical scripture and an African American spiritual. In the Old Testament, the prophet Jeremiah asks, "Is there no balm in Gilead?," referring to, in Seele's words, "a land that was ravaged by plagues, poor health care, racial discrimination, ethnic cleansing, ruthless treatment of women and violence." The spiritual answered the question—"There *is* a balm in Gilead"—with an added layer of New Testament salvation, that the balm of Christ's love will heal "the sin-sick soul." Through the song, she wrote, "Our ancestors . . . gave instructions to go, teach and to take responsibility for each other." "So," Seele says today, "you have a question, you have an answer, and you have the hands that make the work and the activity, make it happen."[23]

It seems unlikely that Seele, who grew up being very active in the church, would not have known about the meaning that the name of her organization would have for Black audiences. But her surprise at discovering the song reinforces the part of her narrative that frames her work as Christian vocation and the very naming of the group as an act of revelation. Seele thus put her personal and professional story, along with her message about AIDS, in a biblical frame, softening any challenge she might pose to pastoral authority on a controversial issue.[24]

Seele's account also places her within the syncretic religious tradition of coastal South Carolina, where her hometown of Lincolnville is found. It was there that a distinct Gullah religious culture formed from a mix of enslaved Africans' spiritual traditions and Christianity. Nineteenth-century observers noted that women played an important role in Gullah slave communities by guiding those who decided to "seek Jesus," as well as by interpreting dreams and visions and predicting the future. Margaret Washington Creel traces this role to the priestess and prophetess traditions of West Africa, which, she argues, became part of Gullah religious culture. By narrating her own story as one of revelation, Seele situates herself within a religious context that is inextricable from the historic wound that she aimed to heal.[25]

During the early days of The Balm in Gilead, Seele also learned to speak in a language that would make sense to major funders. Here she received help and support from some of the gay white men who had been among the first to respond to the epidemic a decade earlier. Rodger McFarlane, the executive director of Broadway Cares/Equity Fights AIDS, a major AIDS fund-raising and grant-making organization based in New York's theater community, gave Seele office space and a salary. Len McNally of New York Community Trust, a public interest funding group, coached Seele in grant writing. After she submitted an initial proposal "full of all this Jesus, religious conversation," Seele says, "Len McNally brought me into his office and said, 'You cannot write no grant like this.' . . . And he taught me how to write a grant, and New York Community Trust gave us our first grant." As Seele recalls, its support anchored the fledgling organization while she moved from work at Harlem Hospital to the nonprofit sector: "These are all gay white men in New York, the founders of Gay Men's Health Crisis and the founders of the movement . . . and they kind of called me and said, 'Hey, let me help you out here.'"[26]

Within a few years, The Balm in Gilead had grown to include two paid staff members in addition to Seele, who remained the organization's public face and spokesperson. In 1993, The Balm in Gilead launched a national Black Church National Day of Prayer for the Healing of AIDS, an annual day of AIDS-themed worship in Black churches around the country, using the Harlem Week of Prayer as a model. Even as The Balm in Gilead developed a national profile, Seele maintained professional ties in Harlem, serving as the vice president of Harlem Congregations for Community Improvement (HCCI), an interfaith neighborhood revitalization group, for which she developed and managed social services and public health programs. By 1994, when Seele left HCCI, The Balm in Gilead could claim to be *the only organization* addressing HIV prevention that has been endorsed by *every* major national African American church denomination and caucus."[27]

Broad support from Black religious leaders allowed Pernessa Seele to present The Balm in Gilead as an ideal partner to public health officials, given the organization's ability to bridge the gap between science and faith. Seele married her understanding of "Black folks' relationship to the church . . . to Jesus or Mohammed or whoever they're calling on . . . [and] the power of prayer" to her background in immunology and medical research. In this way she promised to bring accurate information about HIV risk and transmission to Black faith communities through prevention programs rooted in sound public health practice. The Balm in Gilead also benefited from Seele's professional contacts; faculty at Columbia University's Mailman School of Public Health served on the organization's early board of directors and helped to write grants and design programs. Joyce Moon Howard, Angela Aidala, and Robert Fullilove, all members of Mailman's faculty, acted as program evaluators for The Balm in Gilead.[28]

Policy makers, for their own part, saw value in supporting The Balm in Gilead. On February 28, 1994, President Bill Clinton's Office of National AIDS

Policy and The Balm in Gilead together convened a conference of fifty-six Black clergy from nineteen denominations at the White House for a conference, the African American Clergy Summit on HIV/AIDS. The following year, the CDC also supported The Balm in Gilead's efforts to replicate the Black Church Week of Prayer model nationwide by sponsoring a workshop at Emory University in Atlanta for representatives from six cities. In March 1996, each of those cities held its own Black Church Week of Prayer for the Healing of AIDS, with the involvement of local congregations, community groups, and state officials. Such partnerships arose from the need for culturally competent programs in the fight against AIDS in Black America, as well as from the federal mandate for HIV prevention community planning that the National Task Force on AIDS Prevention helped to secure.[29]

The White House's Office of National AIDS Policy also saw the African American Clergy Summit as an opportunity to deepen cooperation between the federal AIDS bureaucracy and the Black religious community. The ministers signed "The African American Clergy's Declaration of War on HIV/AIDS," which pointed to the church's "long and distinguished tradition of leading its people to light in times of great suffering" while acknowledging that the church "has been too long negligent on the most pressing subject of AIDS/HIV." The clergy promised to "wage a war on fear and ignorance of AIDS/HIV" through prevention and education, as well as through "consciousness-raising sermons about AIDS prevention and compassion for all, regardless of sexual orientation, drug dependency, or lifestyle choices."[30]

Phill Wilson, who had adapted the *Hot, Horny and Healthy!* playshop for Black gay men, addressed the summit. He argued that the AIDS crisis in Black communities stemmed from a lack of care for those most affected by the epidemic: "The truth is we have babies with AIDS today, because we didn't care enough about their mothers yesterday. The truth is we have women with AIDS today, because we didn't care enough about their addicted partners yesterday. The truth is AIDS is running rampant in our neighborhoods and families today, because we didn't care enough about gay men yesterday. The truth is we are all going to be affected tomorrow . . . if we don't care enough today! And most importantly, the truth is no amount of caring will be enough if it is not joined by action!"[31]

Although the problem of AIDS may be new, Wilson argued, the solution was familiar to those versed in the history of the Black freedom struggle: a firm commitment to justice for all. But whereas earlier phases of the movement had often sidelined women's issues and marginalized gays and lesbians altogether, winning the fight against AIDS would require understanding "that racism, sexism, classism, homophobia and heterosexism are inextricably connected."

## A Proclamation from
# THE BALM IN GILEAD, INC.
*An Organization Dedicated to Healing the African American Community Through Prayer, Health Education and Advocacy*

## THE AFRICAN AMERICAN CLERGY'S DECLARATION OF WAR ON HIV/AIDS

**The time has come today** to face the depth of devastation caused by AIDS in the African American community; to recognize that African Americans are the most disproportionately represented community of color with respect to HIV/AIDS; that AIDS continues to be the leading cause of death nationwide of African American men between the ages of 35 and 44, and of African American women between the ages of 25 and 44; that the number of teenagers infected with HIV nearly doubles each year; and that each and every American knows someone, or in the next 12 months will know someone who has died of AIDS.

**The African American Church** has a long and distinguished tradition of leading its people to light in times of great suffering, and of caring for its parishioners. It has a proud history of pastoral activism and has proven itself a formidable mobilizer of congregations. But the time has come today to recognize that as far as our churches have come in the night, there are steps yet to go before dawn; that the African American religious community, despite this legacy, has too long been negligent on the most pressing subject of AIDS/HIV. The church's godly mission is to minister love and support to its congregations, and to forsake no one, yet, until today, it has not assumed its proper mantle of responsibility in this time of chaos caused by the ravages of AIDS to mind, body and soul of our people.

**Now, therefore, we,** leaders of African American churches in America, deem it necessary to acknowledge by means of this proclamation that only through stalwart commitment, strength of mind and courage of heart on the part of the religious community can we ever hope to combat the AIDS epidemic. By this proclamation, we declare our intent to do all in our power to eradicate the scourge of AIDS in our time; to wage a war on fear and ignorance of AIDS/HIV, from the pulpit and in our institutions, until such a time as AIDS is no longer a threat to the lives of the people, and we call upon our fellow clergy, men and women, to do the same.

**We, members of the clergy** of African American churches in America, recognizing that as long as one human being remains uneducated, as long as one human being suffers from AIDS, it is one too many; we vow to develop comprehensive AIDS prevention programs for our youth; to develop effective AIDS awareness and prevention strategies for and with our congregations and communities; to provide supportive counseling to Persons Living with AIDS and to their non-infected families and loved ones; and to preach consciousness-raising sermons about AIDS prevention and compassion for all, regardless of sexual orientation, drug dependency, or lifestyle choices.

**We furthermore affirm** our commitment to working with grassroots organizations, corporations, and governmental bodies on the federal, state and municipal levels to secure generous financial support of AIDS awareness and prevention and to educate our congregations in those programs; and to work throughout our own institutions, the seminaries and schools of theology, to combat silence on the subject of AIDS and promote an enlightened, non-judgmental clergy, unimpeded in the war on AIDS by nonproductive biases.

**We furthermore affirm** our commitment to identifying tangible goals and means of assessing progress on those goals, formulating policy, and engaging in advocacy on behalf of our communities with respect to the issues around AIDS.

**We furthermore affirm** our support for The Black Church National Day of Prayer for the Healing of AIDS as a vehicle for mobilizing African American religious institutions to fight AIDS through prayer, education, and advocacy nationwide. And in this resolve advocate for universal health care.

**We furthermore affirm** that from this day forward, we resolve to open our eyes and acknowledge those persons among us living with AIDS and their families and loved ones, and to encourage others to see; to open our ears to their voices among us, and to insist that others hear; to open our hearts in compassion, and expect others to do the same, and in so doing, cast off the denial that has hindered our churches in the past, and in so doing move forward with a sense of divine mission to educate our communities, our congregations and our fellow clergy about AIDS, and in so doing, say at last,

Surely, there is a *balm in Gilead.*

**In witness whereof,** we have hereunto set our hand this twenty-eighth day of February, in the year of our Lord nineteen hundred ninety-four, on the occasion of the first African American Religious Leaders Summit on HIV/AIDS, convened by The Balm In Gilead, Inc., at The White House, in Washington, District of Columbia.

Perhaps seeking to win over those who were reluctant to make room for gays or drug users in the "Beloved Community," Wilson linked the fight against AIDS to the civil rights movement by riffing on a quote from Southern Christian Leadership Conference leader and Freedom Rider C. T. Vivian ("Those who hate, don't discriminate"): "Those who hate me because I'm Gay... hate all of us because we're Black. Those who opposed Choice ... oppose Gay Rights, rational AIDS funding and Civil Rights. People who gay-bash ... also burn crosses and wear white hoods."[32]

But the most challenging part of Wilson's address came in his description of what it was like to live with—and die of—AIDS. Wilson himself had been living with HIV for fourteen years and was unsure of how much longer he had left to live. He quoted the AIDS activist Chris Brownlie about the visceral experience of late-stage AIDS: "It is waking up wet, so wet, wetter than you were at birth. It is having your skull split by its swollen lining. It is changing your pants again because at the critical moment you couldn't tell the difference between gas and excrement. It is changing your sheets because the stench woke you up." Wilson went on to describe Brownlie's feelings of sorrow in seeing his own pain reflected in his grieving partner: "It is bearing the unbearable, enduring the unendurable, and hoping in the face of hopelessness. It is the haunted look in your lover's eyes when a new crisis begins. It is mourning together. It is mourning alone. It is holding him in your arms and in your heart. It is crying because your heart is breaking over leaving him behind. It is the sweet pain of knowing that you are dying, and the overwhelming sadness for those who will kiss you into their dreams."[33]

With Brownlie's words, Wilson took the discussion of AIDS out of the abstract and made it concrete. He presented gay love as real and worthy of respect. What he did not tell the audience (or at least not in the printed text of his address) was that *he* was the one who looked hauntedly into Brownlie's dying eyes and kissed Brownlie into his own dreams. Chris Brownlie had been Wilson's partner for nine years, until his death in 1989.[34]

The White House summit and declaration marked both a growing willingness among Black church leaders to use their influence to combat HIV and AIDS and The Balm in Gilead's growing national influence. Still, some viewed the group's work with skepticism. Gary Paul Wright, a Black gay man and then administrative coordinator of education and international programs for the American Foundation for AIDS Research, criticized churches for taking "the approach of the ostrich": "There is a lot of squawking going on about compassion and love and outreach, but when it comes down to hands on caring and support, heads get buried in the sand."[35]

Indeed, ministers' desire to address HIV and AIDS from the pulpit would take them only so far. To spur them to action, The Balm in Gilead would also need to train faith leaders to incorporate messages about the disease into their ministry. The Harlem Week of Prayer included educational workshops for clergy who wanted to develop AIDS programs at their churches, but the Day of Prayer's much larger scale called for a different form of clergy education. Thus The Balm in Gilead set out to show Black churches what "consciousness-raising" worship might look like in the context of HIV/AIDS.

## Jesus Is Alive and Living with AIDS

In 1995 The Balm in Gilead published *Who Will Break the Silence?*, a resource guide that stressed the power of prayer as an avenue for the "healing of AIDS." Here prayer was not a "magic wand" that would bring an end to the devastation wrought by HIV and AIDS but a conversation with God, one that could yield "support, insight and guidance." Through the book's prayers and worship services, congregations could come to realize the ways that people living with AIDS had been marginalized within the community and resolve to make AIDS services a part of the regular ministry.[36]

With *Who Will Break the Silence?*, The Balm in Gilead aimed to make the Black church into a "safe space" both for people with HIV and AIDS and for gay people more generally. The book thus reflected the group's anti-stigma approach to the epidemic. In a letter of support to the Paul Rapoport Foundation, which supported LGBT and HIV/AIDS programs, Colin Robinson of GMAD praised the group for "help[ing] open many doors which had been closed to any possibility of healing discussions about homosexuality within the Black Church." He also noted that The Balm in Gilead possessed a "unique ability to attract ecumenical African American religious leadership," which "has long been a pivotal point of consciousness change in African American communities." Robinson had firsthand knowledge of the group's success, as GMAD had conducted workshops for the Harlem Week of Prayer.[37]

To make such "healing discussions" available to churches around the country, The Balm in Gilead convened a group of eight men and women, including people with AIDS, "biblical scholars, poets, musicians, heterosexuals, lesbian and gay persons," to write *Who Will Break the Silence?* The authors, referred to as "the Prayer Group," highlighted scripture that stressed God's universal love and Jesus's advocacy of the poor and sick. In this way they turned the logic of AIDS stigma in the church on its head, reframing the church's rejection of gay and HIV-positive members as sin. The "sin-sick soul" that would be healed by

The Balm in Gilead was sick not from the sins of sex or drug use but from the sins of exclusion and rejection.

In addition to prayers and services, *Who Will Break the Silence?* also included transcripts of the Prayer Group's exegetical conversations, in which they interpreted relevant pieces of scripture. The transcripts explained their scriptural readings and legitimized their efforts by showing the authors' deep knowledge of the Bible and church history. They also served to educate readers by "reveal[ing] some of the challenges, growth and healing experience by the Prayer Group," similar to those that participating churches might encounter through their own involvement in the Day of Prayer. Out of their Bible study and conversations, the group members produced both a set of prayers and outlines for entire services showing that the Black church could "break the silence" on AIDS, sexuality, and drug use. In this way the Prayer Group members took part in the long tradition of using the Bible to both make sense of their own experiences and to call for justice. In other words, they created their own language-world for the Black church's fight against AIDS.[38]

In her introduction to *Who Will Break the Silence?*, Pernessa Seele also situated the book in the arc of Black history. She compared members of the Prayer Group to other "silence breakers," from Harriet Tubman to Langston Hughes, Martin Luther King Jr., and Malcolm X. She thus claimed the fight against HIV and AIDS as a Black political issue, on par with earlier freedom struggles. Some in the Prayer Group saw their work through this lens as well. Discussing a verse from Jeremiah, one group member protested that the imagery of dance and praise seemed disconnected from the gravity of the epidemic, in which "babies are dying faster than they're living now, and mothers are sicker than they've ever been." Another member of the group pointed out that the roots of the church itself lay in another period of immense hardship, "in slavery times, times when women are being raped and used . . . [but] we had to rejoice. The other option is death."[39]

For the Prayer Group, the title of *Who Will Break the Silence?* carried multiple meanings. Silence, when it meant "denial and ignorance and fear and isolation," could be an impediment to leveraging the church's power and influence to address AIDS in the community. The answer to the title question came from Mark 1:29–39, in which, the Prayer Group summarized, "the disciples hunted for Jesus and brought Jesus back to all the people." Just as the disciples had spread the gospel throughout their known world, The Balm in Gilead could interpret the gospel in the context of the AIDS epidemic for *all* people, regardless of the stigma of disease, sexuality, or addiction. However, silence could also carry a positive connotation and function as "the listening silence." This "active silence" could mean listening to others in the congregation, as with the testimony of people with HIV and AIDS, or it could be the silence of meditation and prayer. In this context, the title could refer to the end of reflective prayer, after which churches and their members would translate the "Spirit of God" they received into action against the epidemic.[40]

*Who Will Break the Silence?* includes two prayers based on Genesis 9:8–17, in which God sets a rainbow in the sky after the Great Flood to symbolize his covenant with Noah and "every living creature." Here, the rainbow represents hope in a time of great hardship, calling on the congregation to confront AIDS and to accept the church's gay members. In one prayer, the pastor recites, "In the midst of the storms of our lives, God sets a rainbow," and then in the next line, "In the midst of the pandemic of HIV and AIDS, God sets a rainbow." The parallel between "the storms of our lives" and the disease establishes AIDS as a problem for the entire congregation, regardless of the praying individual's HIV status. At the end of the prayer the entire group responds, "We remember God's covenant with all," signaling that the church—like God—includes everyone.[41]

In the second prayer, "For Safe Space," congregants ask the "God of the healthy and God of the sick . . . God of the gay and God of the straight . . . God of the sober and God of the addicted" for an end to silence, "so that the healing of HIV and AIDS may begin." The "safe space" for which the prayer asks is one "free from our judgments of others and ourselves," in which people are "free to live without requiring lies of each other." The rainbow, as a symbol of gay pride since the 1970s, also represents the acceptance of gay congregants. One of the worship services outlined in *Who Will Break the Silence?* instructs church leaders to distribute rainbow ribbons or stickers for everyone in attendance to wear and to hang a rainbow banner at the front of the sanctuary. The significance of incorporating a symbol of gay identity so thoroughly into the service could not have been lost on the Prayer Group; two (presumably gay) members noted the importance of the rainbow as a symbol for "our community." However, they agreed that the rainbow also symbolized inclusiveness, or "the universality of God's care." Placed at the beginning of the sample service, the rainbow and the covenant—with "all of the earth, all creatures, with no exceptions"—would provide a "spiritual foundation" for the church's AIDS ministry.[42]

The authors of *Who Will Break the Silence?* carried forward the theme of healing through prayer. They saw prayer as a "fulcrum" around which "demons" of denial, homophobia, and judgment could be cast out from the community. "Prayer of a Black Gay Christian" reads,

God, I'm tired of our ways being hidden,
    of our rights being disregarded.
You may know me and love me
    but the church is hiding the truth.
God, you know that I am gay,
    but the church doesn't want to admit it,
    and I'm tired of waiting.
The youth are fainting;
    ignored, we feel powerless, and we are weary.
Not only does our strength need to be renewed,
    God, we need some changes.
        We need some changes now.[43]

In the conversation about Isaiah 40:21–31 that produced "Prayer of a Black Gay Christian," the Prayer Group addressed the sense of powerlessness among people who had been "denied membership, denied access, denied leadership roles, denied period" in the church and the "transference" through which such people might perceive rejection from the church as rejection from God. However, in the context of the epidemic, Black gays and others affected by HIV in the church were "learning new ways to move beyond that powerlessness into being powerful, and giving voice is one of them."[44]

The Prayer Group also offered prayers that framed HIV and AIDS as an illness that had infected not just individuals but the entire church and Christ himself. While prayers invited congregants to meditate on their individual role in creating a "safe place" within the church, they also constructed a sense of collective struggle against the epidemic. People with AIDS could be less easily ostracized from a church understood to be "living with" the disease. "A Prayer to Celebrate Healing" also highlighted specific people with AIDS, putting them in a biblical context:

O God of Abraham, Sarah and Hagar
O God of Jesus and Mary Magdalene
O God of Arthur Ashe and Magic Johnson
O God of Mother Hale and her children . . .

The prayer later reinforced the need to embrace those who had been stigmatized, thanking God for "the privilege of coming before your throne as family, not divided between those who are sick and those who are well, not divided between those who are addicted and those who are recovering, not divided between straight and gay."[45]

One worship service featured a series of short "role plays" that addressed AIDS denialism in Black communities. Characters in the role plays dismissed grim statistics as "another racist plot to make us look bad," eschewed condoms, or shifted the blame for AIDS and other community problems onto drug dealers. In each case, a member of the congregation was to interrupt the dialogue by walking across the altar, holding a sign that read "Jesus Is Alive and Living with AIDS." The Prayer Group members wrote in the introduction to *Who Will Break the Silence?* that the image of a little girl with such a sign running to the front of the sanctuary had come to them during their prayer and discussion, an example of the "ways in which we heard the Spirit of God speak to our group." As with Seele's sense of being called to her work with The Balm in Gilead, those in the Prayer Group ascribed their insight to divine revelation.[46]

Despite the radical content of *Who Will Break the Silence?*, the book's format, with prayers presented both individually and as part of complete services, held open the possibility that churches would avoid more controversial passages. The ways that churches received and used *Who Will Break the Silence?* is difficult to measure. According to The Balm in Gilead, the book has been sent to tens of thousands of individual congregations. Although the exegetical transcripts were dropped from the later edition of the book, the prayers and services remain almost entirely unchanged, suggesting that they have not met with significant opposition from participating churches.[47]

As we will see in the next chapter, the advent of protease inhibitors in the middle 1990s, along with the free trade policies of the Clinton administration, intersected to put "global AIDS" at the front and center of national conversations about the disease. Amid this growing interest, Seele and The Balm in Gilead leveraged their experience working with Black churches in the United States to broaden their efforts "from the villages of Harlem to the villages of Africa." As they modified programs to fit both the religious beliefs of African churches and the reality of the epidemic there, Seele and The Balm in Gilead nevertheless based their claim on the essential similarity of people of African descent, no matter where they lived.[48]

## "Black People Do Black Church All Over the World"

In 2001, The Balm in Gilead secured a cooperative agreement with the CDC to replicate its training and education in sub-Saharan Africa, where the epidemic raged nearly out of control. Over the next five years, the organization worked with faith leaders in Côte d'Ivoire, Tanzania, Kenya, Nigeria, and Zimbabwe to develop HIV prevention programs and AIDS services through the countries' churches and mosques. The Balm in Gilead's international effort grew in part from Pernessa Seele's belief that religious experience united Black people around the world. As early as 1995, in an essay in *Anglican Theological Review*, Seele framed HIV among African Americans as part of the larger epidemic within the "African global community." She argued that the epidemic had reached crisis proportions among Black people worldwide because "African peoples, regardless of nationality," suffered from "sub-standard living conditions under which sickness and disease are more apt to spread," lack of health care, and inadequate education. And with sexual contact being the primary mode of HIV transmission among African and African-descended peoples, she insisted, "we must be able to talk about sex with our children and face realities concerning their level of sexual activity . . . examine our own sexual behaviors and put to rest the vestiges of sexual myths." Seele pointed to a solution, one that she knew quite well. The church, as "the cornerstone of the African global community" and "the only institution that has the ability to mobilize the masses and disseminate appropriate information," would have to use its power to educate people about HIV transmission and provide comfort and care to those who had already become infected. Quoting the now-familiar spiritual, she concluded that if religious leaders accepted their role in fighting the AIDS epidemic, the church could "indeed be the balm 'that heals the sin-sick soul.'"[49]

At the same time, The Balm in Gilead's growing profile attracted international attention. According to a report submitted to the Ford Foundation in 1998, the organization had received requests for assistance in establishing church-based HIV prevention programs from throughout Africa and the Caribbean. The Balm in Gilead planned to apply for funds the following year to develop relationships with groups abroad through a "state-of-the-art" website and a series of meetings for Black religious leaders from around the world.[50]

Seele's interest in taking The Balm in Gilead overseas intersected with a broader shift in interest toward "global AIDS" in the late 1990s and early 2000s. In his address for World AIDS Day in 1998, President Bill Clinton highlighted the number of children orphaned by AIDS worldwide and commissioned Sandra Thurman, his AIDS policy adviser, to undertake a fact-finding mission on the impact of the epidemic on sub-Saharan Africa. In her report, Thurman told the White House that AIDS had taken a heavy toll on the region's "fragile health care systems," including traditional support networks based on family and village ties. She also stressed the disease's potential to wipe out "decades of progress on a host of development objectives," such as increased life expectancy. Moreover, the prevalence of HIV among military officers and government officials threatened to undermine political stability in the region, making AIDS a security concern as well as a public health issue. Finally, sub-Saharan

Africa, where the epidemic was already "entrenched," portended developments elsewhere, particularly India and the post-Soviet republics of Eastern Europe and Central Asia, where HIV was also rapidly spreading.[51]

The concern with AIDS as a threat to global security carried over into the George W. Bush administration. Bush had campaigned on a platform of "compassionate conservatism," which included proposed funding for faith-based programs. Soon after taking office, Bush established the Office of Faith-Based and Community Initiatives, which some saw as a rather cynical ploy to draw off churchgoing Black voters from the Democratic Party while further privatizing key social services. Reverend C. Mackey Daniels of the National Baptist Convention, for example, described the move as "an effort to muffle the prophetic voices of the African American Church." In this context, The Balm in Gilead entered into a cooperative agreement with the Centers for Disease Control to expand its programs to Côte d'Ivoire, Tanzania, Kenya, Nigeria, and Zimbabwe under the auspices of the Africa HIV/AIDS Faith Initiative.[52]

In building programs abroad, The Balm in Gilead used models it had developed for Black churches in the United States. From its perspective, stigma around the disease and "health beliefs and practices in general" were similar enough that "the African American community provided a frame that could definitely be used in an African context." The groups, they believed, shared a deep investment in spiritual beliefs and religious institutions, as well as linked histories of "slavery, apartheid, colonialism, racism, health disparities, poverty and now the pandemic of AIDS." African churches in sub-Saharan Africa cut across social lines to reach a large number of people representing a cross-section of society, just as they did "within Black communities globally." Like their counterparts in the United States, Black African churches and faith leaders established the moral values and social norms for their communities, positioning them to influence both the behaviors that spread the virus from person to person and the stigmatizing attitudes about HIV that allowed people to think of AIDS as a disease of the abject.[53]

In Côte d'Ivoire, Tanzania, Kenya, Nigeria, and Zimbabwe, The Balm in Gilead representatives planned to bring leaders from different denominations together to form national offices that would coordinate faith-based AIDS efforts in their respective countries. The leaders of The Balm in Gilead worried that, without national direction, "local faith-based HIV programs [would] become fragmented efforts that are often stigmatized for their work." Just as it had gained endorsements of major Black churches in the United States, The Balm in Gilead worked to establish an HIV/AIDS desk in the national offices of the major denominations in all five countries. By winning support from national religious leaders, it argued, the organization could "establish a spiritual consciousness that every local church or mosque would become involved in some type of AIDS programming because it is the right (spiritual) thing to do." To challenge popular belief that AIDS represented punishment for a person's sinful behavior, it tried to substitute an alternative morality, that to ostracize people with the disease or ignore the epidemic was a dereliction of religious duty. Moreover, national faith leaders who had been trained by The Balm in Gilead "to speak intelligently about HIV disease issues . . . not from a place of fear and stigma, but from a place of compassion and facts," could in turn train local priests and imams, magnifying the organization's efforts throughout each country. Using this model, The Balm in Gilead could help deliver information about AIDS to a large number of people using relatively few resources.[54]

In early 2002, The Balm in Gilead convened representatives from the governing national bodies of major religious denominations in each of the five countries for a conference in Tarrytown, New York, twenty miles north of Manhattan. African Catholic, Protestant, and Muslim leaders met with the president of the Caribbean Council of Churches, officials from leading African American denominations, and representatives from the CDC and the Gates Foundation to discuss the impact of AIDS in their home countries and to develop strategies for addressing the epidemic based on conditions on the ground. The Balm in Gilead also hoped to secure the cooperation of its African guests, who would return to the governing bodies of each denomination to cement their partnership in the Africa HIV/AIDS Faith Initiative.[55]

Following the Tarrytown meeting, The Balm in Gilead sent a delegation that April to tour the five Faith Initiative countries, assessing both existing programs and each denominational office's capacity for future initiatives. Aisha Satterwhite, a specialist in nonprofit communications and fellow with the Academy for Educational Development and the Ford Foundation, kept a travelogue of the trip for The Balm in Gilead's website. Judging from Satterwhite's account, Pernessa Seele frequently emphasized the connections between African Americans and Africans during their travels. At a worship service in Youpougon, Côte d'Ivoire, she told the congregation, "I love the worship experience of Black people. We are joined by our faith, our belief in God, and by our praise. We praise God alike. We sing alike. Even though we are singing in different languages, we are saying the same things. Black people do Black church all over the world." Seele compared the present experience with HIV and AIDS to the scourge of slavery in the past, recounting the role that the African Methodist Episcopal Church had played in the lives of African Americans. Although Seele spoke through a translator, Satterwhite wrote, "the congregations were incredibly responsive and understanding often before the translation was even completed" because they "felt what Pernessa was saying" and understood that, "just like in days of old, the church must be at the fore-front in the response to HIV/AIDS."[56]

In Nigeria, where The Balm in Gilead aimed to bring Christians and Muslims together to address the country's emerging AIDS epidemic, Seele again found similarities between Africa and Black America: "Harlem and any other black community in the U.S. looks just like Nigeria. There is a church on every corner." She referred to herself as an "Ibo woman," highlighting her own likely ancestral ties to the country, where Igbo-speaking[57] people had been enslaved centuries earlier before being shipped to colonies across the Atlantic, including Seele's birthplace in the South Carolina Lowcountry. Despite the separation of time and space between "the African American faith community [and] their brothers and sisters in Nigeria," Seele insisted that they could come together to fight HIV and AIDS through the church, because even though "we don't know each other, we don't speak the same languages, . . . we love the Lord." The Nigerian hosts also appeared to share Seele's sense of kinship with their visitors from the United States. Satterwhite reported that at an Anglican reception in Lagos, "throughout the singing and the speech-making, the phrase 'welcome home' was often heard."[58]

Seele also framed the epidemic as a singular challenge to Black communities around the globe, stemming from similar forms of oppression experienced by people of African descent, whether in Nigeria, Negril, or New York. "This epidemic is 100% preventable and 100% out of control in black communities everywhere," she lamented. Responding to those who blamed Black people, rather than anti-Blackness and inequality, for their own suffering in the epidemic, she continued, "There is nothing wrong with us. There are conditions we've been living with—poverty, denial, miseducation, no education, limited resources, and no resources—that help keep this disease spreading." She also warned audiences that Black people the world over had "confused our theological and religious beliefs with the facts. HIV/AIDS will not be stopped by our beliefs. We respect these beliefs, but this will not save our brothers, sisters, mothers, and fathers. Education will."[59]

At Chishawasha Seminary outside of Harare, Dr. Randall Bailey of Atlanta's Interdenominational Theological Center led students in a Bible study centered on scripture in the context of AIDS. He told students, "Our theology silences us and doesn't allow us to acknowledge that we have options" in using biblical principles to stem the rising tide of the epidemic. Reversing the moral stigma and judgment of people with AIDS back onto the church, he continued, "Abandoning people is a sin. We've missed God if we turn our backs on people." He implored the seminarians to advocate for people with AIDS, invoking Jesus's example of "being in solidarity with those whom no one wants to be in solidarity with." A priest at St. Leo's Church in Lagos, Nigeria, conveyed a similar message in his sermon, referencing Matthew 25:40 as he chastised those who would ignore or condemn people with HIV and AIDS. With words that sounded as though they might have come straight from *Who Will Break the Silence?*, he preached, "That person who is infected could be Jesus. Show them hatred, ridicule, and contempt, and you are doing it to Jesus."[60]

Others struck a very different chord. At the end of the delegation's visit to Côte d'Ivoire, Methodist, Catholic, and Pentecostal leaders held a press conference with The Balm in Gilead to announce their intent to address the epidemic through their ministry. To signify their intent, they signed "The Côte d'Ivoirean Clergy's Declaration of War on HIV/AIDS," a document almost identical to "The African American Clergy's Declaration of War on HIV/AIDS" signed at the White House in 1994. Aside from switching out statistics on AIDS among African Americans for those on the epidemic in Côte d'Ivoire, the second document eliminated references to "sexual orientation" and "drug dependency," such that the clergy vowed to "preach consciousness-raising sermons about AIDS prevention and compassion for all, regardless of *lifestyle choices.*" The choice to eliminate the references to sexuality and drug use may reflect the conservative views of The Balm in Gilead's partners in Côte d'Ivoire; it may also reflect the epidemiology of AIDS in Africa, where heterosexual sex accounts for much more HIV transmission than it does in the United States. It is certainly possible—even likely—that both factors played a role. But regardless of why, dropping any mention of sexual difference from the Côte d'Ivoirean declaration erased same-sex-desiring Africans from the conversation and reinforced the idea of an essentially heterosexual Africa—the very same idea that GMAD and the men of the Black gay renaissance fought to overturn.[61]

As part of the Africa initiative, The Balm in Gilead also formed an International HIV/AIDS Faith Advisory Board, composed of religious representatives from each of the five African countries plus the United States. In "A Theological Call to Action," released after the board's first meeting in 2004, they drew from both the Bible and the Qu'ran to support a religious intervention against AIDS. The board members pointed to structural and systemic factors perpetuating the epidemic, including "poverty and migratory patterns relating to economic and political conditions . . . famine and war, as well as the search for a better quality of life." But they stopped far short of accepting sexual diversity in their home communities. Although the board resolved that "discrimination is sinful" and affirmed "the infinite worth and value of all persons," they made few direct references to sex at all. They acknowledged that sexuality was among the "very real issues raised by HIV/AIDS" that "confront and challenge all of us in deeply personal ways." The board members noted, perhaps referring to their own deliberations, that "the interpretation of scriptural principles for specific problems tends to be contentious." As with the Côte d'Ivoirean declaration, same-sex-desiring Africans were nowhere to be found in the board's call to action.[62]

During the CDC funding period, The Balm in Gilead also helped revise, reprint, and distribute *Helpers for a Healing Community*, a pastoral care manual for HIV and AIDS originally published in 1994 by Map International, a Christian organization focused on improving the health of people living in poverty worldwide. The book aimed to help African Christian ministers address the epidemic among their congregations through pastoral care. As in *Who Will Break the Silence?*, *Helpers for a Healing Community* stressed the church's moral obligation to provide for the sick and suffering, despite the stigma of AIDS. Along these lines, the authors challenged pastoral counselors to consider whether "our own illnesses of stigmatization and discrimination around HIV/AIDS define us as 'affected,'" framing pastoral counseling itself as a process of healing for the church as a whole.[63]

The authors of *Helpers for a Healing Community* also framed AIDS ministry as the expression of traditional African values in a Christian context. Information, such as the knowledge that AIDS was not a divine punishment, would not by itself change behavior but might impel churches to include people with HIV and AIDS in their fellowship, when delivered in a context that tapped into common values. The authors presented the value of community—the "key to understanding the African continent and Diaspora view of being"—as one framework through which they could deliver information about AIDS. "Communal life," they wrote, "is a single entity, the lung through which we breathe, filled with religious and moral obligation, and without which every person ceases to be." They connected African tradition to African American history, mixing proverbs such as the Zulu saying "A person is a person because of people" with quotes from Sojourner Truth ("I feel the power of a nation within me") and Martin Luther King Jr. ("All people are interdependent"). Here the "mutual and reciprocal presence" of African tradition was also compatible with Christian tradition, which, "broadly defined, professes to be a community of presence." In this context, "our willingness to be present with those who suffer and are violated, who are oppressed and demeaned," represented "a form of the Christian commitment to be present to one another in and out of pain, through sickness and in health, from this life to the next." AIDS ministry thus lay at the intersection of African tradition and Christian community, doubly compelling pastoral counselors to minister to those with HIV and AIDS.[64]

The authors of *Helpers for a Healing Community* also pointed to biblical prophets as people who, not unlike Seele herself, had been "enabled to see spiritual realities that others could not or would not see." Through such stories, the book offered helpers a way to see themselves as spiritual leaders who could reveal the truth of God's ministry to those who ostracized and alienated people with HIV and AIDS. If a congregation took issue with AIDS ministry, the pastor or lay counselor could take comfort in seeing his or her work as of a piece with that of Moses, Jeremiah, and Deborah, each of whom had been a "mouthpiece for God" despite having "no special genius, elite status, or innate talent." A helper should also "look to the prophetic model of Jesus and his disciples . . . in the execution of his/her ministerial duties." Pastoral counselors, embodying the role of prophet, should not only speak the word of God but also act, taking care of social and medical as well as spiritual needs, both "among their own people and beyond the confines of their fellowship."[65]

Although the authors of *Helpers for a Healing Community* encouraged pastors to discuss "God's beautiful gift of love and sexuality," they considered heterosexual sex within marriage to be the only form of sexuality worthy of approval. Whereas *Who Will Break the Silence?* marshaled scriptural resources to encourage Black churches to accept gay parishioners, the authors of *Helpers* avoided any direct mention of homosexuality. The book referred obliquely to those who had contracted HIV through "ungodly acts," including sex with an HIV-positive man or woman, without differentiating among the variety of sexual activities that might expose a person to the virus. Instead, the authors advised that the goal of pastoral counseling for people with HIV should be to achieve repentance and redemption and to help people avoid risky behaviors in the future. The book offered no specific advice on how to counsel men who had contracted HIV through sex with other men or how to help gay men reduce their risk for HIV and AIDS. Even as *Helpers* instructed that "healing, not condemnation, is the goal of pastoral counseling," the guide distinguished the innocent infected from those who had contracted the virus through "irresponsible behavior." Repeated references to Matthew 25:40, which instructs Christians "to offer sensitive and compassionate help . . . 'to the least of these' [emphasis in original]," established that people with HIV, or at least those who had contracted the virus through sinful living, represented the lowest of God's creatures. This attitude was not unique to The Balm in Gilead edition of *Helpers*; the earlier edition informed readers that "the AIDS epidemic has come upon the world primarily because we have left God's plan for sexuality." At the same time, The Balm in Gilead did not temper the message that AIDS was the result of "ungodly acts."[66]

In Africa, The Balm in Gilead faced some of the same challenges in mobilizing churches and mosques against HIV and AIDS as in the United States. Moral and theological conservatism, particularly around "human sexuality, responsibility, vulnerability and mortality," led Christians and Muslims alike to see AIDS as divine punishment. In all five countries of the Africa HIV/AIDS Faith Initiative, The Balm in Gilead found a general lack of awareness about AIDS; in Zimbabwe in particular, it found a "tremendous lack of information regarding AIDS, other sexually transmitted diseases and basic human anatomy." Civil war broke out in Côte d'Ivoire within months of the delegation's 2002 visit, leading to a travel warning for Americans and closure of the CDC country office, crippling efforts there to implement a work plan. Nevertheless, The Balm in Gilead pointed to the formation of the Coalition of Religions against AIDS of Côte d'Ivoire as evidence of some success. More importantly, however, lack of funding crippled The Balm in Gilead's efforts. The initial contract had been small, just $500,000 to build AIDS education and prevention systems in the five Faith Initiative countries and to staff the national offices. In a final report to the CDC in 2005, the group lamented that only CDC-Tanzania had continued its cooperative agreement with The Balm in Gilead. Without funding to support each national HIV/AIDS office and its staff, it reported, "the successes of this initiative are slowly disappearing."[67]

Nevertheless, Pernessa Seele received accolades back home: President George W. Bush invited her to join First Lady Laura Bush during the 2006 State of the Union address, during which he lauded Seele for her work. In some ways, The Balm in Gilead's work in Africa prefigured his administration's approach to global AIDS. The President's Emergency Plan for AIDS Relief that Bush announced in 2003 committed $15 billion over five years to HIV treatment and prevention in sub-Saharan Africa, with significant involvement from evangelical Christian groups. Seele credits Bush with "really help[ing] the world understand why faith was important to the AIDS epidemic."[68]

Today, The Balm in Gilead maintains an office in Dar es Salaam, which coordinates the organization's ongoing efforts to address the AIDS epidemic there through the country's churches and mosques. Seele points out, with some bitterness, that the other four Faith Initiative countries "totally ignored the vast amount of money and tremendous work that had been put in and said, 'Nah, we're going to do something else,' because they could." Perhaps The Balm in Gilead's approach did not appeal to African community partners in the way Seele expected. Perhaps they chafed at the idea that peoples separated by thousands of miles and centuries of history would have much in common at all. Perhaps they resented the way that Seele's president could use America's wealth to dictate African public health priorities, with little to no input from Africans themselves. Whatever the reason, Seele maintains, "When you see these particular countries talking about interfaith work around health issues, it really began with The Balm in Gilead."[69]

AS THE BALM IN GILEAD worked through the Black church in the United States to combat the spread of HIV among African Americans, it aimed to expand the boundaries of Black community through gay-affirming programs. Looking to develop its programs abroad, The Balm in Gilead also highlighted connections between the epidemic in Black America and the one in the "AIDS Belt" of sub-Saharan Africa. Since "Black people do Black church all over the world," Seele argued, churches could help turn the tide of new HIV infections in Black communities on both sides of the Atlantic. In this way The Balm in Gilead claimed a place for African Americans within an essential Black identity, arguing to federal funders and faith partners in the United States as well as in Africa that interventions would work in Harare as they had in Harlem. Government funders had their own interests in promoting the organization's work, and in global AIDS more generally, framing the pandemic alternately as an international security concern and an opportunity to demonstrate the efficacy of compassionate conservatism and faith-based social programs on the world stage.

The Balm in Gilead story differs from others in this book in important respects. Whereas Gay Men of African Descent looked to examples both past and present of same-sex desire in Africa to validate Black gay identity in the United States, The Balm in Gilead seems to have dropped its focus on breaking the silence surrounding homosexuality when it came time to expand into Africa. Perhaps the group's partners on the ground resisted gay-affirming approaches to AIDS education, or perhaps support from the Bush administration came with the understanding that such approaches would be off-limits. Moreover, whereas leaders of the Nation of Islam looked to Africa for a cure for AIDS, Seele looked to the continent as a site for humanitarian intervention and uplift. But while The Balm in Gilead saw African Americans and Africans as united by a global Black identity rooted in religious faith and expression, Africans themselves did not necessarily share this vision.

## CHAPTER 6

# Stop Medical Apartheid from South Africa to Philadelphia

ACT UP Philadelphia and the Movement for Global Treatment Access

O N OCTOBER 6, 1999, hundreds of protesters from the Philadelphia chapter of the AIDS Coalition to Unleash Power (ACT UP) swarmed the sidewalk outside the Office of the United States Trade Representative in Washington, D.C. Some operated a pair of giant puppets that showed the trade representative herself dangling from the marionette strings of a sneering drug company executive. Others lay down in the street to block traffic, holding up tombstone-shaped signs with messages that connected U.S. trade policy to AIDS deaths in Zambia, South Africa, Thailand, and Brazil. A pair of drummers kept time for the group's chants while protesters on the sidewalk held up signs that read, "Stop racist trade policy! Medicine for ALL nations!" The crowd was diverse, consisting of "community organizing dykes, pacifist Quaker activists, and Black drug users who got wise in prison." The story of how this unlikely coalition of activists took on the U.S. Trade Representative connects the histories of African American AIDS activism and ACT UP. It also highlights the ways in which class, along with race, connected African American AIDS activists to their counterparts in sub-Saharan Africa and other parts of the developing world.[1]

By the end of the 1990s, most chapters of the once-powerful ACT UP had disbanded. At its height in the late 1980s and early 1990s, the founding New York chapter had drawn crowds in the hundreds to its weekly meetings. A few years later, however, attendance had dwindled. ACT UP Philadelphia, in contrast, grew in size through the late 1990s and early 2000s, drawing new members from the city's Black community, including large numbers of poor people and recovering drug users. At the same time, the group became increasingly involved in a larger movement for affordable HIV/AIDS treatment in the developing world. So how did a group of mostly poor Black HIV-positive Philadelphians become involved in the struggle for global treatment access when they faced their own daily struggles against discrimination, poverty, and illness?

ACT UP Philadelphia members came to see themselves as having common cause with people with AIDS in the developing world. Whether in South Philadelphia or South Africa, they argued, poor people of color were victimized by neoliberal policies, including welfare privatization, trade rules that valued pharmaceutical profits over public health, and development loans that remade developing economies according to the desires of global capital. Locally, they opposed moves to privatize Medicaid in Pennsylvania and prison health care in New Jersey. They also challenged U.S. trade practices that increased inequality and thus exacerbated the global AIDS epidemic. ACT UP Philadelphia framed these campaigns as part of the same fight against policies that strengthened corporate interests at the expense of poor people's health and well-being. Thus, they "linked the local to the global" to mobilize poor African Americans on behalf of people with AIDS in the developing world, based on their shared relationship to political and commercial power structures. In this way, ACT UP Philadelphia put poor people's politics at the center of the fight against global AIDS.

Thanks in part to the leadership of African Americans in ACT UP Philadelphia, the campaign for global treatment access won remarkable successes. Sustained protests of Al Gore on the presidential campaign trail led to the reversal of a Clinton-era trade policy that limited the ability of countries in sub-Saharan Africa to procure inexpensive generic AIDS drugs. Today, the group also claims at least partial credit for George W. Bush's President's Emergency Plan for AIDS Relief (PEPFAR), a massive funding package for the fight against HIV and AIDS in the Caribbean and sub-Saharan Africa. At the same time, these changes were never as sweeping as ACT UP Philadelphia wanted them to be. Hence this story also points to the ways that overlapping political and corporate interests have constrained the fight against global AIDS.[2]

Studies of ACT UP have, for the most part, not included this later period, which came after most chapters had declined or disbanded. Two feature-length documentaries, *How to Survive a Plague* and *United in Anger*, focus on ACT UP New York during the group's heyday. Deborah Gould documents the work of key chapters in New York, Chicago, and San Francisco during the late 1980s and early 1990s, focusing on the role of emotion in direct action AIDS activism. Raymond Smith and Patricia Siplon do acknowledge the "dramatic rebirth" of ACT UP Philadelphia and the group's role in the fight for global treatment access but do not examine it in detail. To explain the

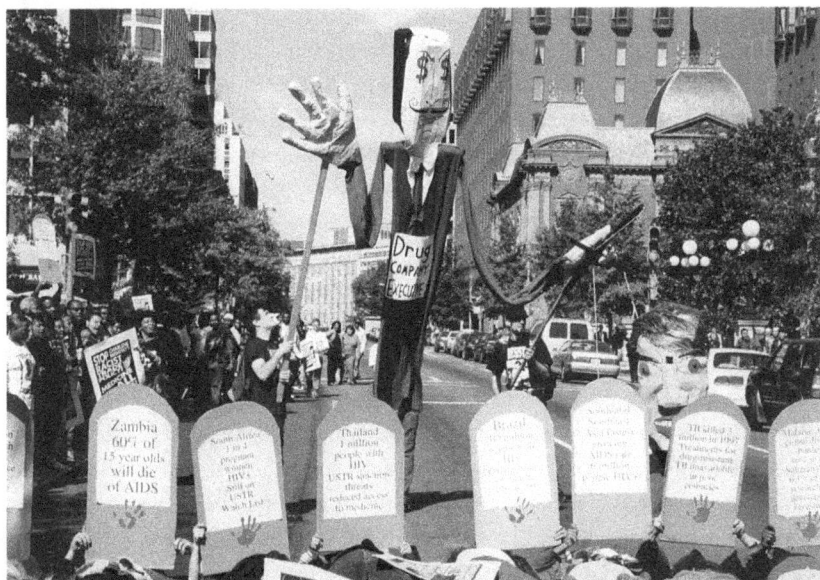

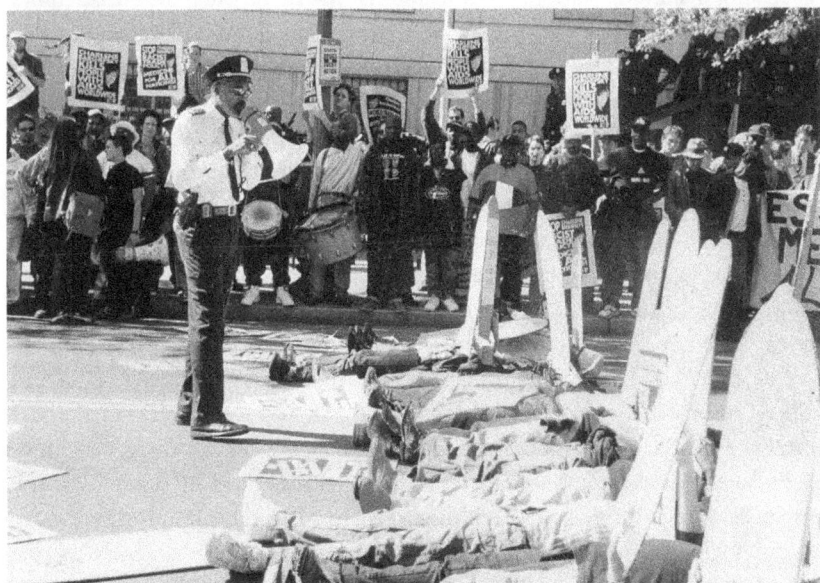

ACT UP Philadelphia protest at the Office of the United States Trade Representative against U.S. actions to limit the use of generic AIDS medicines in developing countries, October 6, 1999. JD Davids Papers, unprocessed, John J. Wilcox Jr. Archives, William Way LGBT Community Center, Philadelphia, PA.

group's advocacy for people halfway around the world, they point to "survivor guilt" and empathy for Africans among veteran AIDS activists, the parallel rise of anti-globalization groups, and the advent of the Internet. As this chapter makes clear, all of these were important factors in the struggle for global treatment access. But looking at ACT UP Philadelphia in detail shows that newer members, who tended to be poor and Black, saw themselves as connected in important ways to people with AIDS in the developing world.[3]

At the same time, Jennifer Brier argues that the epicenter of AIDS politics shifted to the global South in the late 1990s, as South African AIDS activists demanding access to generic HIV and AIDS drugs "succeeded where American activism failed." However, as this chapter makes clear, ACT UP Philadelphia worked with other poverty rights and AIDS groups to challenge what Brier refers to as "capitalist medicine" in Pennsylvania and New Jersey *before* access to generic HIV medicines in South Africa became a major activist issue. The group's many African American members came to see their own struggle as bound up with that of people confronting poverty, racism, and AIDS halfway around the world—not out of "survivor guilt," as Smith and Siplon argue, but because of a shared relationship to capitalist medicine. ACT UP Philadelphia members supported South African efforts by putting domestic pressure on key policy makers. The group also used direct action to push for major funding programs for the fight against global AIDS.[4]

Other African American AIDS activists argued that Black communities in the United States had something essentially in common with their counterparts in Africa and other parts of the diaspora. African American members of ACT UP Philadelphia also maintained that they had something important in common with people in places like South Africa, where AIDS cut a wide swath through the country's Black majority. But they additionally saw themselves as having common cause with people with AIDS in Thailand and Brazil, where capitalist medicine in the form of U.S. trade policy threatened efforts to fight AIDS. In other words, African Americans in ACT UP Philadelphia talked about the fight against global AIDS in terms of global class, although at times they also expressed a sense of racial solidarity with African AIDS activists. The emphasis on class may have been due to the multiracial nature of both ACT UP Philadelphia and the larger global treatment activist movement. The role that veteran white activists played in ACT UP Philadelphia, both in recruiting Black members and in setting an agenda that included global treatment advocacy, raises difficult questions about organizing across gradients of power and privilege. At the same time, ACT UP's African American members changed the group's approach to direct action, while members themselves were changed as they became outspoken AIDS activists.

## ACT UP Still Does

During the late 1980s and early 1990s, the AIDS Coalition to Unleash Power changed the ways that AIDS was diagnosed, treated, and talked about in the United States. The founding New York chapter staged its first protest in March 1987 at the New York Stock Exchange over the high price of AZT, at that time the first and only drug approved to treat HIV in the United States. Over the next six years, more than one hundred ACT UP chapters and similar groups sprang up around the world. Their "zaps"—disruptive protest actions—were often dramatic and confrontational and addressed everything from federal funding for AIDS research, to the Catholic Church's position on condoms, to the way that the CDC's case definition of AIDS prevented women from being diagnosed with the disease. ACT UP proved most successful at achieving its goal of getting "drugs into bodies" by making new treatments available to large numbers of people with AIDS. Those efforts culminated in the protease inhibitors and combination therapies that became available in the middle 1990s. The drugs offered a new lease on life to those who could afford them, changing HIV infection from a death sentence into a chronic, manageable disease. As a movement, ACT UP embodied the activist ethic of empowering people with HIV to challenge the policies that kept effective prevention methods and promising new treatments out of the hands of those who needed them.[5]

Nevertheless, around 1992 ACT UP as a nationwide movement began to decline. This was in part a function of the group's success. Some members made inroads into the worlds of policy making and research. Others had by this point spent five years fighting public apathy toward AIDS while their friends continued to die of the disease. With protease inhibitors and combination therapies still several years off, a deep sense of despair made continued organizing difficult. Solidarity among members also grew untenable, as divisions of race, class, and gender amplified disagreements over ACT UP's agenda. State surveillance and repression also likely played a role in the group's decline. Demonstrations often provoked a violent police response, and Freedom of Information Act requests later showed that the FBI collected a large file on the group. And many simply did not make it, as AIDS claimed some of the group's best and brightest.[6]

But as other chapters declined, ACT UP Philadelphia grew in size and strength by focusing on those who lived at the margins of the AIDS community in the City of Brotherly Love. Just as Rashidah Hassan predicted years earlier, the AIDS epidemic had "settled" among Philadelphia's disenfranchised, even as the overall picture of the epidemic began to improve. Advances in treatment led to a dramatic decline of 23.5 percent in AIDS-related deaths among

Philadelphians between 1995 and 1996. But the improvement in survival rates was not evenly shared: AIDS-related deaths dropped by 41 percent for whites but only by 13 percent among African Americans. Deaths also decreased far more dramatically among men who contracted HIV through sex with other men than among those who contracted the virus through intravenous drug use, and deaths *increased* slightly among people who contracted HIV through heterosexual sex, a group composed mostly of women of color. While protease inhibitors extended the lives of Philadelphians with AIDS, African Americans, including large numbers of women and IV drug users, benefited far less than did whites.[7]

ACT UP Philadelphia confronted this deepening inequality within the AIDS epidemic head-on. Members recall that the group was always relatively diverse, but in the middle 1990s they made a concerted effort to organize recovering drug users and ex-prisoners, who were disproportionately poor and Black and disconnected from the social services and medical care that they needed. To this end, ACT UP Philadelphia members conducted teach-ins at local drug recovery houses such as One Day at a Time and ran a monthly group at We the People, a local coalition of people with AIDS with many members who were also poor people of color. Those who led this shift included a core group of veteran activists who were white and HIV negative. Nonetheless, they were committed to building power among people with HIV and AIDS, and especially among those who had been left behind by the larger AIDS movement. These veteran activists included JD Davids, who had been a member of ACT UP Philadelphia since 1990; Paul Davis, who came from the Tenants Union in Seattle; Kate Krauss, who came from ACT UP Golden Gate in San Francisco; and Asia Russell, who had joined ACT UP Philadelphia as a teenager in the early 1990s.[8]

As they brought new members into the group, ACT UP Philadelphia veterans recognized that poverty itself might be a barrier to activism. Accordingly, they began offering food and subway tokens at meetings, held every Monday night in the basement of St. Luke's Episcopal Church in Center City. Earl Driscoll, a white recovering drug user who joined ACT UP Philadelphia in the early 1990s after visiting the group's needle exchange program, describes these small material incentives as a gateway to activism: "Someone could come for two tokens and a piece of a hoagie and some iced tea . . . and by hearing what they hear when they're there become an advocate and become someone active."[9]

Project TEACH (Treatment Education Activists Combating HIV), a peer education program geared toward poor people of color with HIV, also helped to shift ACT UP Philadelphia's membership. JD Davids and Jeff Maskovsky developed the program in 1995, out of "the belief that people have a right to know about their own bodies and to determine their own health care." In 1998 they added a version of the program in Spanish to reach Philadelphia's Puerto Rican community as well. By 2000, Project TEACH had produced over 250 graduates, most of them African Americans who had struggled with substance abuse. Each of these graduates then became a peer educator who could counsel people in their communities about the disease. The support of a peer educator, program organizers found, often made "the difference between an individual remaining in, or dropping out, of care."[10]

Project TEACH also introduced participants to AIDS activism. According to Val Sowell, a white queer woman who became involved with ACT UP Philadelphia in 2000 and served as Project TEACH's office assistant, the program connected people with AIDS to needed services and helped them to see that those services were "fought for and we have to continue to fight to keep [them] from being taken away." As one of their assignments, participants attended an ACT UP demonstration for an "activist inoculation." While not all Project TEACH graduates went on to become "core" members of ACT UP, the program introduced them to direct action AIDS activism and to ACT UP Philadelphia as a group committed to improving the lives of poor people of color living with HIV.[11]

As ACT UP Philadelphia expanded, the group prioritized issues that mattered to new members. ACT UP Philadelphia had been instrumental in starting Prevention Point, the city's needle exchange program, in 1991. The program operated illegally for its first year before being legalized by Mayor Ed Rendell through an executive order. By the middle of the decade, ACT UP Philadelphia was pushing to repeal a ban on federal funding for needle exchanges. As part of that campaign, participants organized a demonstration in September 1997 targeting Health and Human Services secretary Donna Shalala, who would implement the new federal policy should President Bill Clinton decide to lift the funding ban. That protest, billed as a "National Day of Reckoning," shows how the campaign for federal needle exchange funding swelled the number of African Americans within ACT UP Philadelphia, who in turn reshaped the group's tactics and culture.[12]

During planning meetings leading up to the National Day of Reckoning, ACT UP Philadelphia members went through the usual process of working out the details of the protest. Veterans of the group, some of whom had been involved with Prevention Point for years, suggested that syringes should be part of the campaign's imagery. Newer members who had joined ACT UP Philadelphia while in recovery from drug use objected to the idea. Some worried that it would validate the misconception that needle exchanges promoted drug use. Others insisted that the images would be a painful reminder to those recovering from addiction, making it difficult to mobilize other former users. So instead of syringes, the group constructed a twelve-foot papier-mâché model of a human spine, suspended from a wooden frame. By delivering it to Washington, D.C., they intended to give Clinton and Shalala the "moral backbone" to stand up to opponents of needle exchange.[13]

On the day of the action, hundreds of demonstrators boarded buses from Philadelphia, Pittsburgh, Williamsport (in Pennsylvania), and Baltimore to the nation's capital. Most were African American and many were also either in recovery from substance abuse or still actively using drugs. Once they arrived in Washington, the group marched several blocks to the Health and Human Services building, where they used the spine to barricade the front doors while members testified about the need for needle exchange programs. For John Bell, a Black HIV-positive recovering drug user and Vietnam War veteran, the National Day of Reckoning action marked a turning point in his own commitment to ACT UP Philadelphia and AIDS activism. Bell would become one of the group's most visible and outspoken African American members.[14]

Bell and other members who came to ACT UP Philadelphia from recovery programs changed the culture of the group, as many of them had embraced religious faith as a key step in overcoming addiction. Veteran members saw nothing wrong with iconoclasm; ACT UP Philadelphia—as well as ACT UP New York—had famously targeted the Catholic Church over opposition to condom use during the late 1980s and early 1990s. When in 1991 the church opposed a plan to distribute condoms in Philadelphia schools, a hundred members of ACT UP Philadelphia gathered at the Cathedral Basilica of Saints Peter and Paul on Logan Square to protest. During Archbishop Anthony Bevilacqua's homily during a service for people affected by AIDS, a member sprinkled condoms at the prelate's feet, shouting, "These will save lives—your morals won't." But when Paul Davis proposed interrupting an appearance by Shalala at a church in nearby Bryn Mawr in April 1998, Bell objected. He insisted that Davis, by proposing to loudly disrupt a church event, risked alienating newer members. Instead, the group stood up in unison during Shalala's speech, turned their backs, and whispered, "Donna Shalala, you killed my brother. Donna Shalala, you killed my sister." Around the same time, ACT UP added a gospel choir to its protest repertoire, connecting AIDS activism to the long musical tradition of the Black freedom struggle.[15]

Nevertheless, some in the Philadelphia AIDS community saw contradictions between the group's avowed commitment to "democratic pro-cess [sic], self-education, and the empowerment of [people with HIV]" and the reality of its organizing. Key members such as Davids, Davis, Russell, and Krauss, who all frequently served as spokespeople for the group, were white and HIV negative, with years of activist experience. They themselves sometimes wondered about the ethical dilemmas that their work raised. According to Kate Krauss,

"If they're in a recovery house, they have to do what the recovery house head tells them to do. . . . Are you manipulating them? . . . And then there is another case to be made that . . . you're still in recovery, you're still in active treatment so you may not have done anything good in this world for a really a long time, and to help a cause that you believe in, which a lot of people do here, even if you're . . . required to do it, it's sort of interesting." Roy Hayes, a Black gay recovering drug user from West Philadelphia and a longtime ACT UP Philadelphia member, also saw the recruiting tactic as a problem: "If they [those in a recovery house] don't go on [an] ACT UP demonstration they'll get thrown out of the house. That should not be. These people should want to go and fight for the cause, [because] they really feel something."[16]

ACT UP Philadelphia at times seemed to fall short of its goal of grassroots political empowerment among the city's poor and disfranchised residents. In notes from a group discussion held just before a demonstration and lobbying session in April 1999, members expressed a desire to "deepen involvement with some of the groups we work with, rather than just doing turn-out for protests." Apparently, some who took part in actions complained of never finding out what happened as a result, suggesting a disconnect between the members who planned actions at Monday night meetings and those who turned out to execute them. John Bell likewise recalled that the purpose of demonstrations sometimes seemed unclear to newer activists: "If a newspaper reporter comes up to Paul Davis and asks him why he's at a demonstration[, then] . . . this person in this recovery house, this African American who's come all the way from Philadelphia, he should be able to say the same thing that Paul says. And if that doesn't happen, then there's a mistake somewhere along the line."[17]

Some of the very people whom ACT UP Philadelphia sought to mobilize also felt alienated by the group's culture. Project TEACH cofounder Jeff Maskovsky conducted over seventy interviews in the Philadelphia AIDS community between August 1996 and March 1998 for his doctoral dissertation on We the People. He interviewed one poor Black person with AIDS who recalled his impression of white ACT UP members like Davids, Davis, and Russell, who lived in "Not Squat," a group house in West Philadelphia: "I took it as a slap in the face when I went to visit one of their houses. They chose to live in a place with windows missing, no clean bathroom, and a hole in the living room floor . . . and that is offensive to people who have to live that way, who don't have rich parents, and who can't go home to the Main Line [a wealthy Philadelphia suburb]." Another interviewee decided, after attending a handful of ACT UP Philadelphia meetings, "I can't do it with them, because . . . they don't get the poor black thing. When they talk to us they talk to us in a patronizing, condescending way. And when they talk to each other, the dialogue is between people who are pretty well educated, but they treat us in really simplistic terms, like we don't understand anything past a two syllable word."[18]

John Bell also recalled feeling excluded by white middle-class members when he first began to attend ACT UP Philadelphia meetings. According to Bell, "Rebecca Ewing, Asia Russell, Paul Davis, [JD] Davids would say things, but they would say them fast, and they would say them sharp, and they would say them under their breath, and I didn't get it. . . . That bothered me." However, he also recalled that at least some of the white members worked to make the group more welcoming to people from different backgrounds. After Bell approached Davids about his misgivings, Davids reiterated the group's goal of empowering people affected by HIV—particularly poor people of color—at the next meeting. Over the objections of another member, he insisted, "It's important that we usher other people in, so therefore they have to understand what's going on, if they're going to take on the work."[19]

ACT UP Philadelphia did indeed try to find ways for newer members to "take on the work." The group held its own trainings on meeting facilitation, "to increase and diversify our pool of meeting facilitators," and sent members to organizer trainings hosted by the Midwest Academy and the Center for Third World Organizing. ACT UP Philadelphia member Waheedah Shabazz-El praises Davis and Davids for their commitment to empowering others, because "they would take you to a certain point and then they would step back. . . . I was taught early on from them that a good organizer works themself out of a job. . . . You build leadership as you go." Shabazz-El, a Black Muslim woman and former postal worker, came to ACT UP Philadelphia in the 2000s after testing HIV positive while briefly incarcerated on a drug charge. Bell, by then working for Philadelphia FIGHT, a local AIDS service organization, visited Shabazz-El in prison to make sure that she would enter Project TEACH upon release. Although she would later come to see Davis and Davids as mentors, it was Bell, a Project TEACH graduate and peer educator, who started her on a path to political education and activism. After her release, she went through Project TEACH and joined ACT UP Philadelphia. She credits the group with not only helping her overcome her "internal stigma" but also enabling her "to speak truth to power, and to still be able to come home and talk to my peers and meet them where they were, until they were able to come and speak to power with me."[20]

## HealthChoices Is Neither

In 1995 ACT UP Philadelphia became involved in one such campaign, in which the group spoke directly to power on issues that impacted poor communities of color. Here members fought as part of a coalition of AIDS groups, advocates for the poor, programs for the homeless and people in recovery, and others to stop HealthChoices, a program that would privatize Medicaid, first in Philadelphia and its surrounding counties and then across Pennsylvania. They lobbied state lawmakers to improve HealthChoices, particularly when it came to care for people with HIV and AIDS, and organized protests that included large numbers of people whose health care was under threat. By fighting back against the displacement of the welfare state into the "free market," along with overall cuts to public spending on health care, they challenged a system of capitalist medicine that valued profits over the very lives of poor people living with HIV and AIDS.

The proposed HealthChoices program began under Governor Bob Casey, a Democrat. Faced with steeply rising state Medicaid costs in the late 1980s and early 1990s, in 1993 Casey proposed to expand HealthPass, a pilot program in South and West Philadelphia that provided recipients with managed care in lieu of traditional medical assistance. With HealthPass, which operated like an HMO, the state paid a fixed monthly rate for Medicaid recipients to see doctors within an approved network of providers. Under the older Medicaid model, patients could receive care from any doctor or hospital, which the state would then reimburse according to their services. Advocates of managed care argued that reform would both cut costs and deliver better care to people on welfare. Those on Medicaid would receive preventive care from a regular physician; as a result, fewer would end up in the emergency room with advanced medical conditions that were expensive and difficult to treat. And because the state would pay a flat rate for those in the program, costs would be lower and more predictable than they had been in the recent past. The new program, which the Casey administration dubbed "HealthChoices," would cover all of Philadelphia along with five nearby counties.[21]

While the state of Pennsylvania hoped to save money from the move to Medicaid managed care, insurance companies stood to profit handsomely. They prepared to bid on state contracts to provide coverage under HealthChoices, estimated to be worth a total of $2 billion each year. While a state audit found that HMOs serving HealthPass clients made "exorbitant profits," insurance executives defended the massive transfer of public funds to the private sector. The head of one company argued, "We're able to take those dollars and allocate them in a way that makes sense to provide better outcomes. Better outcomes [mean] healthier people." But managed care did not always lead to "better outcomes." Insurance sales representatives used aggressive—sometimes underhanded—tactics to push poor clients to enroll in their plans. These patients sometimes found themselves with private plans that delivered far less than promised; some who went to the hospital seeking treatment that had been covered under Medicaid left with stacks of medical bills that they were unable to pay.[22]

The fight against HealthChoices was explicitly about medical care for poor people in Pennsylvania, but it was also shaped by national political events. AIDS activists had hoped that the election of Bill Clinton in 1992 would finally bring national health care to the United States; their hopes were dashed first when Clinton proposed a less radical plan to reform the health care system and again when even that plan fell to congressional opposition. Political backlash swept Republicans to power in the 1994 midterm elections, where they won majorities in both houses of Congress along with the governorship in Pennsylvania. Governor Tom Ridge picked up the mantle of managed care for the state's poor, even as he ejected hundreds of thousands of people from the welfare rolls in the name of fiscal austerity. Likewise, toward the end of his first term Clinton made good on his promise to "end welfare as we know it" by signing the Personal Responsibility and Work Opportunity Act. In doing so he replaced the decades-old Aid to Families with Dependent Children program with the far more stringent Temporary Aid to Needy Families, effectively unraveling a key piece of the American social safety net.[23]

These developments in turn reflected even bigger trends. As historian Daniel Rodgers has observed, over the last quarter of the twentieth century, "market ideas moved out of economics departments to become the new standard currency of the social sciences." Consequently, "protean, spill-over words like 'choice' were called upon to do more and more work in more and more diverse circumstances." This market logic also found its way into arguments for the sweeping welfare reforms instituted by Bill Clinton, a Democrat, and Tom Ridge, a Republican. As Rodgers points out, in both cases the effect was "to precipitate the welfare poor into the market to do its work: incorporating, disciplining, assorting, punishing, and rewarding." This was also the idea behind the move to managed care: the private insurance market (with public dollars) would distribute health care better and more efficiently than the old system had. In this way the market-based Medicaid reform dubbed "HealthChoices" and promoted by Pennsylvania politicians on both sides of the aisle seems very much of its time.[24]

ACT UP Philadelphia opposed the plan. The group pointed out that people with HIV and AIDS were expensive to treat, which made them unattractive customers for the insurance companies moving into Philadelphia's Medicaid market. According to ACT UP Philadelphia, since profit-driven "HMOs use a variety of tactics to reduce care, and therefore, save money," they would offer substandard care to people with HIV and AIDS or discourage them from enrolling in the first place. Major changes to Medicaid might also disrupt the treatment and care of people with HIV and AIDS, with deadly results. Interruptions in health coverage, such as for those forced to change insurance plans, might lead to gaps in treatment and thus to drug-resistant strains of HIV. Others might find that changes to the system would disrupt their care by making them ineligible to see a trusted doctor. While HealthChoices may have seemed like an unstoppable force, ACT UP Philadelphia pushed for changes that would improve the way it treated poor people with HIV and AIDS.[25]

At the same time, ACT UP Philadelphia fought against Republican plans to unravel Pennsylvania's social safety net. In early 1996, Ridge announced his plan to reduce welfare spending in the state not only through managed care but also by kicking over 150,000 "able-bodied" people out of the state's medical assistance program. The governor further proposed deep cuts to the state's Special Pharmaceutical Benefits Program, which provided HIV and AIDS drugs to poor Pennsylvanians.[26]

ACT UP Philadelphia and other advocacy groups attacked Ridge's plan, arguing that the price of its short-term savings to the state would be increasing misery among the poor and rising costs over the long term. At a budget hearing in February 1996, state officials defended the plan, saying that those cut from the Medicaid rolls would be expected to either obtain health insurance from their employer or earn enough money to purchase their own in the private market. Advocates countered that many of those who stood to lose medical assistance already worked low-wage jobs or were looking for work but had trouble finding it. Moreover, they pointed out, shrinking Medicaid would force those who lost coverage to delay medical care until their ailments became difficult and expensive to treat—exactly the situation that HealthChoices was supposed to prevent. Those suffering from otherwise treatable ailments might find themselves unable to work as a result of their lost medical coverage. As Tara Colon of the Kensington Welfare Rights Union argued, that coverage "keeps working people off welfare."[27]

At the same meeting, ACT UP Philadelphia members criticized the governor's proposed cuts to the Special Pharmaceutical Benefits Program, which came at precisely the moment that promising new treatments were becoming available. Without such programs, the gap between haves and have-nots in AIDS treatment, which closely tracked racial disparities in the epidemic, would only get worse. For threatening to withhold the treatments from poor people with HIV and AIDS after fifteen years of false hopes and disappointment, Steven Parmer of ACT UP Philadelphia accused the state officials of "ignorance or darkness of heart."[28]

As the Pennsylvania General Assembly wrangled over Ridge's budget, ACT up Philadelphia organized a phone campaign in support of the Special Pharmaceutical Benefits Program. Ridge had based his cuts on expenditures from the previous year, which left almost a third of the program's budget unspent. ACT UP Philadelphia members warned that the high cost of new medications and rising demand would lead to a much greater need for funding in the near future. Their phone calls saved the Special Pharmaceutical Benefits Program budget, and the group extracted promises from the state to hold HealthChoices HMOS to an HIV/AIDS standard of care and that people with HIV would be able to choose a doctor experienced in treating the disease. However, the broader effort to prevent Medicaid cuts failed. Although ACT UP Philadelphia and its allies sent "hundreds of bus loads of demonstrators" to the capitol, state legislators passed a budget containing many of Ridge's original cuts. As a result, an estimated 250,000 Pennsylvanians lost their health coverage.[29]

ACT UP Philadelphia continued to protest HealthChoices throughout the fall and winter. In November, participants staged a short march from Washington Square Park to the Liberty Bell, with tombstone-shaped posters and a die-in to dramatize the program's predicted effect. On December 1, they took advantage of press coverage for World AIDS Day to draw attention to the campaign with an action called "Day without Health Care." In the past, ACT UP Philadelphia had commemorated World AIDS Day by covering the city's iconic *LOVE* sculpture with a black shroud. For the Day without Health Care, members draped the Center City home of Feather Houstoun, head of the state's Department of Public Welfare, with a twelve-foot banner. Giant letters spelled out "RAGE" in the "LOVE" configuration, while a longer message skewered privatization advocates' rhetoric of consumer choice: "HealthChoices is neither—People with HIV/AIDS need real choices!"[30]

As the February enrollment deadline for HealthChoices loomed, ACT UP Philadelphia found that the state was not holding up its end of the bargain on care for people with HIV and AIDS. Benefits counselors staffing a HealthChoices hotline did not advise people with HIV of their right to select a specialist as their primary doctor, and a phone survey conducted by the AIDS Law Project further found that none of the HealthChoices HMOS could refer callers to HIV-experienced doctors. Meanwhile, the Department of Public Welfare and HMOS refused to make public a list of practitioners specializing in HIV/AIDS. In response, We the People protested at two South Philadelphia welfare offices, demanding release of the list. The Welfare Department relented, agreeing to make a partial list, put together by local AIDS organizations, available upon request. Still, ACT UP Philadelphia reported that when the February deadline arrived for the first round of managed care enrollment, welfare recipients "[lost] their doctors by the hundreds."[31]

In March 1998, ACT UP Philadelphia staged one of its last HealthChoices actions at the Pennsylvania State Building to demand that two new drugs be covered by the state's Special Pharmaceutical Benefits Program and to call for an increase in the city's per capita reimbursements to HealthChoices HMOs to meet higher rates offered elsewhere. Over a hundred protesters, most of them African American, carried coffins and a twenty-foot-tall grim reaper puppet with Ridge's face, chanting, "HealthChoices is a lie. They don't care if people die." Joyce Hamilton, a Black recovering drug user who had joined ACT UP Philadelphia after seeing an earlier HealthChoices demonstration, reiterated the group's critique of Medicaid managed care as a form of capitalist medicine. In a press release for the action, she stressed that, under the program's market-driven logic, "HMOs have a financial incentive to provide less care." Two years later, care for people with HIV and AIDS under HealthChoices had not improved. Project TEACH peer educators continued to find that HealthChoices clients with HIV and AIDS "frequently had gaps in medication access due to pharmacy problems or rejection of prescriptions by the HealthChoices HMOs . . . and that their clients were confused about whether or not they could see an HIV specialist as their primary care doctor, even though this remains their right."[32]

Alongside the HealthChoices campaign, ACT UP Philadelphia fought other moves to privatize health care. Beginning in early 1996 the group protested New Jersey governor Christine Todd Whitman's plan to outsource medical care for the state's prison system to Correctional Medical Services, a St. Louis-based firm, as well as a New Jersey state law requiring prisoners in the state to pay for their own health care. Gregory Dean Smith, an HIV-positive Black gay ACT UP Philadelphia member, served as the group's connection to the New Jersey prison system. At the time, Smith was serving a twenty-five-year sentence for attempted murder after allegedly biting a Camden County Jail guard on the hand. Smith posted his newsletter, *Tales from behind the Wall*, on the ACT UP Philadelphia website. He criticized Correctional Medical Services for its unreliable deliveries, which often arrived late or not at all. "Sorry to say," Smith wrote, "but this company is killing the inmates."[33]

Despite such efforts, ACT UP Philadelphia failed to stop both the shift to Medicaid managed care in Pennsylvania and the privatization of prison health services in New Jersey. Although the group and its allies won some concessions in the HealthChoices fight, those victories were easily undermined by lack of state enforcement. Nevertheless, the campaign strengthened ACT UP Philadelphia's credibility in communities of color. Growing numbers of HIV-positive African Americans joined ACT UP Philadelphia during the campaign because the group agitated for the needs of poor people living with the disease and because of the growing visibility of Black members in the organization. Joyce Hamilton, who joined ACT UP Philadelphia during this time, recalled in a 1998 interview, "When I saw them I said, 'wow! These people are fighting for people with the virus.'" She continued, "I don't think people think of it as a white gay organization anymore."[34]

The HealthChoices campaign also set up the next stage in ACT UP Philadelphia's evolution, as the group turned from fighting Medicaid privatization in Pennsylvania to securing access to HIV medicines for people halfway around the world. In both cases activists took on the bipartisan consensus in American politics that market forces could effectively and humanely distribute health care to the world's poor. Their victories on this front would be frustratingly partial but victories nonetheless as they pushed for a massive expansion of resources in the global fight against AIDS.

## Essential Medication for Every Nation

Those who joined ACT UP Philadelphia around the time of the HealthChoices campaign faced their own daily struggles. Many were living with HIV and dealing with the physical and emotional effects of the virus. Some were also dealing with the side effects of their HIV medication. John Bell, for example, suffered from neuropathy, which produced tingling pain in his right foot. Many were fighting to stay clean and sober, and some were also putting their lives back together after being released from prison. These members hailed from neighborhoods in North, West, and South Philadelphia, where jobs remained scarce and crumbling houses served as a daily reminder of the city's faded glory. In short, ACT UP Philadelphia members faced daily struggles that could easily have consumed their time and attention. So how did they end up deeply involved in a years-long campaign to secure access to HIV and AIDS drugs for people in far-flung corners of the world?

Part of the answer lies in the mentorship that new members received from ACT UP veterans. Project TEACH trained hundreds to become treatment advocates in their own communities, which primed them to fight for access to treatment for people in South Africa, Thailand, and Brazil. Many members also came to see their own struggles as connected to those of other poor people around the world. Jose de Marco, who joined ACT UP in 1996, recalls that he would highlight the similar struggles of poor people with AIDS in Philadelphia and their counterparts in the developing world. At teach-ins he would tell people, "Look how fucked up this shit is. There's no difference between South Philly and South Africa. Folks over there don't have anybody to fight for them, only us." Members also felt a responsibility to advocate for others because they enjoyed access to life-saving medications. John Bell told the *Philadelphia Weekly* in 2001 that his initial response to the campaign was, "'No, we've got to take care of things here.' But then I realized that I had good health today because other people had thought about me."[35]

The connection that ACT UP Philadelphia members felt with people with HIV and AIDS around the world was more than imagined. Veteran members had befriended other AIDS activists at international conferences, and newer members would soon get their own chance to do the same. The growing reach of the Internet also created new connections. AIDS activists in Africa sent emails to ACT UP Philadelphia, describing horrific conditions: morgues in Zimbabwe that stayed open around the clock to handle the sheer volume of dead bodies, HIV-positive men in South Africa who were having sex with virgin girls in hopes that they would thus be cured of the virus, and medical clinics so ill-equipped that they could offer people with AIDS "little more than a bottle of aspirin."[36]

The Critical Path AIDS Project, the brainchild of ACT UP Philadelphia founding member Kiyoshi Kuromiya, also fostered connections to AIDS activists around the world. Since the early 1990s, Critical Path had used the Internet to disseminate AIDS treatment information. At the time of Kuromiya's death in May 2000, the project also provided free web hosting to nearly a hundred activist groups and email addresses to many ACT UP Philadelphia members. Kate Krauss would later tell the *Village Voice* that the global treatment access movement comprised "a network of allies who communicate by e-mails, teleconferencing, and listservs," a network established in part by Critical Path. Kuromiya signaled his view of the epidemic in the banner for his newsletter, a map of the earth by futurist Buckminster Fuller in which all seven continents appear as a single chain of landmass. The image captured the sense of connection that Kuromiya sought to foster through Critical Path because, he explained, "we view AIDS as a global problem."[37]

ACT UP Philadelphia took up the issue of global treatment access as part of a larger conversation about global inequality. Its efforts overlapped and intersected with a burgeoning anti-globalization movement that took on multinational corporations, along with the national governments and international institutions that supported them. Then there were the religious leaders, civil society groups, and celebrities that pushed the International Monetary Fund and World Bank to "drop the debt" held by developing countries. They argued that the IMF and World Bank "put the global economy on a path of greater inequality and environmental destruction" by requiring poorer countries to "adopt belt-tightening measures [that] increase poverty, reduce countries' ability to develop strong domestic economies and allow multinational corporations to exploit workers and the environment." Activists in these allied movements made global AIDS a part of their argument against neoliberal globalization, and ACT UP incorporated issues such as debt repayment into its organizing as well. In this way the movement for global treatment access helped, and was helped by, groups seeking to change the way that the United States and other wealthy nations promoted corporate interests at the expense of the health and well-being of poor people around the world.[38]

The promising new treatments that ACT UP Philadelphia fought to include in the Special Pharmaceutical Benefits Program also played a role in the fight for global treatment access. Although protease inhibitors had previously been available to people with AIDS as experimental therapies, they were announced to the world as a promising new treatment at the Vancouver AIDS Conference in 1996. The clinical trials results presented at the conference brought breathless coverage from the news media, with some going so far as to proclaim the "end" of AIDS. The reaction from activists in Vancouver was far more skeptical. In his remarks at the conference's opening ceremony, ACT UP New York veteran Eric Sawyer warned against celebrating the arrival of protease inhibitors, since they were too expensive for most people with AIDS around the world. "Genocide continues against poor people with AIDS," he insisted, "especially those from developing countries, by AIDS Profiteers who are more concerned about maximizing profits than saving lives. . . . The greed of AIDS Profiteers is killing impoverished people with AIDS." In his report from the conference, Kiyoshi Kuromiya bitterly observed, "'One World, One Hope'—the theme of the meeting—was the big lie of Vancouver. Ninety percent of the meeting concentrated on drug advances that would never reach the ninety percent of PWAS [people with AIDS] who live in the developing world. And in the US, the promise of medical care and access to the new classes of promising drugs for all our citizens is an empty promise."[39]

Although U.S. AIDS activists argued for expanded access to HIV and AIDS drugs at Vancouver in 1996, the mobilization of groups like ACT UP Philadelphia around the issue was still several years off. After the Geneva AIDS Conference in 1998, the activist physician Alan Berkman laid out a "multi-level strategy rooted in grassroots activism" to demand treatment and care for people with HIV and AIDS around the world. His plan led to a series of conference calls in January 1999 among representatives from a range of activist and advocacy movements, out of which the Health Global Access Project Coalition, or Health GAP, was born. Health GAP would come to involve activists across the United States and on both sides of the Atlantic, including the ACT UP chapters in Philadelphia, New York, and Paris, along with Médecins sans Frontières, Oxfam, and South Africa's Treatment Action Campaign. The group existed largely as a "virtual organization," coordinating actions and press releases via phone calls and email. But it also pulled off protest after protest in New York, Philadelphia, and Washington, D.C., arguing for changes to U.S. policy that would deliver life-saving treatments to people in need. These actions succeeded thanks in no small part to ACT UP Philadelphia's ability to mobilize large numbers of African Americans living with HIV.[40]

Health GAP first took aim at the ways in which U.S. trade policy kept HIV/AIDS treatments out of the hands of the world's poor. It argued that the Clinton administration used its outsized influence to prevent other countries from producing or acquiring generic versions of patented medications, even when doing so was allowed under international intellectual property agreements. In this way, the White House put the interests of the pharmaceutical lobby, which opposed any effort to expand drug access, ahead of the millions of people suffering for want of HIV and AIDS drugs.

Evidence of this close cooperation between leaders in Washington and multinational pharmaceutical companies came to Health GAP in early 1999, in the form of a leaked report detailing the Clinton administration's pressure on South Africa over the country's 1997 Medicines Act. The law allowed drugs to be imported from countries with lower prices, a practice known as "parallel importing," and encouraged the use of generic versions of patented drugs, which could be produced with government permission through a practice known as "compulsory licensing." South African leaders insisted that the Medicines Act fell within the World Trade Organization's agreement on Trade-Related Aspects of Intellectual Property Rights (TRIPS), which allowed member nations to pursue such measures in cases of national emergency. The HIV incidence in South Africa, which stood at over 10 percent in 1997 and was rising quickly, seemed to fit that bill. Nevertheless, a group of thirty-nine drug manufacturers sued the South African government in early 1998. Moreover, as the 1999 report made clear, Vice President Al Gore (as chair of the U.S.-South Africa Binational Commission), the Departments of State and Commerce, and Trade Representative Charlene Barshefsky had "engaged in a full court press . . . to convince the South African Government to withdraw or amend the offending provisions of the law." The report marked a turning point in the global treatment access movement. Asia Russell later recalled, "For the first time, it became clear what the US government role was. . . . It wasn't just that the government was indifferent. It was taking actions that accelerated needless suffering and death."[41]

Armed with this knowledge, ACT UP Philadelphia and Health GAP took aim at U.S. trade policy. In April 1999 they sent eleven buses full of protesters, along with three from New York, to Washington, D.C., for a demonstration and lobbying session to oppose the African Growth and Opportunity Act. The bill, which would liberalize trade between the United States and a number of African countries, enjoyed strong support from both parties in Congress and the Clinton administration. ACT UP Philadelphia argued that the bill, which it referred to as the "African Re-enslavement Act" and the "More AIDS for Africa Act," would provide growth and opportunity not to the majority of Africans but to the "multinational oil, pharmaceutical, mining, and other corporations . . . who would gain the most from it." The bill also made no mention of HIV and AIDS, even as the United Nations estimated that the affected region contained 21 million people with HIV, two-thirds of the world's total. Carrying signs that read "Human Rights, Not Corporate Rights," and "Just Say No to Drug Lobbyists," protesters encouraged lawmakers to instead support Representative Jesse Jackson Jr.'s HOPE (Human Rights, Opportunity, Partnership, and Empowerment) for Africa Act. Jackson's bill promised to cancel U.S.-held African debt while allowing compulsory licensing and parallel imports. The HOPE Act would also prevent the federal government from using taxpayer dollars to exert pressure on African countries over intellectual property rules, as the Clinton administration had done with South Africa.[42]

Health GAP and ACT UP Philadelphia soon found an opportunity to push the South Africa dispute into the national spotlight. When Vice President Al Gore launched his presidential campaign in June 1999, the groups swung into action. They nicknamed his campaign "Apartheid 2000," likening unequal access to AIDS drugs to the system of violent racial segregation only recently overturned in South Africa. A handful of activists from Philadelphia zapped an early rally in New Hampshire by unfurling a banner behind the vice president that read, "Gore Kills, AIDS Drugs for Africa." Weeks later in Philadelphia, hundreds of AIDS activists, along with African American and gay and lesbian community leaders, protested outside one of his $1,000-a-plate fund-raising dinners. They held up a life-size Gore puppet, dangling from the strings of a much taller drug company executive. In a press release announcing the action, ACT UP Philadelphia member Joe West compared the Clinton administration's efforts to roll back the Medicines Act to South Africa's brutal recent history of racial segregation: "We are looking forward to supporting a candidate who will end Medical Apartheid, rather than one who is complicit in this racist application of trade policy." West explained that his interest in the matter stemmed in part from his own racial identity: "As an African American, I will support a candidate who will take strong stands against big drug companies so that millions of lives in Africa can be saved." Some AIDS advocates, however, thought the protesters "missed the mark." Daniel Zingale, director of the lobbying group AIDS Action Council, complained, "The true culprit is not Al Gore but the drug companies." But from the protesters' perspective, Gore was culpable: as vice president he had used his power to protect the drug companies' bottom line at the expense of people in dire need of medicine.[43]

The demonstrations drew attention to the South Africa trade dispute and cast an otherwise arcane and obscure policy issue in stark moral terms. News outlets reported on the protests, as well as on Gore's ties to pharmaceutical corporations and lobby groups. Within a few months, the protests paid off. In September, Trade Representative Barshefsky announced that the United States and South Africa had reached an agreement: in exchange for assurance from South African leaders that the Medicines Act would be carried out in accordance with World Trade Organization rules, the United States agreed to withdraw pressure to change the law. ACT UP Philadelphia and Health GAP hailed the announcement as a victory, albeit a partial one. In a letter to Gore, Eric Sawyer and Paul Davis made their goals clear: "The Health GAP Coalition and its diverse member organizations are seeking an end to interference with access to *all* essential medications for any illness for *any* nation unable to purchase drugs at 'Big Pharma' prices. Although appreciated, a settlement with only South Africa that makes exceptions for AIDS drugs to an otherwise lethal trade policy is not an adequate arrangement." In a press release following the announcement, ACT UP Philadelphia drove this point home, promising that "disruptions and demonstrations will not end until the Administration transforms trade policy to support access to essential medications, rather than the whims of pharmaceutical companies placing profit before human lives."[44]

ACT UP Philadelphia and its Health GAP allies kept their word. Subsequent protests pushed the drug access issue far beyond South Africa, since the United States had also pressured Thailand, Brazil, India, and a host of other countries to stop using compulsory licensing and parallel imports to obtain affordable HIV and AIDS drugs. For a rally in Washington, D.C., on October 6, 1999, they repurposed the puppets from Philadelphia a few months earlier, this time with Barshefsky instead of Gore as the drug executive's plaything. Protesters lay down in the middle of Seventeenth Street, holding signs shaped like tombstones with messages that pushed the drug access issue far beyond South Africa. One read,

Thailand
1 million people with HIV
USTR [U.S. Trade Representative] sanction threats
reduced access to medicine

and another, "Zambia: 60% of 15 year olds will die of AIDS." Protesters had marked the signs with red handprints to make their point clear: the U.S.

government had blood on its hands. On November 17, ACT UP protesters returned to Washington, this time occupying Barshefksy's second-floor office. They hung a banner that read "Essential Medication for Every Nation" from the balcony and rained empty pill bottles and dollar bills printed with Barshefsky's face on the sidewalk below. On November 30, the day before World AIDS Day, they returned to the capital for the third time in two months. They chanted "Medication for every nation!" while marching past the offices of Bristol-Myers Squibb, which was embroiled in a patent with Thailand over compulsory licensing of the AIDS drug ddI. At the White House fence, they presented Bill Clinton with a "Golden Funeral Urn" in absentia to mark the millions of deaths around the world that had resulted from his policy of "corporate welfare for drug companies." Hassan Gibbs, a Project TEACH educator and ACT UP Philadelphia member, criticized the administration for "continu[ing] to play puppet to the pharmaceutical companies" while "millions of people with HIV in developing nations are having essential medication held back from them." The ACT UP Gospel Choir capped off the protest with a rendition of "Amazing Grace."[45]

Again, the protests worked. The following day Clinton announced, "The United States will henceforward implement its health care and trade policies in a manner that ensures that people in the poorest countries won't have to go without medicine they so desperately need." He also promised that Trade Representative Barshefsky would work with the Department of Health and Human Services "to make sure that our intellectual property policy is flexible enough to respond to legitimate public health crises." In meetings with administration officials over the next few months, Health GAP members pushed for the policy to be broadly applied across the developing world. The executive order that Clinton signed in May 2000 to implement the policy came up shy of that goal. Instead, the United States would no longer "seek, through negotiation or otherwise, the revocation or revision of any intellectual property law or policy of a beneficiary *sub-Saharan African country*" (emphasis added). The change also came through an executive order rather than via an amendment to the African Growth and Opportunity Act, which would have codified it as federal law. Still, for AIDS activists the new policy marked a significant improvement over the one that Barshefsky had announced eight months earlier.[46]

ACT UP Philadelphia and Health GAP had succeeded in changing the way that officials within the trade representative's office thought about pharmaceutical patents. Barshefsky later remarked, "We all missed it. I didn't appreciate at all the extent to which our interpretation of South Africa's international property obligations were draconian." The drug companies opposed the change in policy, insisting that it would "dampen research" by cutting into industry profits, and argued that poorer countries lacked the health care infrastructure to deliver medicines to people in need. AIDS activists pushed back against this use of the "R&D [research and development] scare card," pointing out that pharmaceuticals were the most profitable industry in the United States and that many of their products had been developed through publicly funded research. In this light, Health GAP member and consumer advocate Peter Lurie argued, the drug companies' opposition to compulsory licensing and parallel imports arose from "their desire not to have their irrational pricing practices exposed. We suggest that providing potentially lifesaving drugs to residents of developing countries should have a higher priority." After six months of protests, Clinton and key officials in his administration apparently agreed.[47]

Nevertheless, ACT UP Philadelphia still had work to do. On Sunday, April 16, 2000, the group sent eleven buses of "rowdy protesters" to Washington, D.C., for a massive anti-globalization demonstration aimed at shutting down meetings of the IMF and World Bank. ACT UP Philadelphia and its Health GAP allies argued that the institutions, which ostensibly sought to reduce global inequality by lending money to poorer countries, made social crises such as HIV/AIDS worse by requiring those countries to divert their limited resources to debt repayment. Loans also frequently came with "structural adjustment" provisions, which required borrowing countries to privatize key industries and reduce government spending on health care, education, and food subsidies. Both the IMF and World Bank were supported by U.S. policy makers.[48]

As with other demonstrations, ACT UP Philadelphia used people power, creative visuals, and personal testimony to make its point. About five hundred members and allies joined the IMF and World Bank demonstrations on "A16," carrying signs that read, "Poor Nations' Debt 4X Their Health Budget," "Stop Privatizing Health Care," and "IMF: Banking on AIDS Disaster." They marched alongside a 150-pound papier-mâché pig under a banner that read, "IMF/World Bank Start Shakin'. Today's Pig is Tomorrow's Bacon." Asia Russell explained the meaning of the giant prop: "AIDS activists are here today locking down to a giant image of the glutton IMF. . . to call for unconditional debt relief to save the lives of people in poverty living with HIV who are being killed by the policies of the IMF." In a speech on the demonstration's main stage, John Bell put the group's message in the context of his experience as a soldier in Vietnam: "We are fighting against international institutions like the IMF and World Bank that require sovereign nations to reshape their economy to suit the needs of global capital. . . . When I fought in Vietnam, I was told that I was fighting *for* my country, and fighting *for* the poor from another country. Today, I KNOW that I am fighting *against* my country, fighting FOR the poor of other nations." As with the fights over HealthChoices and trade policy,

ACT UP Philadelphia focused on the ways that U.S. public policy supported global capitalism, which resulted in unnecessary suffering among poor people with HIV and AIDS. In the end, protesters failed to stop the IMF and World Bank meetings from taking place but succeeded in getting extensive press coverage for their cause.[49]

In July, ACT UP Philadelphia members once again marched for global access to HIV and AIDS treatment, this time during the International AIDS Conference in Durban, South Africa. There a handful of representatives from the group, including Paul Davis and Melvin White, a Black gay HIV-positive man, went door to door in the city's townships to recruit protesters for a march to demand affordable medicines. Davis later recalled that the experience brought them face to face with the severity of the country's epidemic; during their township organizing, the group witnessed three funeral processions for people who had died of AIDS complications. At the march, South African AIDS activists welcomed their colleagues from Philadelphia and acknowledged their work for global treatment access. In her address to thousands of protesters, Winnie Madikizela-Mandela led a chant of "*phansi!*" (isiZulu for "down") and thanked the activists who had come from "Philadelphia, Guatemala City, and Mumbai to express their outrage at the tyranny of the market and to demand that people come before profit."[50]

For the rest of the summer, ACT UP Philadelphia focused greater attention on the Republican presidential candidate, George W. Bush. Given his pro-business stance, Bush seemed likely to repeal Clinton's executive order on TRIPS, undoing the movement's progress on AIDS drugs for Africa. The Republican National Convention in Philadelphia in late July provided activist groups with an opportunity to co-opt media attention for their cause. For one demonstration, ACT UP Philadelphia joined other activists, doctors, and nurses to demand national single-payer health care. In language reminiscent of the HealthChoices campaign, the group attacked Bush's record of "supporting the profit-driven, care-denying drug companies and insurance firms" and protested a "proposed prescription plan for Medicare [that stood] to line the pockets of drug companies and HMOs." On July 31, the opening day of the convention, ACT UP Philadelphia hung a banner reading, "Bush + Drug Company Greed Kills. Generic AIDS Drugs for Africa Now!" across the face of a billboard next to I-676, a downtown freeway. At another Bush zap less than a month before the election, over five hundred protesters organized by ACT UP Philadelphia marched to the Republican Party National Headquarters, carrying coffins full of empty pill bottles to dump on the building's front steps. In a press release, Paul Davis warned that if Bush rescinded the Clinton executive order on TRIPS, the "reversal will leave millions of Africans for dead, while

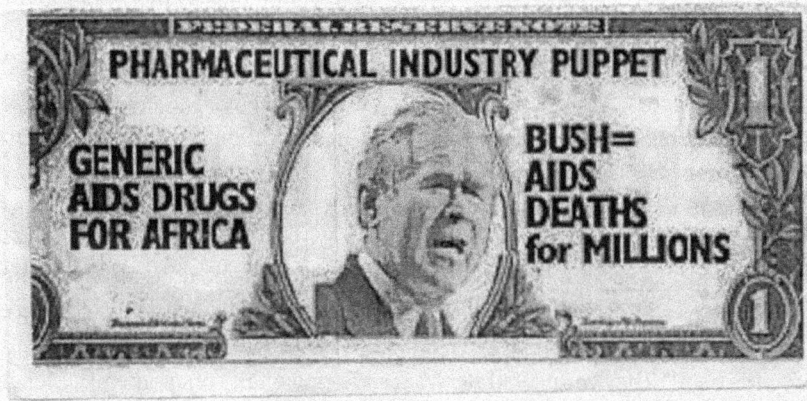

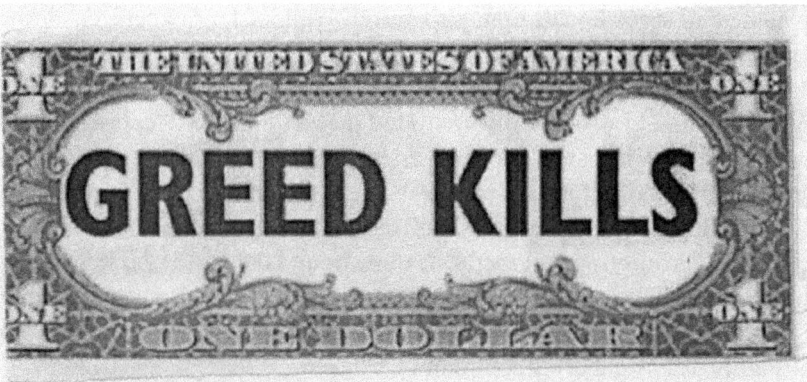

Front and back of a dollar bill prop used as part of ACT UP Philadelphia protests against President George W. Bush, ca. 2002. JD Davids Papers, unprocessed, John J. Wilcox Jr. Archives, William Way LGBT Community Center, Philadelphia, PA.

soaking US taxpayers, [as] Americans will be forced to continue subsidizing the exorbitant profits of the price gouging pharmaceutical industry." In each action, ACT UP Philadelphia argued that Bush's support for capitalist medicine would wreak havoc on the health of the most vulnerable, both at home and abroad.[51]

Bush's contested victory in the presidential election that November brought a mixed bag of policies on global AIDS. The new president did not rescind Clinton's executive order on TRIPS for sub-Saharan Africa, but his administration did file a complaint with the WTO to keep Brazil from supporting compulsory licensing efforts in Africa. Bush also announced that the United States would contribute only $200 million to United Nations secretary general Kofi

Annan's proposed Global Fund to Fight AIDS, Tuberculosis, and Malaria, far short of the $2 billion Annan requested. ACT UP Philadelphia and Health GAP criticized Bush for the paltry commitment, especially in light of his proposed domestic tax cuts. Moreover, the groups feared that such a small donation from the United States would have a "chilling effect" on contributions from other G8 countries, crippling the program.[52]

In June 2001, ACT UP Philadelphia sent buses carrying five hundred demonstrators to a "Stop Global AIDS" rally in New York, where UN delegates gathered for a special session to hash out the terms of the Global Fund. Marching down the Avenue of the Americas through a rain shower, protesters chanted, "Pills cost pennies! Greed costs lives!," and, "We're here, we're wet, it's time to drop the debt!" They connected Bush's trickle-down tax policy, anemic Global Fund commitment, and support for pharmaceutical companies to AIDS deaths at home and abroad, with signs that read, "Trillions for tax cuts, death for people with AIDS," and, "Death by patents, drugs for Africa." According to JD Davids, the activists saw their struggles as the result of the same systemic inequities faced by people halfway around the world. He told reporters, "Our members feel passionate about these issues because they realize that it's the same life-threatening forms of racism and economic injustice that impact their lives here in the United States." Kate Krauss similarly described the "searing experience" of meeting other activists from around the world who were dying for lack of medication. She told the news site *Salon*, "It's not much of a jump from caring about your local community which is being ravaged by AIDS to caring about a neighboring community."[53]

After the terrorist attacks of September 11, 2001, ACT UP Philadelphia and Health GAP members worried that the emerging "war on terror" would sap momentum and resources from the fight against global AIDS. Two months after the attacks, the group held a town hall meeting at the Church of the Advocate in North Philadelphia to discuss their work "in the midst of a new storm." A flyer for the meeting highlighted the daily worldwide death toll from AIDS, over double the number of fatalities in the attacks on Washington and New York, and "primarily in African nations suffering from intense debt burden and the impact of US-led international trade policies that benefit big companies, not people in need of medication." The flyer connected imposed austerity in the developing world and "our communities and cities . . . struggling for resources for health, education and housing, while leaders in Washington, DC cry out for more tax cuts for the rich to promote 'stability.'"[54]

At the same time, AIDS activists around the world celebrated the outcome of the Doha WTO ministerial in Qatar in November 2001, where member countries affirmed that "the [TRIPS] Agreement can and should be interpreted and implemented in a manner supportive of WTO Members' right to protect public health and, in particular, to promote access to medicines for all." The Doha Declaration made clear that developing countries would be able to use compulsory licensing and parallel imports to increase access to essential medicines, including through the importation of generic drugs produced under compulsory licenses in countries such as India and Thailand. As a result, the price of HIV drugs dropped significantly over the next few years.[55]

With the victory at Doha on compulsory licensing and parallel imports, ACT UP Philadelphia pressured Bush to step up the United States' commitment to the Global Fund. In the fall of 2002, as the drumbeat for war with Iraq intensified, the group planned another protest in the capital. The November 26 march on the White House, which would draw demonstrators from New York, Philadelphia, and Baltimore, played on the administration's hawkish rhetoric. One sign read, "AIDS: Code Red Emergency," playing on the color-coded terror alert system introduced after 9/11. Tymm Walker, a Black gay ACT UP Philadelphia member, compared global AIDS to the nuclear, chemical, and biological weapons that administration officials insisted were being stockpiled by Saddam Hussein: "It's a weapon of mass destruction and it's being ignored." Flyers advertising the march implored, "Money for AIDS/Not for War."[56]

March organizers also proposed a "Presidential AIDS Initiative" to expand global treatment access through a sustained, multibillion-dollar annual "investment" by the United States to fight AIDS and other infectious diseases in the developing world. Their plan would offer treatment to three million people with HIV and AIDS worldwide within three years, including generic medications for countries lacking the capacity to produce their own. In addition to a vastly expanded treatment program, the plan called for a "fair-share US contribution to . . . comprehensive HIV prevention in low- and middle-income countries," including "effective economic, social, and public health strategies aimed at women and girls" and support for "children orphaned or left vulnerable by the AIDS pandemic."[57]

Throughout the month following the White House demonstration, ACT UP encouraged supporters to keep up the pressure on Bush by calling, faxing, emailing, and sending letters to the White House. Nevertheless, it came as something of a shock when, in his 2003 State of the Union address, the president called on Congress to enact an Emergency Plan for AIDS Relief. The $15 billion, five-year program would treat and prevent AIDS in the developing world, with a focus on the Caribbean and Africa. AIDS activists welcomed the news. On its website, ACT UP New York linked from Bush's announcement to the page for the White House action with the caption, "THIS DID NOT HAPPEN IN A VACUUM!" On the same page, an anonymous commenter wrote, "The White House

AIDS Initiative bore some fruit. For real: congrats, folks." Indeed, elements of Bush's plan reflected ACT UP's proposed "Presidential AIDS Initiative," including a major increase in AIDS spending in Africa, attention to AIDS orphans, and a larger contribution to the Global Fund.[58]

Nevertheless, AIDS activists remained wary. Some noted that the annual price of medications that Bush had quoted in his address reflected generic pricing for the drugs and wondered if the president thus signaled that the United States would use compulsory licensing and parallel imports to procure drugs for PEPFAR. In a press release, Robert Weissman, codirector of Essential Action, a progressive consumer lobby group, charged that the administration was pushing for restrictive intellectual property rules in its bilateral and regional trade relationships, in violation of an earlier agreement. Activists also criticized the plan's paltry commitment to the Global Fund, with only a billion new dollars for the program, in contrast to the $2.5 billion annual contribution that activists proposed.[59]

Implementing PEPFAR proved complicated. Congressional negotiations stalled over whether funds would be used to perform abortions and the relative weight given to condoms versus abstinence for HIV prevention. Legislators settled on an "ABC" plan that stressed "abstinence" as a primary mode of prevention (with abstinence-only programs receiving a third of the program's prevention dollars) along with "being faithful" for married people and "condoms" as a third option only "when appropriate." Bush initially exempted PEPFAR from the "Global Gag Rule" that bars foreign organizations that provide abortions or abortion referrals from receiving U.S. aid but later reversed his stance. Randall Tobias, who served as global AIDS coordinator for the program's first three years, had also been CEO of the drug manufacturer Eli Lilly, pointing up the president's ties to the pharmaceutical industry. ACT UP Philadelphia and Health GAP had criticized the Clinton administration for strengthening global industry at the expense of the world's poor; even with increased funding for global AIDS through PEPFAR, Bush appeared to do the same.[60]

Still, PEPFAR made significant headway in its first phase, which ended in 2009. HIV treatment was initially slow in coming due to the prohibitively high cost of branded medications. However, PEPFAR countries were able to treat a growing number of people as the program progressed, after a reformed approvals process made cheaper generics available. Scientists estimate that by the end of 2007 the program had saved the lives of 1.2 million people with HIV and prevented perinatal transmission of HIV for almost a quarter-million babies. The program was reauthorized in 2008, 2013, and 2018, and has contributed over $90 billion to the fight against AIDS. Even Bush's critics have praised the program, considered to be the president's "greatest legacy."[61]

ACT UP Philadelphia today counts PEPFAR as one of its major victories, even as current and former members express mixed feelings about the program. Although Kate Krauss later came to think of PEPFAR as a "very sincere thing," she at first saw the program as an effort by the administration "to keep its fingers on the money and use it as leverage in political battles." She felt that "the money should go to the much less political Global Fund, which was international and not bilateral." Jose de Marco credits ACT UP Philadelphia's "constant chasing [Bush] around and embarrassing him" with "getting millions of drugs" to "millions of people in South Africa." Val Sowell also points to the group's role in pushing for PEPFAR but remains ambivalent about the program itself, which she refers to as "a mess we can't do without"—necessary, but politicized and redundant with the Global Fund. She also believes that the role of grassroots activists in pushing for the program has been erased. Instead, she says, PEPFAR "gets to be about Bush and not about us."[62]

Of course, other factors also pushed Bush to announce a major AIDS relief program for Africa in early 2003. Bush had touted his own avowed "compassionate conservatism" during the presidential campaign, and Senator Bill Frist, a surgeon who had done volunteer medical work in Africa, reportedly encouraged the president to make global AIDS a priority. According to one account of PEPFAR's origins, Bush had already pushed top American AIDS scientists to "think big" on the pandemic when activists at the 2002 International AIDS Conference in Barcelona forced the issue by interrupting a speech by Health and Human Services secretary Tommy Thompson. Joseph O'Neill, Bush's newly appointed National AIDS Policy director, reportedly told the president, "These are people who are fighting for their lives. . . . In that kind of circumstance, people do act in ways that are not helpful, but you can't let that get in the way of doing the right thing."[63]

However, by the time of Bush's 2003 State of the Union address, ACT UP Philadelphia had spent four years protesting U.S. policies on AIDS in the developing world and demanding major funding and generic medicines to fight HIV in Africa—both of which became part of U.S. foreign aid policy under PEPFAR. ACT UP Philadelphia also helped change U.S. trade policy toward South Africa. Early actions during the Gore campaign put pithy slogans in front of news cameras, while demonstrations in Philadelphia and Washington showed the global treatment access movement's ability to mobilize large actions, thanks to hundreds of protesters from ACT UP Philadelphia. The group's greatest strength was the people—many of them poor African Americans who were in recovery or who had been incarcerated, or both—whom it empowered to advocate for the rights of similarly disfranchised people around the world.

AS ACT UP PHILADELPHIA EVOLVED during the late 1990s and early 2000s, the group kept alive an activist phenomenon widely presumed to have died out and shifted its center of gravity from middle-class white gay men to poor people of color. Locally as well as globally, the group sought to increase access among the poor to medications that would extend and improve the lives of those living with HIV and AIDS. Members challenged forms of capitalist medicine that restricted access to health care, from managed care and cuts to Medicaid in Pennsylvania to pharmaceutical price gouging in the global South. In both cases, they used grassroots, direct-action protest to win life-saving treatment for people in need. However, their victories left the architecture of Medicaid managed care in place, and the security of trade allowances for generic medicines is tenuous at best.[64]

In a sense, then, ACT UP Philadelphia won numerous battles to improve conditions for people living with HIV and AIDS but failed to reshape the larger political and economic structures in which those people live. Nevertheless, ACT UP Philadelphia's story speaks to the possibility of interracial organizing against AIDS, however fraught that work may be. Together, activists from very different walks of life and around the world imagined and promoted humane alternatives to neoliberal globalization. Whereas other groups linked AIDS in Black America to AIDS in sub-Saharan Africa through the lens of diaspora, ACT UP Philadelphia more often stressed the importance of global class in linking South Philadelphia to South Africa, along with Thailand, Brazil, and other nations that aimed to put people and public health over profits.

## CHAPTER 7

# The South within the North

## SisterLove's Intersectional Approach to HIV/AIDS

IN MANY WAYS IT MAKES SENSE to end this book with the story of SisterLove, an Atlanta-based organization founded by Dázon Dixon Diallo,
which is dedicated to fighting HIV/AIDS among African American women.
For one, the epicenter of the HIV epidemic in the United States sits squarely
in the Deep South, as it has for some time. There, as in Black communities
across the nation, women remain especially vulnerable to the disease and underserved when it comes to both HIV prevention and AIDS care. But it is also
home to some of the most interesting and progressive organizing in the fight
against HIV/AIDS in the United States, which points toward the possibility of
an end to AIDS. As Dixon Diallo herself has said, "For everything that the men
have done to forge the fight on this epidemic, to open the door, it will be the
women who close the door on this epidemic."[1]

The story of SisterLove also runs alongside all of the stories that have pre-
ceded it here. Dixon Diallo became involved in AIDS education and activism
right about the same time that Rashidah Hassan delivered her challenge to
AIDS vigil marchers in Philadelphia and that Black gay men in New York were
starting to organize as Gay Men of African Descent. And because of Sister-
Love's longevity, its more recent history parallels The Balm in Gilead's move
to develop AIDS education in African churches and Health GAP's "AIDS Drugs
for Africa" campaign. There are other connections as well—for a time, Dixon
Diallo even served on Health GAP's board, alongside Jose de Marco of ACT UP
Philadelphia.

Many features of this story will also sound familiar. The frustration that
Dixon Diallo came to feel with white pro-choice activists resembles Rashidah
Hassan's experience with the Philadelphia AIDS Task Force. As with GMAD,
Dixon Diallo and others in SisterLove drew intellectual sustenance from Third
World feminism and advanced a holistic vision of Black women's health and

AIDS politics. And as was the case with the other groups profiled in this book, SisterLove's funding struggles at times threatened to scuttle the organization.

Yet SisterLove's story also adds important layers to the larger narrative. It allows us to see that AIDS activism is connected not only to the women's health movement but specifically to the *Black* women's health movement.[2] Dixon Diallo and SisterLove also took part in a global conversation about women's rights, sexuality, and reproductive health, which shaped their approach to fighting AIDS in Georgia and South Africa. They adopted a consciously intersectional approach, which meant thinking through the ways that power worked along many different axes: not only race, gender, and class, but region and nation as well. As an organization based in the "South within the North," SisterLove fought an uphill battle against neglect, apathy, and vitriol when it came to the health of Black women in the heart of the former Confederacy. But SisterLove also recognized the need to think carefully about the imbalance of power between itself and its community partners in the global South and worked to mitigate it.

Through its work in South Africa, SisterLove mapped a relationship between Black women in the United States and their African counterparts that recognized their differences as well as their similarities. They also worked to make a place for queerness within Blackness, although not in quite the same way the National Task Force on AIDS Prevention or GMAD did. In focusing its AIDS education efforts on women who had been marginalized, including sex workers, incarcerated women, and women on welfare, the group pushed at the boundaries of respectable Black identity to make room for those in need of sister-love.[3]

IT'S NO ACCIDENT that Dázon Dixon Diallo has spent the majority of her life fighting for Black women's sexual and reproductive well-being. While she was growing up in Fort Valley, Georgia, the adults in her life nurtured her passion for the health sciences. Dixon Diallo's parents were both biologists and an aunt worked as a public health nurse; her mother was also her biology teacher. She counts all three as important influences on the path she would take later in life.[4]

Dixon Diallo arrived at Spelman College in the early 1980s. Those years witnessed a succession of important works by Black feminists and other feminists of color. The Combahee River Collective had issued its influential manifesto on "Black feminism as the logical political movement to combat the manifold and simultaneous oppressions that all women of color face" in April 1977. In 1981 Barbara Smith—herself a founding member of Combahee—published

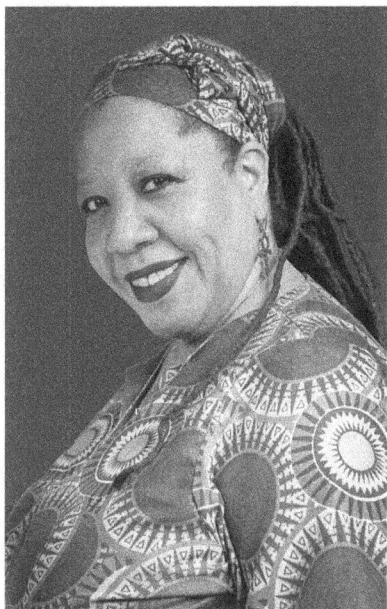

Dázon Dixon Diallo, the founder and president of SisterLove, Inc. Her purple earrings are in the shape of Prince's "love symbol." Photo by Katy Beltran. Courtesy of SisterLove, Inc.

*Home Girls: A Black Feminist Anthology*, with poems and prose examining the many dimensions of Black women's experience, including their sexuality. *This Bridge Called My Back: Writings by Radical Women of Color* came out the same year, giving voice to Latina, Asian American, and Native American women authors as well. Both books were published by Kitchen Table: Women of Color Press, started by Barbara Smith and Audre Lorde. Lorde had also examined women's erotic potential as both an instrument of their oppression and the key to their liberation in her 1978 essay "Uses of the Erotic."[5]

If Dixon Diallo found at Spelman some of the intellectual tools that would ground her work as a sexual health activist, she also found them in her favorite music. Dixon Diallo's teen years coincided with Prince's rise to musical stardom, and she quickly became a devoted fan. A Black feminist analysis of the multiple and intersecting oppressions that made African American women vulnerable to HIV would find its way into SisterLove's programs, but so too would the Purple One's celebration of female sexuality. To this day, Dixon Diallo often incorporates purple—as a scarf, headwrap, lip color, or earrings shaped like the Prince "love symbol"—into her outfits. She sometimes features his music in her presentations as well. When she emceed a plenary session at the 2017 United States Conference on AIDS, she used "Erotic City," which she considers to be her "theme song," as her introductory music.[6]

Spelman also connected Dixon Diallo to the burgeoning Black women's health movement. In 1983 the college hosted the National Conference on Black Women's Health Issues. The conference was sponsored by the National Women's Health Network, a predominantly white feminist organization, and organized by Byllye Avery, a Black feminist health activist who had grown frustrated at the lack of attention to the specific needs of women of color within the larger women's health movement. The conference would give birth to Avery's own organization, the National Black Women's Health Project. It would also be formative for Dixon Diallo. She recalls "seeing all of these incredible black women that I knew from my studies, that I knew from my readings, that I knew from . . . exposure through my mother's work. Here they are, right here in my presence, and I just had to join and see what was happening. I played hooky from work for a whole week to hang out with this incredible movement of women through the National Black Women's Health Project." The conference sparked an interest in the problems of violence and teenage pregnancy that women in the community surrounding Spelman College faced on a daily basis. Dixon Diallo began "to look more specifically into where I might be able to make a difference with other women of color or other women's needs." That interest, in turn, led her to a job at the Feminist Women's Health Center (FWHC).[7]

The conference also gave rise to self-help as a guiding ideology for the National Black Women's Health Project; Dixon Diallo would later adapt it to her work with SisterLove. In the context of the women's health movement, "self-help" meant making women more familiar with their bodies through cervical self-exams. But coming out of the Spelman conference, "self-help" came to mean a therapeutic collective conversation about Black women's experiences. Through the stories of individual women, groups would begin to undo the internalized racism and sexism that contributed to Black women's poor health. As Toni Bond, who became involved in the movement during the 1980s, would later write, "Many of us have so internalized this oppression that it has transformed into a self-hatred and seeps into and impedes our ability to work collectively. . . . In essence, many of us believe the lies we have been told." By healing Black women's internalized oppressions, self-help promised to spark a broader movement for social justice.[8]

The self-help model would become a key piece of SisterLove's approach to HIV/AIDS in Black women, as Avery and others would become mentors to Dixon Diallo. "When I first thought about doing SisterLove, [Byllye Avery] along with Ama Saran, who was also a stalwart sister from National Black Women's Health Project, sat me down. And we had a conversation about what this would look like when you start doing organization work and organizing and building, that you're really doing movement work. And you have to understand that this isn't just about you trying to do a thing. It isn't about just starting a nonprofit, or even it's not just about putting a program into the community. But it is about using what you can do to help women change their own lives."[9]

## Is Your Love Healthy?

Dixon Diallo traces the origins of the "Healthy Love" party to 1985 and the revelation that famed actor Rock Hudson was sick with AIDS. Although Hudson was gay, he had been in the closet for the entirety of his decades-long career. News of the matinee idol's illness sparked a wave of concern about heterosexual HIV transmission. Worried women flooded the hotline at AID Atlanta, where Dixon Diallo was a volunteer. Clearly, there was a need for women to learn how to protect themselves from HIV.[10]

Dixon Diallo and a group of other concerned women gathered to discuss the possibilities for women's AIDS education. These included Sharon Kricun of AID Atlanta; Mary Lynn Hemphill of the FWHC; Sandra McDonald of Outreach, Inc., an AIDS education project targeting African Americans; and Delores French, "a well-known madam in the Atlanta community" and founder of Hooking Is Real Employment (or HIRE), an advocacy group for sex workers. AID Atlanta already had its own safer sex party intervention titled "P.S., I Love You" (the "P.S." stood for "play safe"), which had been developed for gay men. Dixon Diallo and the others adapted the existing workshop for use with women and piloted the first "Do It Safe" party in February 1987.[11]

The party soon became a regular part of the FWHC's offerings, and the Women's AIDS Prevention Project—with Dixon Diallo at the helm—found a home at the center. As with other safe-sex party interventions, Do It Safe emphasized knowledge about HIV transmission and eroticizing safer sex. Women were encouraged to craft sexual fantasies that would also carry little risk of HIV transmission. In one activity, the "Box of Safe, Erotic Potential," participants were asked to use a variety of household items (suggestions included a turkey baster, a jar of honey, and a feather duster) to "conjure their own ideas of a potential safe sex experience." Other activities taught participants how to put on a condom, introduced them to dental dams, or had them role-play negotiating safer sex with a partner.[12]

However, at the same time that Dixon Diallo was getting the Women's AIDS Prevention Project off the ground, the FWHC became a target for anti-abortion activists. Randall Terry and his group Operation Rescue took advantage of the media platform offered by the Democratic National Convention in the summer of 1988, staging three days of direct action against Atlanta abortion providers, including the FWHC. The three-day campaign turned into a months-long ordeal, as anti-abortion activists refused to give their names to police, instead remaining in jail. Meanwhile, Operation Rescue continued its campaign of intimidation.[13]

The blockades took their toll not only on the FWHC's clients and staff but on the clinic's finances as well. Fighting Operation Rescue in the courts while protecting the clinic from the threat of violence meant hiring lawyers as well as off-duty police. In the end, FWHC cofounder Lynne Randall estimated that Operation Rescue had cost the clinic $100,000. That cost meant that staff and programs, including the Women's AIDS Prevention Project, had to be cut.[14]

Dixon Diallo recalls that from the "practical side" of the FWHC's finances, cutting the Women's AIDS Prevention Project was completely justifiable. But from her perspective, it also revealed a central tension within the organization: AIDS was not a concern for the middle-class white women who ran the FWHC, nor was it a particular problem for those women—others like themselves—whom they imagined as their clientele. According to Dixon Diallo, "That was the perception for those of us women of color in the community: that AIDS is not their issue, but it is ours, and we'd better do something about it."[15]

When Dixon Diallo left the FWHC, she renamed the Do It Safe program "Healthy Love" and revised the curriculum "to capture the interest of women at high-risk, specifically African-American women and other women of color." AIDS prevention remained the focus of the party but within a broader set of issues that impacted participants' lives. The manual opened not with a discussion of the disease but with a series of questions: "If you love someone who beats on you and yells constantly, is your love healthy? If your partner is using drugs, and you may have tried them because you love him/her, is your love healthy?" "Healthy love" meant not only supportive relationships with significant others but also "the kind of love that one has for herself so that she may live healthy and feel empowered to make decisions." From this sense of empowerment, healthy relationships would follow.[16]

Other revisions to the Healthy Love curriculum emphasized the self-help discussion model as well. Facilitators were instructed to create an atmosphere in which women would be comfortable sharing personal experiences and to have the group sit in a circle to signal that everyone was on equal ground. The curriculum emphasized that this was important for "bring[ing] in the self-help approach to AIDS prevention and education." In turn, self-help could be "a catalyst for change in women's condition and women's lives."[17]

As the epidemic grew, Dixon Diallo worried about the impact of HIV among poor and rural Black women. She encountered women in the first group through her work as a counselor at the Grady Hospital Infectious Disease Clinic, where many received their HIV diagnosis. She knew women in the second group through her ties to Fort Valley, which was also home to the historically Black Fort Valley State College (now Fort Valley State University). In 1990 the town of just around eight thousand was in the midst of twin epidemics of drug use and sexually transmitted infections. Dixon Diallo got the idea to tackle AIDS among both groups at once. With funding from the American Foundation for AIDS Research, she partnered both with the Center for Black Women's Wellness, a program of the National Black Women's Health Project housed in McDaniel-Glenn Community, one of Atlanta's public housing projects, and with the Fort Valley chapter of Delta Sigma Theta sorority. Under the name Women United for Women at Risk, she trained women in both places to facilitate their own Healthy Love parties. As with similar programs by GMAD and the NTFAP, Women United for Women at Risk was built on the idea that training vulnerable people to educate their peers about safer sex could change sexual norms in the community as a whole.[18]

The experience of facilitating HIV education with women through Women United for Women at Risk uncovered a deep need for the program, along with formidable challenges. SisterLove reported to the American Foundation for AIDS Research that the women involved felt the work was "long overdue" and were "starving for this kind of support and attention." But AIDS prevention and care was just one way in which the women had been ignored and overlooked, and HIV was "just one of many problems that they have." Some tailored the program to their context, as with a group of women in public housing who used "a 'street team' approach with 'familiar folk' to recruit women into their groups." However, some of the same women lacked the ability to read and write, which made evaluating the success of the program through responses to a written survey difficult.[19]

As the work with women in McDaniel-Glenn made clear, poor Black women in Atlanta were dealing with more than just HIV. Many also struggled to find stable housing, were raising children on their own, or had been caught up in the carceral system. HIV made these problems worse, and vice versa. Women who tested positive or developed AIDS were shunned by their families, and homelessness made it difficult for HIV-positive women to take care of their health.

But the clinical definition of AIDS handed down by the CDC was based on the way that the disease presented in men and left out the opportunistic infections commonly experienced by HIV-positive women. Because federal agencies used the CDC's definition to determine eligibility for disability and housing benefits, many women with AIDS were left to fend for themselves. Being based in Atlanta, SisterLove was well situated to join the coordinated effort to force change at the CDC by a coalition of groups advocating for women with AIDS. But not only was the campaign about winning social benefits; it was also part of the same fight for Black women's sexual autonomy that animated all of SisterLove's work.

## Opening Pandora's Box

During the first decade of the epidemic, few women with AIDS could be diagnosed as such. Doctors diagnosed patients with AIDS using the CDC's case definition, which consisted of a number of opportunistic infections. A patient who presented with several of these at once would receive an AIDS diagnosis. But the definition was based on how the disease presented in gay men during the early years of the epidemic and did not include many of the opportunistic infections typically seen in women with advanced HIV disease. Without an AIDS diagnosis, women could not access any of the social benefits or services available to people with the disease. Since women of color, and Black women in particular, were more likely to be infected with HIV than their white counterparts, they suffered disproportionately as a result of being excluded from the CDC definition. It would take a sustained campaign led by women, including the National Women's Committee of ACT UP, the Women's Caucus of ACT UP New York, and Terry McGovern of the HIV Law Project, to change the definition. Women of color, including Dixon Diallo, would play an important role in that campaign.

The campaign combined legal strategy with direct action tactics. Terry McGovern of the HIV Law Project filed a class action lawsuit against Secretary of Health and Human Services Louis Sullivan, claiming that the means for determining "HIV-related disability were arbitrary, capricious and contrary to the mandates of the Social Security Act." Meanwhile, ACT UP and allied groups rallied hundreds of people at a time at the offices of the CDC, responsible for the AIDS case definition, and the Department of Health and Human Services, which oversaw the welfare programs denied to women with the disease. Chanting "CDC, you can't hide, we charge you with genocide" and "Murder by omission, change the definition," they staged die-ins, occupied agency office buildings, and, during one demonstration at the CDC, draped a black banner with the message "CDC KILLS" over the side of the building. Dozens, if not hundreds, were arrested at each demonstration. While being dragged into paddy wagons they shouted, "Women die, they do nothing!" and "Act up! Fight back! Fight AIDS!"[20]

In flyers and policy documents, ACT UP placed the redefinition campaign at the intersection of race, class, and gender. Participants argued that "the CDC refuses to expand the definition to reflect what is currently known about the manifestation of AIDS in communities other than white, middle-class, gay men." Additionally, they pointed out, many women with HIV/AIDS were also poor, and three-quarters of those who *had* been diagnosed with AIDS under the CDC's definition were women of color. As Terry McGovern recalls, "The original AIDS definition was not looking at the concept of converging epidemics. So tuberculosis wasn't in it; bacterial pneumonia wasn't in it. So it wasn't just women; it was lots and lots of poor people, if you had to pick a denominator."[21]

Direct action tactics gave poor women of color with AIDS the opportunity to speak—outside of federal agencies, through a bullhorn—truth to power. At one demonstration at the Department of Health and Human Services in Washington, D.C., Phyllis Sharpe, a formerly homeless African American woman from Brooklyn, told her story of being denied disability benefits despite being unable to work due to fatigue and repeated urinary tract infections. Iris de la Cruz, a Puerto Rican former sex worker, described women with AIDS dying of preventable, treatable infections after being denied access to Medicaid: "I don't want to die. I don't want to die of PID [pelvic inflammatory disease]. I don't want to die of AIDS." Katrina Haslip was there too, holding a tombstone-shaped sign that read, "Women with HIV Get Cervical Cancer" above her head, her short dreadlocks gathered into pigtails. While incarcerated at Bedford Hills Correctional Facility, she had converted to Islam, came out as HIV positive, and helped to found AIDS Counseling and Education. She would die from AIDS-related illness just a month before the CDC officially changed its AIDS definition in January 1993.[22]

Living in Atlanta, Dixon Diallo was well positioned to participate in protests at the CDC headquarters. At the first, in January 1990, she delivered a short speech in which she put the demand to change the AIDS definition in the context of other forces that endangered the lives of women of color, who "endure more violence within our communities and relationships, are subject to more crimes, are more vulnerable to the drug epidemic, have poorer health care, survive more rape and incest experiences, have fewer sexual and reproductive health choices, and die faster of most terminal diseases." Those problems predated AIDS, but the disease had "opened a gigantic Pandora's box of the social ills and oppression that women of color are existing or surviving through." The epidemic, she argued, had revealed "the western, white, male dominated culture in its true form": one content to watch people die "in the name of investment and profit, poor healthcare planning, and lack of interest in those lives most affected by AIDS."[23]

Protests continued at other federal agencies throughout the year, returning to the CDC in December 1990. For World AIDS Day on December 1, SisterLove's Community AIDS Resource and Education Fair included a teach-in by ACT UP. Two days later, on Monday, December 3, ACT UP marched on the CDC in pouring rain to again demand that the definition be expanded to include women. Maxine Wolfe, a veteran of leftist movements and member of ACT UP's Women's Caucus, recalls, "It was the most pouring rain day I've ever seen in my life. It was not to be believed. And people stayed out there. Women with HIV stayed out there. It was just really powerful."[24]

At one point during the demonstration, ACT UP members pushed their way into the building and occupied CDC offices before being arrested. Available footage suggests that the overwhelming majority of those who did were white activists; Dixon Diallo hints at why by pointing to the history of violent retribution against African Americans who dared to challenge the status quo in the Deep South. Riffing on the message that "we have to no longer be silent, and that silence kills"—reflected in the "Silence = Death" T-shirts worn by many in ACT UP—she recalls that "as southern women and black southern women, we learned for generations that silence will save your life, because if you talk back, they might kill you. The more angry you get, the worse your punishment will be, not the better." Although Dixon Diallo and SisterLove worked with ACT UP Atlanta and others to change the CDC's definition of AIDS, not everyone in the coalition could afford the risk of adopting ACT UP's confrontational tactics and angry tone.[25]

The problems facing women with HIV went far beyond the CDC. For Dixon Diallo and other feminist activists, the case definition was just one way that sexism shaped the study and treatment of AIDS. Women of childbearing age were excluded from clinical trials of experimental AIDS drugs, out of concern that the medications might harm any fetus they could conceive in the future. Pregnant women with HIV were counseled to have abortions on one hand but denied services by abortion providers on the other. At the same time, news media reported on women with AIDS as "reservoirs of disease" waiting to infect male partners. Furthermore, the notion of woman-to-woman transmission was nowhere to be found in the AIDS science agenda, as noted in the ACT UP chant "CDC, can't you see? Lesbians get HIV!" All in all, women with HIV were treated only as vectors of disease that might infect (straight) men or the unborn, but not as people deserving of a healthy life in their own right.

The larger issues of gender, racial, and medical justice at play in the campaign to redefine AIDS were laid out in *Women, AIDS, and Activism*, a volume of short essays that started out as a booklet for ACT UP's women and AIDS teach-in and was published by the ACT UP New York Women and AIDS Book Group in 1990. The book included Dixon Diallo's speech, along with essays by Iris De la Cruz; Sunny Rumsey, an AIDS educator of Afro-Caribbean and Native American descent; DiAna DiAna and Bambi Sumpter, who offered AIDS education to Black women through DiAna's hair salon; and Charon Asetoyer, who would go on to become a founding member of SisterSong, a women of color reproductive health collective that also included SisterLove.

The assertion of the right of women with HIV/AIDS to make choices about their health and reproduction connected feminist AIDS activists not only to the reproductive rights movement but specifically to the ways that movement took shape among women of color. At a time when many feminists of color were frustrated by the narrow focus of middle-class white feminists on access to abortion, contributors to *Women, AIDS, and Activism* highlighted the larger issues of bodily autonomy at play. They linked the status of women of color and poor women with AIDS to histories of eugenics and forced sterilizations, which had been used for generations to rob Black, Latina, and Native American women of the right to have children. They argued that the ways in which women of color had historically been denied bodily autonomy were perpetuated in the testing and treatment of women with HIV, the majority of whom were women of color.[26] As Dixon Diallo put it in a 2009 oral history, "I want access to abortion, but I also don't want to be discriminated against by people who want to force abortion on me as a choice because they don't believe in HIV-positive women's sexuality and ability to parent."[27]

As Dixon Diallo and others in the campaign to redefine AIDS made clear, the deadly intersection of racism, misogyny, and poverty meant that Black women with HIV died faster than perhaps any other group affected by the disease. But if AIDS was an outgrowth of the "Pandora's box" of oppression that Black women faced, then Dixon Diallo might make some headway by striking at the root of the problem. Many of the programs that SisterLove developed over the next several years would do just that.

## Building a Movement

Just as women with HIV played a key role in the campaign to redefine AIDS, so too did they shape SisterLove's programs. This was born out of the ethic of Black feminist self-help, with its focus on giving women the space to speak and be heard. Dázon Dixon Diallo recalls that she "would just start going to the [Grady Hospital Infectious Disease Clinic] on Fridays, when they would host the Women's Clinic, and would just sit in the waiting room. . . . I would turn off the TV, you know, Phil Donahue was still on back then . . . and start talking with women about what was going on with them. . . . Other than health needs, what did they need?"[28]

Dixon Diallo's recollection of talking to women in the Grady clinic waiting room distills the Black feminist foundations of SisterLove's work to an archetypal scene. Within the walls of the hospital, historically a space of both white male authority and Black women's trauma, Dixon Diallo invited Black women not only to talk about their experiences (and in this telling literally silenced an authoritative white man) but to act as experts on their own health and care. Dixon Diallo continues, "Out of that same support mechanism[—]just by listening to women's stories and how common the experiences of discrimination, or just being treated differently by their families, or being put out of their own homes, of losing their housing, or being at risk of losing their housing . . .[—] just by listening to the women's stories and ideas about what they might need, we ended up creating the first transitional housing program for women with HIV and their children in the South."[29]

That program was LoveHouse, which began in 1992 when a SisterLove supporter offered her condominium to women living with HIV. SisterLove managed the lease and provided support services for the women living there, but the small, shabby space could hold only four single women. Dixon Diallo knew that there were more HIV-positive women, including those with children, who needed a place to live while getting back on their feet. LoveHouse would need to expand.[30]

Dixon Diallo got a lead on two adjacent homes, owned by another advocacy organization, in a predominantly Black section of southwest Atlanta. Set back from the road and surrounded by a thicket of tall trees, the two-acre property would offer residents peace and privacy. SisterLove began leasing one home, which housed seven single women, starting in June 1993. The following year it purchased both properties, which increased its capacity to ten single women and five of their children. SisterLove submitted grants to cover the purchase of the properties and start-up costs for the program and received funding from the Metropolitan Atlanta Community Foundation, the Atlanta Women's Fund, and the City of Atlanta's Housing Opportunities for People with AIDS.[31]

LoveHouse was meant to be a transitional space where HIV-positive women could stay while receiving "support and resources to transition from dependency to independence." But SisterLove's clients needed more than just housing. Many came from backgrounds marred by poverty and violence and required "specialized support and training to address needs such as substance addiction, sexual abuse recovery, domestic violence and effective parenting techniques." In this way, SisterLove aimed "to develop the overall quality of women's lives, and not just focus . . . on their HIV status." Several years later, the group would reflect that "incorporating a holistic framework of social service delivery and advocacy . . . had [a] historical impact on improving the lives of women at risk and living with HIV/AIDS, as well as their families."[32]

SisterLove's other programs promoted the same goal of giving women with HIV agency over their own lives, as well as over the group's AIDS advocacy agenda. Beginning in 1992, SisterLove organized OurTime, an annual "private healing retreat" to St. Helena Island in South Carolina. The women on the retreat, who were drawn from the HIV-positive women's support group at the Grady women's clinic, determined the program for the retreat.[33] The advice that Dixon Diallo received from Byllye Avery and Ama Saran about "using what you can do to help women change their own lives" echoes through a 1993 proposal for a grant to fund the following year's OurTime retreat: "The beginning of finding some solutions to address HIV+ Women's needs is to provide time, space and support for the women to share some of their ideas, with each other first, and with SISTERLOVE next." Indeed, the proposal argued, women from previous retreats had "solidified a system of support for a program which has become mostly their own."[34]

The setting for OurTime also suggests that, as with GMAD, a connection to Black history and diaspora could empower and heal in the context of AIDS. The retreat was held at Penn Center, the historic site of a school for African Americans established after the liberation of the South Carolina Sea Islands during the Civil War. It was also home to an annual festival celebrating Gullah culture, which is notable for preserving the traditions of enslaved West Africans brought to what is now the southeastern United States during the eighteenth century. Moreover, women on the retreat could visit Oyotunji African Village, an "intentional community in North America, based on the culture of the Yoruba and Dahomey tribes of West Africa."[35] While not explicitly connected to the weekend's discussion about HIV treatment or living with AIDS, the choice to hold the retreat at a site steeped in the preservation of Black history and tradition was no accident. Rather, it was an integral part of SisterLove's mission of healing and empowerment.

## Forming a Collective

Just as the feminism that grounded her work in founding SisterLove was international in scope, the horizon for Dixon Diallo's movement building lay far beyond Georgia. Before they called themselves "women of color," writer-activists like Barbara Smith and Pat Parker called themselves "Third World women" to capture the solidarity they felt with the global South and their opposition to the capitalism and militarism of the United States and its allies. Likewise, feminists from the global South shifted the international conversation about population and development from a focus on population control, which sought to limit women's fertility in order to spur economic development, to reproductive and human rights, which enabled women to decide whether and when to have children. This effort to center the global development agenda on the human rights of women, with input from a diverse set of feminist voices from around the world, was spurred on by the announcement of the United Nations Decade for Women, designated from 1975 to 1985.[36]

The same international conferences that helped to foster a global feminist movement driven by women from the global South also shaped Dixon Diallo's activism. The first of these was a 1988 trip to Belize for a conference on reproductive health and self-help with Byllye Avery. They traveled "with bags full of speculums and the Chux mats and the mirrors and the flashlights and the K-Y Jelly" that they used to teach women to do cervical self-exams. She recalls how "it was the most empowering experience to share that . . . sense of power that came from knowing this most intimate part of yourself." Although she was not yet bringing messages about AIDS to global audiences of women, the same emphasis on women's sexual autonomy and empowerment would ground her later efforts to do so.[37]

Two years after Belize, in 1990, Dixon Diallo traveled to Quezon City in the Philippines for the Sixth International Women and Health Meeting. That experience highlighted both the limitations of the U.S. women's movement and the need to bring AIDS into the global women's health agenda. In the first instance, Dixon Diallo found herself in Quezon City as one of only a handful of women of color from the United States in a much larger delegation. In the second instance, "there was very little, if any, inclusion of HIV/AIDS in the agenda or in any overall platforms around reproductive health and rights." The experience made clear to Diallo that women of color in particular needed to claim a place at the table when it came to discussions of women's health and reproductive rights, to make sure that intersectional issues like HIV/AIDS would not be overlooked. Thereafter she "started making a way of forming delegations to get to all of these meetings and meet with women who were dealing with HIV and AIDS and other reproductive rights issues, and learn from what they were doing, how they were challenged by some of the issues on the ground, and how they were responding and what that was like and what we could learn and what we might be able to share."[38]

Dixon Diallo organized delegations to key international conferences on women's and reproductive rights, advocating at every turn for HIV/AIDS to be on the agenda. Those meetings included two watershed moments in the history of the global women's health movement: the 1994 International Conference on Population and Development in Cairo and the 1995 Fourth World Conference on Women in Beijing. The Cairo meeting was notable for the "unprecedented involvement in . . . drafting the Program of Action," which urged "governments to restructure their population policies to address such issues as the reduction of maternal mortality, the prevention and treatment of sexually transmitted diseases, including HIV/AIDS, the prevention and treatment of unsafe abortion, and, above all, the empowerment of women." The 1995 meeting in Beijing built on the Cairo framework, adding language about women's sexual rights: "The human rights of women include their right to have control over and decide freely and responsibly in matters related to their sexuality, including sexual and reproductive health, free of coercion, discrimination and violence." Although language regarding sexual orientation was struck from the final consensus document, Dixon Diallo recalls that the SisterLove delegation incorporated sexual diversity, along with issues of violence and sexual autonomy, into the conference's HIV/AIDS workshops: "We did present a lot of the workshops that were focused on HIV and AIDS, and we brought in the many different intersections. So we had even a section on HIV and lesbians. We had a section on HIV and violence. We had safer sex and how women can negotiate in difficult spaces."[39]

Alongside and in conversation with the global movement for women's rights, women of color within the United States had built their own movement for gender justice. As historian of feminist politics Jennifer Nelson has observed, these women argued, beginning in the 1970s, that "freedom from simultaneous sexual, racial, and class oppressions could only be achieved with voluntary reproductive control." The conversations about women's rights as human rights taking place in Cairo and Beijing also shaped the way that women of color were thinking about their work within the United States. A few months before the Cairo meeting, a group of Black women, including representatives from the National Black Women's Health Project and the Chicago Abortion Fund, gathered informally at a conference sponsored by the Illinois Pro-choice Alliance. They shared their frustrations with the mainstream abortion rights movement: with its narrow focus on "choice," the movement alienated women to whom an even more fundamental freedom to make choices about their reproduction had been denied. These included women who had been sterilized or given contraceptives without their consent, those who lost children to the high rates of infant mortality that plagued poor communities of color, and those who "chose" to terminate otherwise wanted pregnancies because they lacked the resources to raise a child. The women in the Chicago group had tried, with mixed results, to bring these issues to majority-white feminist groups. Loretta Ross, who had served as director of Women of Color programs for the National Organization for Women before moving to the National Black Women's Health Project in Atlanta, had experienced these frustrations first-hand.[40]

But Ross and the others were also well versed in the work that women activists, from the Combahee River Collective to feminists in the global South, had done to put individual health in a broader framework of social justice. There they found "a connective framework that ties economic justice, human rights, reproductive rights, immigration rights . . . together." In time, they would label this "reproductive justice." At the Cairo meeting they "fortified" this approach "by heeding women of the Global South who used the human rights framework to make stronger claims for sexual and reproductive autonomy, emphasizing the dialectic between individual and group rights." Ross recalls that "the primary consensus reached at Cairo was the link made between development, poverty and reproductive health. . . . The lack of sexual health for women results from poverty as well as gender inequality, particularly in sexual relationships, such as with HIV/AIDS and violence against women." In years to come, advocates for reproductive justice would look for ways to "Bring Cairo Home" to the United States. Ross would do so through her organization, the National Center for Human Rights Education, which became a founding member of SisterSong.[41]

The SisterSong collective began in 1997 with meetings in New York and Savannah, Georgia, organized by the Latina Roundtable on Reproductive Health and Rights. Made up of sixteen organizations, SisterSong aimed to address reproductive tract infections (RTIS) among African American, Latina, Asian/ Pacific Islander, and Native American women. RTIS include sexually transmitted infections such as HIV, as well as yeast infections and complications from unsafe abortions and other negligent medical care. Women of color suffer disproportionately from RTIS, which often go undiagnosed and untreated, leading to infertility, disease, and death. SisterSong articulated a platform for collective advocacy around RTIS among women of color that would encompass the needs of the four constituent communities while building up organizations that addressed those needs at the grassroots level. Self-help philosophy would guide the women's work along the way, while workshops on human rights and reproductive justice would help the whole collective place the health needs of U.S. women of color within a larger conversation about the rights and status of women worldwide.[42]

Officials at the Ford Foundation were also interested in translating the global women's movement to a domestic context. During the late 1980s and 1990s the feminist leaders within Ford had sensitized it to the perspectives and approaches of women's rights activists in the global South, particularly as they concerned the fight against AIDS. At the same time, Alexandrina "Reena" Marcelo, a program officer in Ford's Human Development and Reproductive Health program, wanted to channel funding to reproductive rights groups for women of color, including the kinds of organizations that would not normally be considered for major grants. She dedicated her entire portfolio, totaling around $4 million, to SisterSong.[43]

Work as part of the collective fit well within SisterLove's mission and ethos. Just as Dixon Diallo had worked to put HIV in the broader context of women's sexual rights and well-being, SisterSong did so with RTIS. SisterSong's mission also focused in part on helping smaller organizations to grow ("capacity building," in the language of nonprofits), which resembled the "movement building" work that Byllye Avery and others had encouraged Dixon Diallo to do. The other African American member organizations were also connected to SisterLove in more ways than one. Dixon Diallo served as program director for Ross's National Center for Human Rights Education, and Ross sat on SisterLove's board. Another member group, the California Black Women's Health Project, was a branch of Avery's National Black Women's Health Project, which had inspired Dixon Diallo to focus her work on Black women's health years earlier. And the final African American group was Project Azuka, an AIDS service organization in Savannah, Georgia, that began as a "chapter" of SisterLove.[44]

Membership in SisterSong was attractive for other reasons as well. In the late 1990s, SisterLove was going through tough financial times. Dixon Diallo had left the organization in 1995 to pursue a master's degree in public health at the University of Alabama. The woman she had hired to replace her as executive director neglected to file tax returns and proved unable to manage the group's public grants. SisterLove racked up a $45,000 tax debt, and Dixon Diallo "returned to SisterLove to keep her doors open, [as] the IRS was preparing to close them." In order to pay down the debt, Dixon Diallo was forced to trim the group's budget, which meant "collaborat[ing] with other women's and AIDS organizations to meet the needs of our constituents/clients that we cannot provide." SisterSong was one such collaboration, and SisterLove received over $600,000 in grant money from the Ford Foundation through the project.[45]

SisterLove's money troubles were not unique. As Dixon Diallo wrote to Marcelo, the group was "struggling with very common problems as a grassroots organization run by women of color." In an oral history recorded in late 2004 and early 2005, Loretta Ross called this "the classic funding trap," in which organizations receive "program money but not capacity building money." In her words, "We get paid on how many trainings you do around [Healthy

Love] parties but then they won't pay the staff person to do the [Healthy Love] parties, or pay to help you develop your financial records or your board of directors [and] then accuse you of bad financial management. You know, it's just—it's an endless cycle of contempt, how women of color often are treated by foundations." With this in mind, SisterSong leaders successfully argued that the first three years of Ford funding to the collective should focus on capacity building. As a result, all of the member groups obtained 501(c)3 status and were able to pay consultants to show them "how to do organizational development and do fund-raising and leadership development."[46]

At the same time, member groups continued their specific work on HIV and other RTIs. SisterLove revised the Healthy Love party curriculum to include RTIs other than HIV and trained new facilitators to present the program at colleges, with community groups, for Atlanta Job Corps trainees, and at Dekalb County Jail. The California Black Women's Health Project likewise presented Healthy Love to women at the Well, its resource center in South Central Los Angeles, as well as at local women's shelters. It also joined the Alliance of Black Women Organizations, a coalition group chaired by Congresswoman Maxine Waters and "committed to spreading the word about the changing faces of HIV/AIDS." For its part, the National Center for Human Rights Education developed a workshop titled "HIV Is a Human Rights Issue," putting the disease in an explicitly moral and political framework that focused on the rights and well-being of the sick, as well as on the larger social and political context in which they lived.[47]

According to Loretta Ross, the initial three-year capacity-building grant was to be followed by a second grant phase, in which member groups would focus more on developing their programs. But when it came time in 2001 to renew the Ford Foundation's funding for SisterSong, conditions had changed. Most importantly, Chukwudi "Chu Chu" Saunders had taken over for Reena Marcelo as the program officer in charge of the collective. The SisterSong grant files are vague as to why Saunders terminated SisterSong's funding after the initial funding period. Dixon Diallo wrote in a memo to Saunders that she appreciated the other woman's "candor" about SisterSong, suggesting that she took a critical view of the program. Saunders likewise referred elliptically in internal memos to "lessons learned from the SisterSong initiative." Loretta Ross recalls that Saunders's tenure at Ford, though short, "was so destructive in that year and a half, it was just amazing." She adds that Saunders "didn't believe in collectives [and] certainly didn't believe in SisterSong."[48]

Whether or not Saunders "didn't believe in collectives" is likewise unclear from the Ford Foundation files, but Saunders *did* elect to fund a new women of color collective just as SisterSong's grant was ending. It is also clear that reproductive justice principles became part of Ford's thinking about the reproductive health portfolio. In presenting this new grant, named the Paths to Health Justice Initiative, Saunders described the same problems cited by reproductive justice activists: the narrow scope of the U.S. abortion rights movement and the need to connect it to the broader human rights agenda laid out at Cairo and Beijing.[49]

After the end of Ford funding, SisterSong considered disbanding, but according to Ross the group recognized "that we could only do together things that we couldn't do individually." Instead, it started planning a national conference to be SisterSong's "public debut" and to "bring together what we thought was the missing voices of women of color who worked on reproductive health issues." The SisterSong Women of Color Reproductive Health and Sexual Rights National Conference at Spelman College in November 2003 (twenty years after the conference that birthed the National Black Women's Health Project) drew over a hundred speakers and at least four times as many participants. SisterSong was here to stay.[50]

Despite the painful end of the Ford Foundation funding for the collective, support for SisterLove through SisterSong helped to sustain the organization as it struggled to get back on its feet. During this time SisterLove entered a new phase in its development. Building on the global vision of sexual health and rights for women and a reproductive justice movement among women of color, SisterLove would travel halfway around the world to South Africa, where the HIV epidemic threatened to undo a fragile experiment in multiracial democracy.

## SisterLove Goes Global

Dázon Dixon Diallo developed connections to AIDS prevention in Africa early on in her time with SisterLove. In 1991 she applied for funding from the International Center for Research on Women to support a collaboration with the Society for Women against AIDS-Nigeria. Dixon Diallo had met the group's president, Dr. Ibironke Akinsete, while conducting AIDS education workshops in the country. Dixon Diallo argued that a set of common challenges warranted a partnership between the two groups, despite the thousands of miles that separated them. "In the United States," she wrote, "most of the women of color are living below the poverty level, and in many cases, survive situations similar to women in 'developing' countries around the world." If poverty, powerlessness, stigma, and denial affected Black women on both sides of the Atlantic, Dixon Diallo proposed, then the Healthy Love program could empower women in Lagos to protect themselves against HIV, as it had for their counterparts in Atlanta. The project went unfunded, but key elements of the proposal—partnership between SisterLove and African AIDS groups, a sense of common experience among women of African descent in different parts of the world, and an emphasis on self-help as a means of AIDS prevention—would be features of SisterLove's later endeavors into Africa as well.[51]

By the end of the decade, as the U.S. government came to see global AIDS as a threat to security and stability in the global South, federal money became available for the type of partnership that Dixon Diallo had proposed years before. In 1999 the CDC and the United States Agency for International Development funded SisterLove to develop the Women's HIV/AIDS Resource Project in partnership with the National Center for Human Rights Education and three South African groups: Positive Women's Network, the Society for Women against AIDS-South Africa, and the Township AIDS Project. The first two groups had been founded by Prudence Mabele, one of the first women in South Africa to publicly reveal her HIV-positive status, whom Dixon Diallo had met during the 1995 Beijing women's conference. Like SisterSong, the Women's HIV/AIDS Resource Project combined education about HIV and other reproductive tract infections with discussions about women's human and reproductive rights.[52]

The project was one of several in the CDC's Linkages Program, which paired AIDS groups in the United States with counterparts in the global South. As part of this work, SisterLove produced a manual for transnational AIDS partnerships, which evinced the influence of Black feminism on the way the group thought about its partnerships with organizations in the global South.[53]

Written by M. Bahati Kuumba, a professor of women's studies at Spelman College, the manual emphasized that in transnational partnerships between organizations in the global North and their counterparts in the global South, agencies should "avoid posing a North → South bias and ... place emphasis on the mutual learning and symbiotic relationship of transnational partnerships." A "'South within the North' NGO" like SisterLove, which served clients marginalized by race, gender, and class within the United States, still needed to think about its own power relative to partner groups in poorer countries. In an interview with Kuumba, SisterLove staffer Seseni Nu remarked that the project "is about sharing knowledge in a horizontal manner rather than a vertical manner. You have to be careful when you are a primary grantee ... [of taking] on the donor mentality of dictating what the sub-grantees [do], or even [of using] that term 'sub-grantee' ... You have to be mindful of your ... assumptions that you may make in terms of what capacities or what capabilities our sister[s] have in South Africa." In other words, even a group like SisterLove needed to take pains to avoid seeing its partners through a colonial lens.[54]

As with SisterSong, SisterLove used self-help to overcome "conflicts and tensions" that arose with the other organizations in the Women's HIV/AIDS Resource Project. The partnerships manual likewise offered the discussion model as a "vehicle for participants to tell their personal stories, to process . . . what it will take for black women to work together on black women's health issues under conditions of stress and oppression." Here Kuumba and SisterLove carried forward the intellectual legacy of the Black women's health movement, offering insights to other agencies working in the global South as well.[55]

But making headway against global AIDS would take more than individual healing; the context in which SisterLove operated would need to change as well. Kuumba emphasized that the group's work responded to "the most lethal manifestations of capitalist-driven globalization." This was true in South Africa as well as in Atlanta, since "austerity programs, trends towards privatization, and economic polarization . . . made health and other basic services more difficult to obtain" for women of color worldwide. Whether they lived in the glimmering "New South" Atlanta of CNN and right-to-work laws or in the "New South Africa," where the afterlife of apartheid haunted the political landscape, SisterLove's clients grappled with the worst effects of global profit-seeking.[56]

At the same time, Kuumba stressed that the partnership between Sister-Love and the South African groups represented "grassroots globalization." Here activists had leveraged communications technology, international conferences, and the global nature of the epidemic into "a growing and dynamic transnationalism." Based on a shared concern for human life and dignity, this other side of globalization pointed toward a more humane alternative to the neoliberal post–Cold War international order.[57]

Indeed, the "lethal manifestations of capitalist-driven globalization" were on full display at the site of SisterLove's next South African initiative, the Thembuhlelo HIV/AIDS Capacity Building Project. Funded by the CDC's Global AIDS Program beginning in 2001, the project would help local community groups focused on preventing mother-to-child transmission of HIV and HIV among youth in the Mpumalanga province to develop all aspects of their organizational infrastructure, from writing grants and managing finances to evaluating the effectiveness of their own programs.

Mpumalanga sits between Johannesburg and Pretoria to the west and borders Mozambique and Swaziland to the east. In the late 1990s Mpumalanga had the second highest HIV infection rate (27.3 percent) in South Africa, surpassed only by KwaZulu-Natal, which lies just to the south. According to the project's South African staff, the local mining industry fueled the spread of HIV in the province. Young men from the surrounding countryside came to

Witbank (later renamed Emelahleni) to work in the mines, along with the truck drivers who carried their products to market. Away from the surveillance of their home communities, the miners and truckers used part of their income to pay for sex, which was in ready supply thanks to the area's grinding poverty. Here, on South Africa's industrial frontier, HIV flourished.[58]

The staff's account of HIV in Mpumalanga fit by then familiar narratives of AIDS as a disease of globalization. In popular and academic accounts alike, the virus spread around the world through human mobility, whether through commercial air travel or along long-distance trucking routes. But HIV in Mpumalanga was spread not simply through a disembodied process of globalization. Rather, specific policy choices made by South African leaders in the name of economic development made conditions of daily life in the province worse for many, in ways that also made them more vulnerable to HIV.[59]

In the mid-1990s, the newly elected democratic government embarked on a program to attract international investment through massive development projects. One of these, the Maputo Development Corridor, ran right through Mpumalanga. Composed of many different infrastructure projects executed through public-private partnerships and linking South Africa's industrial centers in Gauteng to the Mozambican port of Maputo, the development corridor was imagined as an engine of prosperity that would create jobs and help lift the young democracy's citizens out of poverty. But according to critics, the project was developed with the state acting as no more than a "'transmission belt' for transnational capital" with little, if any, attention to "holistic, environmentally sustainable and people-centered . . . aspects." For example, the project developed the N4 national highway as a toll road, which meant that local residents now had to pay a fee to commute to school, work, and shopping centers. The N4 redevelopment also displaced women fruit-sellers from along the roadway; as one member of the South African Commission on Gender Equality remarked, "The only industry that appears to be working for women is sex work that has sprung up along the highway." And while the state devoted a share of its (already limited) capacity to such projects, key positions in local and provincial health and social services departments went unfilled. In other words, South African leaders (including President Nelson Mandela) had pushed forward a project that enriched foreign investors at the expense their constituents.[60]

As SisterLove staff pointed out, Mpumalanga's HIV crisis was also rooted in the country's apartheid past. The municipalities where SisterLove worked had been part of the Ndebele "homeland" designated by the apartheid regime, and their residents had been subjected to forced removal, dispossession, and labor exploitation. The underdevelopment of the Black homelands as a matter of white nationalist policy left residents impoverished, in poor health, and ill-equipped to deal with a deadly new epidemic.[61]

Early in the project, SisterLove found that there were no groups focused on preventing mother-to-child transmission (MTCT) in Mpumalanga and so broadened its focus to include a wider range of groups addressing HIV/AIDS. Many provided home-based care to the sick and consisted largely of volunteers "who got together to work on HIV/AIDS because they saw the need." SisterLove helped them register as nonprofit organizations with the South African government, which allowed them to seek new sources of funding. SisterLove also established local forums, where representatives from HIV/AIDS groups in each municipality could share information and begin to collaborate on prevention and education programs. By some measures, these efforts were a success. According to SisterLove South Africa staff member Busisiwe Baloyi, the capacity-building assistance produced a noticeable "change in the way that some of the organizations do things, the way they talk about their organizations, and most of them have gained confidence in themselves and their organizations."[62]

SisterLove also adapted the Healthy Love curriculum for a new program, South Africa's Training of Trainers, geared toward youth HIV/AIDS organizations in Mpumalanga's rural districts. This "Enhanced Healthy Love Model" was designed to serve young men as well as women and aligned with the national Life Skills Education curriculum so that successful trainees could become certified as health educators and expand their outreach into schools. Through this peer education program, SisterLove hoped to spark a shift in the way that young people in Mpumalanga thought about sex and HIV/AIDS.[63]

At least some of the Thembuhlelo project's successes owed to the nonhierarchical approach outlined in SisterLove's transnational partnership manual. First, SisterLove deliberately hired local staff for the South Africa office. Although Dázon Dixon Diallo and others from the Atlanta office flew in for periodic evaluations, the South Africa staff members were responsible for managing the project's day-to-day operations. In the same vein, SisterLove used a culturally competent approach, tailoring its programs to the local context. One local government official observed that SisterLove "would work with the people and accommodate whatever level of literacy and education there was." SisterLove also took care to involve local groups in the project's planning stages, and the organizations in turn "reported that they appreciated being asked what their needs were and participating in the feedback process and inputting on strategic planning . . . [which] led to them feeling a sense of shared ownership in the project." This collaborative relationship stood in contrast to the way that other foreign agencies had conducted similar projects in the past. A member of one local organization reported that SisterLove "wanted to know from us what the organization [has], what we receive from other organizations, our needs, how they can strengthen our organizations. Not the way other people have done before, when they come with their things and leave us."[64]

Even as SisterLove stressed the commonalities between the "South within the North" and the global South, it recognized that its position as an established AIDS service organization from the United States, supported by both federal and foundation funding, put it on unequal footing vis-à-vis its partners on the ground in South Africa. Although SisterLove tried to even out that balance of power, the South African groups sometimes subverted those efforts, making clear that they saw SisterLove as a "mentor" organization rather than as an equal player. An outside evaluation of Thembuhlelo found that "there is not an equal relationship between the SisterLove and beneficiary organizations. The risk associated with this is an over-dependence on the SisterLove be these organizations to solve all their problems."[65]

The Thembuhlelo project encountered other obstacles as well. Chief among these was that the CDC announced that it would cut off funding two years early, in 2004 rather than 2006, although Dr. David Allen, CDC's South Africa country officer, told the group that he remained supportive of the project. The loss of funding not only shortened the project's time line significantly but also sent SisterLove staff scrambling to make up the difference.[66]

On the ground, low levels of education within local groups also proved to be "a major obstacle in implementing the activities as well as running the organizations. Basic administrative needs such as job description, role clarification and organizational structures [are] non-existent in most of the organizations." In some cases, the lack of education extended to the groups' knowledge about the disease, as some requested more training from SisterLove in "Basic HIV/ AIDS." This was a problem particularly with the youth organizations, where SisterLove found that trainee facilitators lacked the basic HIV/AIDS knowledge they needed to teach the Healthy Love program. Although a handful were able to translate the curriculum from English into their first language, the majority of those trained were unable to become certified as facilitators.[67]

Poverty in the region likewise challenged SisterLove's efforts. An analysis of community groups in Greater Marble Hall and Greater Groblersdal, two rural districts along the border between Mpumalanga and the Limpopo province to the north, found that the local communities requested basic necessities, such as "food, water, housing and clothing." SisterLove would become "engaged in poverty alleviation indirectly" by assisting such groups, but for those who lacked access to such basic necessities as food and water, AIDS might nevertheless seem like a secondary concern.[68]

Navigating their relationship with local and provincial officials also proved difficult. SisterLove staff found government departments dealing with health and social services to be disorganized, with key positions unfilled at the start of the Thembuhlelo project. For their part, community groups reported interference and a lack of respect from local and provincial officials, who handed out government grants as political favors. At the end of the project's first year, SisterLove reported that "establishing the necessary relationships and gaining buy-in and support from key stakeholders has taken a significant amount of . . . time." But officials could not simply be bypassed. In order for local groups to grow, they would need government support.[69]

Government officials, for their part, begrudgingly praised SisterLove's efforts. Catherine Molsepe, manager of community services for Marble Hall municipality, told SisterLove intern Morgan Dooley that she "was truly impressed by how the [SisterLove] staff would work with the people . . . and accommodate whatever level of literacy and education there was." However, she complained of being "completely uninformed initially about the project," perhaps because she had taken her position in March 2004, as the project was winding down. Sonto Mlangeni, the health promotion coordinator for Thembisile municipality, similarly complained that SisterLove "only involved us in the initial phases and excluded us as time went on." He was also bothered that the community groups seemed to have gotten the idea "that they are independent of the government and no longer need us." But whereas officials like Mlangeni found this development troubling, local organizations reported that one of the benefits of receiving help with capacity building was that they had "become independent from the Department of Health and Department of Social Services."[70]

Perhaps the biggest obstacle to conducting an MTCT prevention program in South Africa is referred to only elliptically in the archive. SisterLove reported "facing several issues around PMTCT [preventing mother-to-child transmission] that include: providing full support and services, adoption of a holistic approach." Despite the country's high rate of HIV infection and the proven effectiveness of AZT and nevirapine in preventing the transmission of HIV from mother to child, the South African government under Thabo Mbeki resisted their use. Only after the South African Constitutional Court ruled that the government had violated citizens' right to health by limiting access to antiretrovirals during pregnancy did the Mbeki government make them more widely available. Yet this was not only a problem at the highest levels of the South African government. As the Women's Health Project reported in its evaluation of the Thembuhlelo project, "The politics of working in the area of HIV/AIDS in the Mpumalanga province was seen as a challenge especially by the US staff. The Provincial Department of Health has been slow in the roll out of programs such as PMTCT."[71]

As the Thembuhlelo HIV/AIDS Capacity Building Project was wrapping up in 2004, Dixon Diallo formed the Thembuhlelo Trust Cooperative, a 668-acre farm in Mpumalanga where staff and volunteers combined AIDS prevention with poverty alleviation. They acquired the land through South Africa's land reform program, which aimed to transfer 30 percent of white-owned agricultural land in the country back to local Black communities. Along with providing HIV testing and education, they raised cows, chickens, and vegetables to meet some of the region's basic needs while selling the surplus as a source of income. Dixon Diallo argued that "when women are poor and economically dependent on men they are vulnerable to HIV," and so by providing local women with some means of economic security, the cooperative would also help them protect themselves from the disease. For those already affected by the disease, the farm would offer "empowerment and independence and help restore dignity and a sense of self."[72]

SisterLove's turn toward cooperative agriculture in Mpumalanga offers yet another connection between the Black freedom struggle and the fight against AIDS, both in Black America and in Africa. After all, collective farming has long been part of the fight for Black freedom, especially in the Deep South. Dixon Diallo makes that connection explicit: "In the South, where we are, we have a lot of the same issues, even if it's a different set of economies, right? We have a lot of poverty and violence and lack of access and opportunity that increase women's risks for HIV and AIDS. . . . And we need to learn how to do that community-development bridge building between service delivery, advocacy, and growing and developing communities so that individuals, families, and whole neighborhoods are able to do what they need to do to solve their own problems." In this way, SisterLove's work in South Africa circled back to its work at home, in the "South within the North," even as that work drew on a longer history of Black women's activism.[73]

Yet Dixon Diallo's comment speaks to a set of diminished expectations as to what kind of resources might be marshaled to combat an ongoing public health crisis in Black America. Low expectations would certainly be justified. As AIDS in the United States became more and more a problem of poor communities of color, and especially of poor women of color, Americans seemed to care less and less. During the 2004 vice-presidential debates, moderator Gwen Ifill—who herself broke barriers as a Black woman in journalism—asked about the government's role in fighting "AIDS right here in this country, where Black women between the ages of 25 and 44 are 13 times more likely to die of the disease than their counterparts." Vice President Dick Cheney touted the administration's response to AIDS *in Africa* before admitting, "I have not heard those numbers with respect to African American women."[74]

Cheney's response is probably more typical of Americans, in 2004 as well as today, than many would like to admit. It points to the way in which we have collectively turned our backs on an ongoing public health crisis because we don't care enough about the people who are dying. From this perspective, the language of grassroots empowerment makes sense: if others can't be bothered to care about the lives of Black women, then they must care for themselves. But this logic devolves responsibility for ending the epidemic to those who have the fewest resources and the heaviest burden to bear. Without dramatic change to the political and economic systems that make Black women more vulnerable to HIV, no amount of individual empowerment is going to change the course of the epidemic. Ending AIDS will require us to deal seriously with the problems of poverty, white supremacy, and misogyny in the United States, to say nothing of everywhere else. And those problems seem to be getting worse, not better.

SisterLove's story is in many ways remarkable. While other Black AIDS service organizations have faded or closed their doors entirely, SisterLove weathered difficult times. It continues to serve women on two continents, with offices in Atlanta and South Africa, and boasts a large corps of staff and volunteers. All the while, its commitment to building a movement of Black HIV-positive women—particularly of those in public housing, at risk of homelessness, and otherwise on the margins of respectability—has never faltered. In fact, SisterLove has put an intersectional approach at the center of its fight against AIDS among Black women, taking into account the ways that class, nation, sexuality, and many other forms of difference combine to produce not just one experience of Black womanhood but a multitude of them.

But that success has been hard-fought, and SisterLove's victories have been won in spite of the environment of hostility and indifference in which it operates. In recent years HIV has reached epidemic proportions in Atlanta. Patients at Grady Hospital are regularly diagnosed with HIV infection and AIDS *at the same time*, which means that too many people are falling through the cracks when it comes to HIV testing and treatment. Overwhelmingly, those people tend to be poor and Black. Atlanta doesn't need SisterLove; it needs a hundred SisterLoves.

# Conclusion

## Generations of Activism

THERE IS NO neat and easy way to bring this story to a close; the HIV/
AIDS crisis is still unfolding in Black communities across the United
States and around the world. As the epidemic rages on, we can learn
from the activists who confronted it—how they won their victories,
how they pushed through their defeats, and how they kept fighting. In other
words, how they made a way out of no way.

We can begin by learning to look at AIDS outside of a narrow biomedical
framework. To be sure, African American AIDS activists fought for access
to the drugs that treat HIV and research into new medical therapies. As the
Kemron story shows, African Americans wanted to see "natural" remedies
included in AIDS drug research and were deeply critical of the high price of
the medicines that were available. Likewise, ACT UP Philadelphia pushed for
global access to HIV and AIDS drugs; its success helped to prevent an untold
number of new infections. But these battles over treatment access were part
of a larger war to change the social determinants of health that put Black
communities at risk for HIV in the first place. Here the National Task Force
on AIDS Prevention and Gay Men of African Descent fought the racism and
homophobia that harmed Black gay men, while The Balm in Gilead used
Christian teachings to make a safe space for queer sexuality within the Black
church. Blacks Educating Blacks about Sexual Health Issues and SisterLove
took the fight against AIDS to street corners and public housing facilities,
where the intersection of race, gender, and class formed a triple threat to
Black women's health. African American AIDS activism thus points to a more
radical vision of AIDS politics, beyond the quest for a "magic bullet" and
toward remedies for the deep inequities that have shaped the course of the
epidemic.

Including African American AIDS activism in the larger story of the epidemic also expands our view of political responses to AIDS backward in time.

It forces us to recognize that grassroots responses to AIDS not only grew out of queer liberation and gay health activism but also fit into a much longer trajectory of the Black health movement. The stories in this book also illuminate some of the connections between African American AIDS activism and earlier struggles, from Dázon Dixon Diallo's work in the abortion rights and Black women's health movements, to the connections between Black feminism and the Black gay renaissance, to Pernessa Seele's effort to bring the organizing experience of Black churches to bear on the AIDS epidemic. At the same time, recognizing African American AIDS activism brings our time line up to the present day. Many histories of AIDS activism in the United States end in the middle 1990s, around the time that most ACT UP chapters disappeared or went into decline. And yet, most of the groups in this book are still around today, continuing the fight against AIDS in Black communities in one form or another.

We can also see these lessons clearly in the fight to protect the Affordable Care Act, signed into law by President Obama in 2010, which mobilized a broad coalition of activists, including some of the African American AIDS activists who appear in this book. After winning the electoral college in November 2016, Donald Trump came to the White House with a promise to repeal his predecessor's signature legislative achievement "on day one." The law, which prohibited insurance companies from discriminating against customers with preexisting conditions (such as HIV) and led to the expansion of Medicaid in roughly two-thirds of states, dramatically expanded medical coverage of people with HIV *and* reduced racial health disparities in the country as a whole. On the day of Trump's inauguration, the pages for the Office of National AIDS Policy and the National HIV/AIDS Strategy were ominously removed from the White House website. All signs pointed to a giant step backward in the fight against AIDS, especially in communities of color.[1]

But even before Trump took office, activists began to mobilize. Veteran AIDS activists traveled the country, training local groups to fight back against Trump's health care agenda. Soon congressional Republicans faced community meetings and town halls full of angry constituents eager to share everything that they stood to lose with the end of the Affordable Care Act. That summer, as senators considered a bill to repeal the law, a broad coalition of health and disability activists traveled to Washington, D.C., to stop them. They occupied the offices of Senate Republicans, telling stories about lives that had been saved by affordable health care and lives that would be lost without it. Photos and footage of activists being led or carried away in handcuffs by Capitol Hill police were splashed across the front pages of newspapers and featured on nighttime cable news shows. Few imagined they would win, but they were determined not to go down without a fight.

I know this story because I was there. Over the course of eight years of researching and writing about AIDS activism, I didn't expect to become an activist myself or to engage in the nonviolent civil disobedience that I understood on paper but not in practice. I had a lot to learn, from the nervous energy that you get from walking into a building knowing that you'll leave in handcuffs, to the fast friendships that form while waiting in detention for hours, to the frustration of talking to congressional staff who don't even pretend to listen to a mother's story about how even small changes to health care policy will mean death for her medically fragile child. I also saw how difficult it is to get activism right—to navigate our collective effort across lines of race, gender, sexuality, and ability. I was deeply engaged in this work only for a few months; I can't imagine doing it for years, let alone decades.

At the same time, even as the HIV/AIDS epidemic continues to rage around the world, we as human beings face another existential threat: irreversible climate change. Scientists warn that we are nearing the "point of no return" beyond which a dangerously warming planet is inevitable, and according to the United Nations, one million species face the threat of extinction.[2] As with HIV/AIDS, those who are already the most vulnerable will be among the hardest hit. Where I live in South Florida, sea-level rise is already speeding up the gentrification of historically Black neighborhoods and displacing residents from parts of the city now seen as desirable by wealthier home buyers and real estate developers. Poor communities throughout the United States will likewise suffer the worst effects of climate change, as will countries in the global South. According to the World Bank Group, climate change could send more than 140 million refugees to look for new homes in the next several decades. Worsening cycles of scarcity and drought in the Middle East and Africa are already fueling recruitment by extremist groups such as Boko Haram and the Islamic State. Without radical action, climate change threatens us all.[3]

And just as African American AIDS activists pointed to all the ways that AIDS was not just a biomedical crisis, we need to think about the climate crisis in terms of the social, political, and economic systems that drive it. The orthodoxy of deregulation that has become commonplace in recent decades, allowing just 100 companies to contribute almost three-quarters of global greenhouse gas emissions, must go. So too must the system of unrestrained global capitalism that allows the wealthy to shift risk—whether it's the risk of stock market speculation, the risk of climate catastrophe, or risk for HIV—onto poor communities of color.[4]

The stories in this book also show us that activism can take many different forms and show up in unexpected places. Turning back the clock on climate change will require action from all kinds of people, including faith leaders, policy makers, the poor and the middle class, the global North and the global South. Those who are veterans of other movements need to help cultivate new generations of activists to carry out a grassroots movement of unprecedented size and scope. At the same time, those veterans must listen to their younger allies, who will live the majority of their lives dealing with the environmental damage that has already been done. As stories of African American AIDS activism show, the people who are most affected by climate crisis need to have a seat at the table to make sure that our solutions do not leave behind, but instead lift up, those who are the most vulnerable.

In writing this book I have often marveled at how people fought relentlessly for years in the midst of a devastating crisis. How did they not lose hope? How did they not give up? Some were literally fighting for their lives, while others felt a tremendous sense of responsibility toward friends and lovers, people in their communities, and others whom they had never met. We can learn from their example and act as though we're fighting our own lives and for everyone else's—because we are.

# ACKNOWLEDGMENTS

Writing these acknowledgments is a surreal experience, giving a sense of finality to a project that at times seemed like it would never be completed. I have worked on this book, in one form or another, for over a decade. Thinking back on all those who have helped me along the way is a welcome, if daunting, task. I hope very much that I haven't forgotten anyone, although I'm fairly certain that I have.

Everyone should have a mentor like Beth Bailey. She guided, challenged, and supported me throughout this project, pushed me to make this a human story with "people doing things," and read draft after draft of the chapters in this book. I'm lucky to know her and even luckier to call her a friend. David Farber had a hand in this project from the *very* beginning, when I started it as a paper in his research seminar on social movement, and he continuously pushed me to ask big questions and make big claims. Bryant Simon gave me a model for what it looks like when social justice suffuses a historian's work, and I know a lot more about Bruce Springsteen for having worked with him. When I first reached out to Alondra Nelson about this project, I didn't fully realize what a big deal she was. I'm glad I didn't, because otherwise I might not have sent her an email. She is the rare kind of person whose warmth touches everyone she comes in contact with, and this book was made much better by her involvement. Finally, Heather Thompson gave me endless encouragement, helped shape this book, *and* gave it a home in this series.

During my years at Temple, Richard Immerman was supportive not just of my work but of the work of countless young scholars. I owe Seth Bruggeman for introducing me to the field of public history, which makes my work (for me, anyway) far more exciting than it would be otherwise. I'm also grateful to the Center for the Humanities at Temple for providing me with generous financial support. Its biweekly seminars helped me see my work in a broader interdisciplinary context. The coffee wasn't bad, either. Thanks go especially to Peter Logan, Liz Varon, and (again) Heather Thompson, who nurtured so many young scholars there. I'm also grateful to the Center for Historical Research at Ohio State University, and particularly to John Brooke and Chris Otter, for giving me the time and space to devote a full academic year to work on this project, which now seems like an unimaginable luxury. I appreciate

Lilia Fernández and David Staley for welcoming and supporting me during my time in Columbus.

Thanks go to the John Hope Franklin Research Center for African and African American History and Culture at Duke University, the Phil Zwickler Memorial Research Grant program in the Division of Rare and Manuscript Collections at Cornell University, the African American Episcopal Historical Collection at Virginia Theological Seminary, the Robert L. Platzman Memorial Fellowship program at the University of Chicago Library, and the University of North Texas Special Collections Fellowship program for providing me with research travel funding at different stages of this project. Joanna Black, Wesley Chenault, Bobbie Finck, Steven Fullwood, Josue Garcia, Julia Gardner, Morgan Gieringer, Maggie Grossman, Polina Ilieva, Rebekah Kim, Susan Malsbury, Brenda Marston, Jennifer Thompson, Joseph Thompson, and Tom Whitehead helped me find excellent archival material at their respective institutions. John Anderies and Bob Skiba deserve special recognition for developing and sustaining the John J. Wilcox Jr. Archives at the William Way Community Center in Philadelphia. Throughout this process they have shared their deep knowledge of Philadelphia's LGBTQ history and connected me to new collections that have enriched this project in important ways.

Likewise, I'm grateful to the folks at the University of California, Berkeley, Oral History Center (formerly the Regional Oral History Office) for opening up to me an entirely new avenue of research. Thanks are due Emily Hamilton, Robin Li, Martin Meeker, and Sam Redman for sharing their insight and wisdom and for setting me on my path as an oral historian. In the same vein, I am forever indebted to those who took the time to share their stories with me through the African American AIDS Activism Oral History Project: Rashidah Abdul-Khabeer, Wesley Anderson, Leon Bacchues, Chris Bartlett, Reginald Brown, Linda Burnette, Victoria Cargill, Fernando Cruz, JD Davids, Jose de Marco, DiAna DiAna, Earl Driscoll, David Fair, Robert Fullilove, Bambi Gaddist, Helene Gayle, Norman Green, Aundaray Guess, Roy Hayes, Michael Hinson, Amanda Houston-Hamilton, Cullen Hunter, Mark E. Johnson, Durell Knights, Kate Krauss, Kevin McGruder, Laura McTighe, Andrew Moses, David Paterson, Robert Penn, Joey Pressley, Pernessa Seele, Waheedah Shabazz-El, Tyrone Smith, Val Sowell, Louis Sullivan, Duncan Teague, Curtis Wadlington, Phill Wilson, Freddie Wright, and Terence Young. I hope that I have done them justice here.

The group of scholars, practitioners, and activists who met at the Rockefeller Archive Center in June 2017 to talk about the historical intersections of AIDS and philanthropy helped me to push this project in new directions, and

I'm deeply grateful for the insights of George Aumoithe, Jennie Brier, Stuart Burden, Beth Clement, Dázon Dixon Diallo, Kwame Holmes, Vinny McGee, Jack Meyers, Kevin Moseby, Marjorie Muecke, Pat Rosenfield, Michael Seltzer, Barb Shubinski, Jim Smith, and Rachel Wimpee. Special thanks go to the archivists at the RAC—Bethany Antos, Michele Beckerman, Monica Blank, Bob Clark, Meg Hogan, Brent Phillips, Mary Ann Quinn, Tom Rosenbaum, and Marissa Vassari—for their help in navigating such a rich set of collections.

Brandon Proia has been fantastically supportive as an editor throughout this process, and I'm lucky that this project fell into such skilled hands. Many people also offered invaluable feedback on parts of this book: Jessica Adler, Kevin Boyle, Beth Clement, Alex Cornelius, Hilary Jones, Okezi Otovo, Mark Padilla, Val Patterson, Bianca Premo, and T. J. Tallie. Thanks also go to *Black Perspectives, Encyclopedia of Greater Philadelphia, Notches,* and *Nursing Clio*— and especially to Carrie Adkins, Laura Ansley, Jacqueline Antonovich, Justin Bengry, Keisha Blain, Gill Frank, Ibram Kendi, Christina Larocco, Charlene Mires, J. T. Roane, and Adam Turner—for giving me and countless others the space to share ideas and publish our work online. Samuel Kelton Roberts and Marc Stein reviewed the manuscript as a whole; their comments helped me to both sharpen my argument and deepen my analysis.

Others have helped to shape both the African American AIDS Activism Oral History Project and the African American AIDS History Project (the digital archive that accompanies this book). Thanks go to Carlos Abarca, Zachery Baker, Nadja Chin, Rafael Cue, India Ferguson, Eric Gonzaba, Riley Hauser, Gia Jelatis, Jasmine Johnson, Donette Manning, Brittany Martinez, Lindsey Maxwell, Christine Monge, Juan Pozo, Veronica Rushton, Maria Santiago, Keegan Shepherd, and Jovany Vincent for their assistance and contributions.

When I got a new roommate—Melanie Newport—in 2009 through the Grad Café, I couldn't have predicted that we would become like family, but here we are. We've shared Thanksgiving dinners, plenty of gossip, and a lot of beer. We've seen each other at our very best and absolute worst, but I couldn't think of a better conference buddy and all-around friend. I'm glad Max Felker-Kantor, Monica Mercado, and Alyssa Ribeiro are part of our squad. Lindsay Helfman and Alex Elkins saw me through some tough moments as a baby academic, and I'm thrilled to see the life they're building together. Carly Goodman and Andrew Thomas made sure that I stayed fed and introduced me to shishito peppers. For that, and for their friendship, I'm deeply grateful. I'm also grateful to Jess Bird, Alex Bornstein, Susan Brandt, Diane Garbow, Ruby Goodall, Dylan Gottlieb, Patrick Grossi, Matt Johnson, Larry Kessler, Roberta Meek, Brenna O'Rourke, Abby Perkiss, Laura Porterfield, Sarah Robey, Kate

Scott, Seth Tannenbaum, Brittany Webb, and John Worsencroft for making my time at Temple far more enjoyable and intellectually stimulating than it would have been otherwise.

When I moved to Miami and Florida International University in 2015, Shane Landrum opened their home and helped me get oriented to an unfamiliar city and a new institution. Molly Giblin was (and is) a great friend, someone with whom I could exchange knowing looks across the hall without even leaving my desk. There are many others at FIU whom I am grateful to count as friends and colleagues: Saad Abi-Hamad, Whitney Bauman, Heather Blatt, Mike Bustamante, Gwyn Davies, Rebecca Friedman, Jenna Gibbs, Percy Hintzen, Ken Lipartito, Judith Mansilla, Ana Menendez, Jon Mogul, Aurora Morcillo, Jason Pearl, Terry Peterson, David Rifkind, Jamie Rogers, Martha Schoolman, Victor Uribe, Reyni Valerio, and Kirsten Wood.

Academia can be hostile to queer scholars and to queer scholarship, and I am deeply grateful to those who have carved out a space for us through the Committee on LGBT History: Katie Batza, Jonathan Bell, Darius Bost, Julio Capó, Chelsea Del Rio, John D'Emilio, Rene Esparza, Gill Frank, Marcia Gallo, Rachel Guberman, Christina Hanhardt, April Haynes, Emily Hobson, David K. Johnson, Will Kuby, Ian Lekus, Amanda Littauer, Jen Manion, Kevin McKenna, Kevin Murphy, Nic Ramos, Don Romesburg, Gabe Rosenberg, Andrew Ross, Jason Ruiz, David Serlin, Emily Skidmore, Tim Stewart-Winter, Amy Sueyoshi, Nick Syrett, Phil Tiemeyer, Stephen Vider, and Cookie Woolner.

Outside of academia, my Bike & Build family made me the person that I am. Thanks go to Kristin Anderson, Liz Ball, Elana Bannerman, Kelsey Baumberger, Michael Binder, Adam Bohr, Skip Burns, Chris Clark, Claire Collins, Megan O'Brien Conboy, Kevin Dulaney, George Eklund, Ashley Gallo, Liz Garrity, Isabel Gottlieb, Travis Hall, Matt Hartman, Megan Healy, Sonya Hirsch, Mary Ellen Hitt, Kristen Hunt, Rachel Jodway, Katie Karas, Khaki Kraft, Lynn Mandeltort, Libby McCann, Aileen Strickland McGee, Danny McGee, Andrew Morgenthaler, Joe Naughton, Brendan Newman, Dan Oates, Courtney O'Neill, Nathan Palmer, Melissa Panter, Angela Parrotta, Amanda Romsa Polack, Erin Potter, Greg Powell, Amanda Schulte, Kristian Sekse, Natalie Serle, Shibrina, Jake Stangel, Becca Stievater, Derrick Thiel, and Nick Webber. I'm also grateful to the O'Brien family for hosting so many of us year after year and for welcoming me for Thanksgiving when I couldn't make it back to California to be with my biological family. Thanks go especially to Bill and Joanie Webber, who not only supported us through nine years of rides but generously sustained this project through the Chris Webber Memorial Fund. Chris, Paige, Christina, Patrick, Anne—you're always in our thoughts.

I have probably laughed more with Jenny Thai than with anyone else on Earth, and I'll always be indebted to the Thai family for welcoming me into their fold. Nikki, Ha, My Le, Mon, Chan, and Amy are the best gifts with purchase anyone could ask for. Thanks also go to the ladies of the Pine Palace—Lila Hussain, Noelle Trinidad Taylor, Jessica Castellanos, and Rachel Zack—for having me as a roommate and couch-crasher during an extended series of research trips.

And then there are the friends who have made my life happier just by being in it. It's been such a pleasure to see Meg Welsh go from intimidating sculler to formidable scholar. I also have her to thank for my friendship with Catherine Reddick, whom I could not be prouder to know. Naoko Kozuki has known me since we were eight years old, which is a testament to her fortitude and grace, and has opened her home to me during many D.C. protests. I highly recommend Becky Bamberger and Sarah Sridasome as burrito buddies and brunch guests. I don't care to imagine what my life would be like if Evie Caldwell and April Burnette Caldwell had not come into it, but I know that it is immeasurably better because I can count them as friends.

Throughout this process my family has been wonderfully supportive, even when they didn't quite understand what I was doing or why. I could not have asked for a better gift than my aunt Nadine's sense of humor. My grandmother Jean has always been generosity and unconditional love incarnate. Thanks are due my grandmother Junior, my uncle John, and my aunt Belle for welcoming me to Wildwood during summers and for their constant support. My stepmother, Leslie, has been exemplary as both a parent and a friend. I could not be prouder of my sisters, Annelise and Renee, and the deeply caring, thoughtful people they have become. My parents, Melanie and Ed, taught me, both explicitly and by example, about doing what you love, doing it well, and doing it with compassion. They're *still* whom I want to be when I grow up.

Last, but very certainly not least, Darwin has put up with my morning grumps, my library book hoarding, and my endless stacks of notes as I worked to finish this project. I'm so grateful for someone who challenges me at trivia, gives me infinite love and support, knows his way around the European rail system, and is always quick to point out which is *really* Crystal Waters's best track. (No, it's not "Gypsy Woman.") I'm so proud of him and lucky to have him in my life.

# NOTES

## Abbreviations

| | |
|---|---|
| BEBASHI | Blacks Educating Blacks About Sexual Health Issues |
| BOF | BEBASHI Organizational Files, John J. Wilcox Jr. Archives, William Way Community Center, Philadelphia |
| BWMT | Black and White Men Together |
| DTP | Duncan Teague Papers, Auburn Avenue Research Library, Atlanta |
| FFG | Ford Foundation Grant Files, Rockefeller Archive Center, Sleepy Hollow, N.Y. |
| GMAD | Gay Men of African Descent |
| GMAD-SC | Gay Men of African Descent Records, Schomburg Center, New York |
| GMOCC | Gay Men of Color Consortium |
| HSC | Human Sexuality Collection, Cornell University, Ithaca |
| JDP | JD Davids Papers, John J. Wilcox Jr. Archives, William Way Community Center, Philadelphia |
| JJWA | John J. Wilcox Jr. Archives, William Way Community Center, Philadelphia |
| KKP | Kiyoshi Kuromiya Papers, John J. Wilcox Jr. Archives, William Way Community Center, Philadelphia |
| NABWMT | National Association of Black and White Men Together |
| NPAC | News and Public Affairs Collection, UCLA Film and Television Archive, Los Angeles |
| NTFAP | National Task Force on AIDS Prevention |
| NTFAP-GLBT | National Task Force on AIDS Prevention Records, Gay, Lesbian, Bisexual, Transgender Historical Society, San Francisco |
| NTFAP-UCSF | National Task Force on AIDS Prevention Records, UCSF Special Collections |
| ONE | ONE National Gay & Lesbian Archives, University of Southern California, Los Angeles |
| QRC | Queer Resource Center Resource Files, CU-500, University Archives, Bancroft Library, University of California, Berkeley |
| SC | Schomburg Center, New York |

SLR    SisterLove Records, Sophia Smith Collection, Smith College, Northampton, Mass.

SWP    Scott Wilds Papers, Temple University Manuscripts and Special Collections, Philadelphia

## Introduction

1. Mealer, *Muck City*.

2. I capitalize "Black" because, as Lori Tharps has argued, "Black with a capital B refers to people of the African diaspora. Lowercase black is simply a color." Lori L. Tharps, "The Case for Black with a Capital B," *New York Times*, November 18, 2014, https://www.nytimes.com/2014/11/19/opinion/the-case-for-black-with-a-capital-b.html.

3. Hurston, *Their Eyes Were Watching God*, 182; Mealer, *Muck City*; Fred W. Friendly, *Harvest of Shame*, CBS, November 25, 1960, https://www.youtube.com/watch?v=yJTVF_dya7E; Elizabeth Blair, "In Confronting Poverty, 'Harvest of Shame' Reaped Praise And Criticism," *Weekend Edition Saturday*, NPR, May 31, 2014, https://www.npr.org/2014/05/31/317364146/in-confronting-poverty-harvest-of-shame-reaped-praise-and-criticism. For another account of the Belle Glade "AIDS capital of the world" story, see Raimondo, "'AIDS Capital of the World.'"

4. Mealer, *Muck City*; Mike Clary, "Small Town Offers Disturbing Look at Future of the AIDS War," *Los Angeles Times*, January 28, 1993, http://articles.latimes.com/1993–01–28/news/mn-2375_1_belle-glade. Researchers began to document the links between crack cocaine use and HIV in the late 1980s. See Fullilove et al., "Risk of Sexually Transmitted Disease"; and Edlin et al., "Intersecting Epidemics." The story of the Fulliloves' research on the links between crack cocaine and HIV is documented in Levenson, *Secret Epidemic*.

5. Steve Rothman, "Doctor Links Conditions, AIDS Rate," *Palm Beach Post*, April 20, 1985, 1B, and Val Ellicott, "Why Should This Community Have AIDS?," *Palm Beach Post*, February 4, 1990, both in Clippings File, Stonewall National Museum and Archives, Fort Lauderdale, Fla.; Val Ellicott, "Bit by Bit, Route to AIDS Revealed," *Palm Beach Post*, February 5, 1990, 1A.

6. Amy Wilson, "Belle Glade's Last Stand?," *Fort Lauderdale Sun-Sentinel*, August 27, 1989, 1E, Clippings File, Stonewall National Museum and Archives.

7. Clary, "Small Town Offers Disturbing Look."

8. The disproportionate prevalence of HIV below the Mason-Dixon line has been clear for some time. Levenson devoted a significant portion of *The Secret Epidemic*, published in 2005, to the fight against AIDS in rural Alabama. Within the last decade several documentary films, including *deepsouth* (directed by Lisa Biagiotti) and *Wilhelmina's War* (directed by June Cross), have explored southern Black communities' struggles with HIV and AIDS. Writing for the *New York Times Magazine* in 2017, Linda Villarosa focused on HIV among Black gay and bisexual men in Mississippi. See Levenson, *The Secret Epidemic*; Biagiotti, *deepsouth*; Cross, *Wilhelmina's War*; and Linda Villarosa, "America's Hidden HIV Epidemic," *New York Times Magazine*, June 6, 2017, 38–49, http://www.nytimes.com/2017/06/06/magazine/americas-hidden-hiv-epidemic.html. For more on Black gay AIDS activists' response to AIDS in the U.S. South, see

Dan Royles, "Race, Homosexuality, and the AIDS Epidemic," *Black Perspectives* (blog), July 6, 2017, http://www.aaihs.org/race-homosexuality-and-the-aids-epidemic/.

At the same time, rising rates of opioid addiction since the 1990s have fueled a growing problem of injection drug use is rural communities. This has led to clusters of HIV infection in areas where AIDS is seldom talked about and healthcare providers are ill-equipped to deal with new cases. Such was the case in Scott County, Indiana, which witnessed an outbreak of new HIV infections in late 2014 and early 2015. Efforts to control the outbreak by establishing a program to distribute clean syringes were hampered by resistance from Scott County residents and state lawmakers alike; Indiana Governor Mike Pence issued an executive order allowing such a program over two months after the cluster of new cases was detected. Similar outbreaks are likely to occur in the future and may alter the geography of the fight against HIV and AIDS in the United States. See Abby Goodnough, "Rural Indiana Struggles to Contend with HIV Outbreak," *New York Times*, May 5, 2015, http://www.nytimes.com/2015/05/06/us/rural-indiana-struggles -to-contend-with-hiv-outbreak.html; "Pence's Principles Tested during HIV Outbreak among Indiana Drug Abusers," *Seattle Times*, August 7, 2016, http://www.seattletimes.com /nation-world/pences-principles-tested-during-hiv-outbreak-among-indiana-drug -abusers; Steven W. Thrasher, "HIV Is Coming to Rural America," *New York Times*, December 1, 2019, https://www.nytimes.com/2019/12/01/opinion/hiv-aids-rural-america .html.

The current rate of HIV infection among Black women is an *improvement* over recent years, as the number of new diagnoses among Black women dropped by more than 40 percent between 2008 and 2015. "Black Americans and HIV/AIDS: The Basics," *Henry J. Kaiser Family Foundation* (blog), February 7, 2019, https://www.kff.org/hivaids/fact -sheet/black-americans-and-hivaids-the-basics/; Murray et al., "'We Hide . . . '"; "HIV and Transgender People," CDC, April 16, 2019, https://www.cdc.gov/hiv/group/gender /transgender/index.html.

9. Lawrence K. Altman, "Rare Cancer Seen in 41 Homosexuals," *New York Times*, July 3, 1981, A20.

10. Nero, "Why Are Gay Ghettoes White?" In saying that urban gay communities were largely white, I do not mean to erase the existence of queer people of color in those same cities. I do, however, mean that the visible gay communities that formed the frontline response to the AIDS epidemic were invested (consciously or not) in a particular form of white middle-class gayness. Allan Bérubé described the "whitening practices" that produced "the dominant image of the typical gay man [as] a white man who is financially better off than most everyone else" in "How Gay Stays White," 234.

Doctors and scientists reinforced the association between AIDS and gay men, in part as a result of their own bias. Researchers aggressively pursued a "lifestyle hypothesis" of AIDS etiology, positing that drug use and repeated exposure to sexually transmitted infections had overloaded gay men's immune systems to the point of failure. In San Francisco, for example, doctors' focus on patients' numerous sexual partners and drug use obscured the significant presence of poverty as a cofactor for disease among the first reported cases, which included a number of homeless male prostitutes. They would later recount that those early patients had been healthy young men struck down suddenly by crippling illness, even though a significant number had presented with preexisting medical conditions related to their marginalized existence. Moreover, doctors shaped the initial clinical definition of AIDS based on the opportunistic infections most common in gay men, which may have masked the prevalence of cases among African Americans in public health reporting by excluding women from official statistics of people with AIDS. The Centers for Disease Control and Prevention finally revised the case definition to more accurately represent the extent of AIDS among women in 1993, twelve years into the recognized epidemic. See Oppenheimer, "In the Eye of the Storm"; Cochrane, *When AIDS Began*; and Sobolewski, "Study of the 1993 AIDS Surveillance Definition Revision." In *Smearing the Queer*, Michael Scarce also examines the "discovery" of "gay bowel syndrome" in the 1970s as a result of homophobia embedded in the construction on medical knowledge.

11. Donald C. Drake, "AIDS Risk to Blacks Discussed," *Philadelphia Inquirer*, November 14, 1985, B12; Fullilove et al., "Risk of Sexually Transmitted Disease"; Edlin et al., "Intersecting Epidemics."

12. In *Remaking a Life*, her study of how women living with HIV navigate systems of care and support, Watkins-Hayes writes, "I am very deliberate about my use of the term 'injuries of inequality' rather than 'social determinants of health.' I want to emphasize the bidirectional relationship between inequality and health and center the root causes of these injuries: growing economic, social, and political inequities that exact devastating consequences on those with limited power." See Watkins-Hayes, *Remaking a Life*, 230. I have adopted Watkins-Hayes's usage here because it better evokes the harm that inequality causes those who experience it. For a somewhat different framing of disparities of HIV infection "as an effect of racism embodied," see Geary, *Antiblack Racism and the AIDS Epidemic*, 50.

13. For more on the stigma of AIDS in African American communities, see Robertson, *Not in My Family*.

14. Spencer Rich, "Reagan Welfare Cuts Found to Worsen Families' Poverty," *Washington Post*, July 29, 1984, A14. Cohen summarizes the Reagan agenda vis-à-vis Black communities in *Boundaries of Blackness*, 79–83. Marable, *Race, Reform, and Rebellion*, 180 quoted on 82.

Academic research on the ways that injuries of inequality exacerbate the AIDS epidemic among African Americans is extensive. African Americans have consistently had far less access to adequate health care than whites, and the closing of public hospitals during the 1970s and 1980s and shrinking social safety net under Ronald Reagan hit black communities especially hard. The war on drugs, mass incarceration, and the physical destruction of poor urban neighborhoods have also exacerbated the AIDS epidemic in black communities. As lawmakers and police cracked down on city residents caught with clean syringes and other drug paraphernalia, intravenous drug users responded by sharing or renting "works" (slang for a needle and plunger) from dealers or at the shooting galleries where they got high. Policing in black neighborhoods thus drove the spread of HIV and other blood-borne illnesses among intravenous drug users and limited the range of possible public health interventions once researchers identified shared needles as a source of HIV infection. Whereas needle exchange programs have proven effective at significantly reducing HIV transmission in drug users, policy makers in the United States have resisted implementing such measures with the discredited argument that needle exchanges promote drug use. For an overview of the other consequences of mass incarceration, see Thompson, "Why Mass Incarceration Matters." Warwick Anderson offers a brief history of the fight for needle exchange in New York City, including Black leaders' opposition to such a program, in "New York Needle Trial," while Gostin et al. survey the laws governing needle possession around the country in "Prevention of HIV/ AIDS and Other Blood-Borne Diseases among Injection Drug Users."

Punitive drug laws and aggressive inner-city police enforcement have produced ballooning prison populations made up of disproportionate numbers of African Americans. Once in prison, arrestees found themselves confined to a space in which sex behind bars may have been relatively common, but condoms and educational materials about HIV and AIDS were rarely available. Many incarcerated men and women entered prison already infected with HIV and were diagnosed while behind bars. The more far-reaching effect of mass incarceration on AIDS in communities of color has likely come from damage to social networks and sexual relationships. The gender imbalance in African American communities produced by mass incarceration put women at a distinct disadvantage in demanding protected, monogamous sex from their partners, giving rise to sexual networks dense with multiple and concurrent partnerships that spread HIV with deadly efficiency. Finally, widespread arrest and imprisonment, not to mention policing and harassment, inflict lasting psychological and emotional trauma even on those who remain in the community, with long-term implications for drug use and sexual behavior. See Adimora et al., "Social Context of Sexual Relationships among Rural African Americans"; Manhart et al., "Sex Partner Concurrency"; Adimora et al., "Concurrent Partnerships among Rural African Americans with Recently Reported Heterosexually Transmitted HIV Infection"; Adimora et al., "Heterosexually Transmitted HIV Infection among African Americans in North Carolina"; Hammett and Drachman-Jones, "HIV/AIDS, Sexually Transmitted Diseases, and Incarceration among Women"; Khan et al., "Incarceration and Risky Sexual Partnerships in a Southern US City;" and Khan et al., "Incarceration and High-Risk Sex Partnerships among Men in the United States."

Scholars working at the intersection of city planning and public health argue that urban policy had a similarly destructive effect on inner city communities in the decades leading up to the AIDS epidemic. During the 1970s, New York City mayor John Lindsay implemented a policy of "planned shrinkage," cutting essential services, like fire protection, to sections of the city that had been partly abandoned. These areas made up some of the poorest sections of the city, populated mostly by African American and Latino residents. Lindsay's policy of literally letting entire neighborhoods burn to the ground resulted in tremendous social dislocation. As community ties disintegrated, substance abuse and frequent sex proliferated, likely spreading HIV and other sexually transmitted infections throughout poor communities of color. Moreover, the burned-out buildings left by planned shrinkage provided intravenous drug users with accessible spaces to use as "shooting galleries," in which needle sharing among addicts offered another means of HIV transmission. See Wallace, "Urban Desertification"; Wallace and Fullilove, "AIDS Deaths in the Bronx"; Wallace et al., "Will AIDS Be Contained within U.S. Minority Urban Populations?"; and Wallace and McCarthy, "Unstable Public-Health Ecology." Rodrick Wallace also presents some of this research for a popular audience with Deborah Wallace in A Plague on Your Houses.

Even for those communities left more or less physically intact by neglect from policy makers, the residential and educational segregation of people of color produced racially segregated sexual networks. Since people most often (but certainly not always) seek sexual partners from within their social world, the disproportionate prevalence of HIV in Black communities has become a self-perpetuating phenomenon, as African Americans are simply more likely to have sex with a partner who is HIV positive. Moreover, those who have few sexual partners are still more likely than whites to encounter someone with a large number of partners, making them part of a much larger sexual network than their circle of immediate sexual contacts. See Peterson et al., "Multiple Sexual Partners among Blacks in High-Risk Cities"; and Adimora, Schoenbach, and Floris-Moore, "Ending the Epidemic."

15. Cohen, "Punks, Bulldaggers, and Welfare Queens." Woubshet uses the term "disprized" in a similar fashion in *Calendar of Loss*.

16. Here I borrow from the work of Hartman in *Lose Your Mother* in thinking about AIDS in Black communities as part of the "afterlife of slavery," the slave trade as a "wound," and transnational Blackness as a complicated "language of kinship" that aims to heal it.

17. Batza, *Before AIDS*, 131.

18. Shilts, *And the Band Played On*; Fee and Fox, *AIDS*; Treichler, *How to Have Theory in an Epidemic*; Petro, *After the Wrath of God*; France, *How to Survive a Plague*; Cohen, *The Boundaries of Blackness*, 9.

19. Inrig, *North Carolina and the Problem of AIDS*.

20. Woubshet, *Calendar of Loss*; Bost, *Evidence of Being*, 4. See also McGruder, "To Be Heard in Print"; and Duberman, *Hold Tight Gently*.

21. Carroll, *Mobilizing New York*.

22. Chambré likewise ends the narrative portion of *Fighting for Our Lives* around 1993, although she includes a coda discussing how the "AIDS community" has changed in the years since Congress passed the Ryan White CARE Act in the early 1990s. Epstein, *Impure Science*; Brier, *Infectious Ideas*, .

23. Altman, "Globalization, Political Economy, and HIV/AIDS"; Pepin, *Origins of AIDS*; Shilts, *And the Band Played On*; Ted Conover, "Trucking through the AIDS Belt," *New Yorker*, August 16, 1993, http://tedconover.com/2010/01/trucking-through-the-aids-belt/; Dan McDougall, "Truckers Take India on Fast Lane to Aids," *The Observer*, November 26, 2005, https://www.theguardian.com/world/2005/nov/26/india.aids; Tiemeyer, *Plane Queer*; McKay, *Patient Zero*.

24. Altman, "Globalization, Political Economy, and HIV/AIDS," 568. Crane also critically analyzes the public-private transnational research networks that produce a significant amount of our knowledge about AIDS in *Scrambling for Africa*.

25. A. Nelson, *Body and Soul*; David McBride, *From TB to AIDS*; S. Smith, *Sick and Tired of Being Sick and Tired*; Wailoo, *Dying in the City of the Blues*; Gamble, *Making a Place for Ourselves*; Thomas, *Deluxe Jim Crow*; Burrows and Berney, "Creating Equal Health Opportunity."

26. See Meriwether, *Proudly We Can Be Africans*; C. Anderson, *Eyes off the Prize*; Sidbury, *Becoming African in America*; Corbould, *Becoming African Americans*; Batiste, *Darkening Mirrors*; R. Frazier, *East Is Black*; Gaines, *African Americans in Ghana*; Ford, *Liberated Threads*; Blain, *Set the World on Fire*.

## Chapter 1

1. Abdul-Khabeer interview.

2. At the time of the speech, some news sources referred to Hassan as "Rashidah," her Muslim name, and others as "Lorraine," her given name. Since she signed her correspondence "Rashidah Lorraine Hassan," I use the first of the two names. Also, although she has since divorced and remarried, taking Abdul-Khabeer as her last name, I use "Hassan" when referring in the text to the oral history I conducted with her in the present, for the sake of coherence. In citing the interview, however, I use her current name, Rashidah Abdul-Khabeer. When referring to her oral history, as well as to the oral histories of other narrators who are living at the time of this writing, I also use the present tense to differentiate between present recollections and information gleaned from past sources.

3. Abdul-Khabeer interview. A 1990 profile of Hassan in the *Philadelphia Inquirer* suggested that Hassan's conversion from Baptist to Muslim corresponded with her marriage to her first husband, Nimr, but the story she told about her conversion during our interview made no mention of him. Perhaps the *Inquirer* got this sequence of events wrong; perhaps this is how she now prefers to tell her personal religious history. She may also simply remember the story in this way, without conscious preference or intent. Regardless of the reason, the story she told me is no less significant in revealing how she today connects her identity to her faith and her work relating to HIV and AIDS. Lini S. Kadaba, "The Black Warning," *Philadelphia Inquirer Magazine*, July 8, 1990, 12.

4. Abdul-Khabeer interview.

5. Abdul-Khabeer interview. By the middle of 1984, 51 percent of the city's AIDS cases were among African Americans, over ten points higher than their share of the city's total population. Philadelphia Department of Public Health, "Acquired Immune Deficiency Syndrome (AIDS) Cases in Philadelphia and Philadelphia Primary Metropolitan Statistical Area (PMSA) Monthly Report," July 6, 1984, box 4, folder "AIDS in Phila 1984–87," SWP.

6. Shilts focused on events in California and New York and at the Centers for Disease Control in Atlanta in *And the Band Played On*. Other works that examine the history of AIDS in the United States in whole or in part through stories in New York or San Francisco include Cochrane, *When AIDS Began*; Chambré, *Fighting for Our Lives*; Brier, *Infectious Ideas*; Gould, *Moving Politics*; and Carroll, *Mobilizing New York*. On the history of Philadelphia's political economy during the twentieth century, see Wolfinger, *Philadelphia Divided*; Countryman, *Up South*; and Levenstein, *Movement without Marches*.

7. Stein, *City of Sisterly and Brotherly Loves*; Mumford, "Trouble with Gay Rights"; Christopher Hepp, "Gays Take Clout Out of the Closet," *Philadelphia Daily News*, April 23, 1984, 4.

8. De Marco interview; Arnold Jackson, "On the Outside Looking In," *Au Courant*, March 10, 1986, 1, JJWA. In Philadelphia, these complaints were confirmed in 1986 by the release of a two-year study undertaken by a coalition of gay community groups. The report found "pervasive racial and sexual exclusivity in Greater Philadelphia's lesbian and gay bars" and noted that "many patrons tolerate this kind of racial and sexual discrimination." See Tommi Avicolli, "Uniform Carding Policy Urged," *Philadelphia Gay*

*News*, June 20–26, 1986, 35, JJWA. Many chapters of the group Black and White Men Together (BWMT) became involved in local campaigns against discrimination in gay bars. See *BWMT/LA Newsletter*, no. 15, January 1982, Periodicals, BWMT Newsletters, BWMT–Los Angeles 1980–1982, ONE. De Marco (as "Joe DeMarco" also contributed an essay titled "Gay Racism" to *Black Men/White Men: A Gay Anthology*, edited by Michael J. Smith, founder of BWMT.

9. Jackson, "On the Outside Looking In," 9, 13; Jose de Marco wryly notes that "the music was always better" at Black gay bars, anyway. De Marco interview.

10. James Roberts, "Black Gays Speaking for Themselves," *Au Courant*, June 9, 1986, 1, JJWA; Joseph Beam, "Domestic Terrorism: No Cheek Left to Turn to Racism," *Au Courant*, October 27, 1986, 14, JJWA. At this time Beam was living near the intersection of Twenty-First and Spruce, two blocks away from Rittenhouse Square in downtown Philadelphia. See Mark Thompson to Joseph Beam, July 8, 1987, box 4, folder 3, Joseph F. Beam Papers, SC. Beam also recounts his experience working at Giovanni's Room in *In the Life: A Black Gay Anthology*, the collection of Black gay men's writing that he edited. Mumford describes the racism that Joseph Beam encountered in the Philadelphia gay scene, as well as his literary legacy, in *Not Straight, Not White*.

11. Don Ransom, "Taking the Forces to Task for Excluding Racial Minorities," letter to the editor, *Au Courant*, October 13, 1986, JJWA.

12. In *City of Sisterly and Brotherly Loves*, Marc Stein found that gay men reported playing a significant role in gentrifying parts of Center City and the surrounding area. For local newspaper coverage of gentrification, see Barbara Kantrowitz, "Money Pours In, Forcing Some People Out," *Philadelphia Inquirer*, April 26, 1979, 3B; and Howard Spodek, "Gentrification: Don't Forget the Poor," *Philadelphia Inquirer*, July 19, 1979, 11A. Andrew Maykuth mentions "quiche-and-fern bars" in "Challenge to Popular Thinking on Cities," *Philadelphia Inquirer*, June 18, 1984, 1B. For more on gentrification, see Levy, *Queen Village*; and Adams et al., *Philadelphia*. Available census data show that the proportion of white residents in the area just below South Street, including Queen Village, rose significantly between 1970 and 1990. Between 1970 and 1980 the number of white residents in census tracts 15 and 16, which run along the south side of South Street from Broad Street to the Delaware River, increased by 14.4 and 25.4 percentage points, respectively. The wave of gentrification continued moving west between 1980 and 1990, when the proportion of white residents in census tract 15 rose another 12.1 points, and the proportion of white residents in the adjacent tract 14 rose by 19.4 points. In each case the loss in proportion of the tract's Black population was equivalent or greater. While these neighborhoods still experienced population loss between 1970 and 1980, the effect of gentrification along the South Street corridor in the late 1970s may be better captured by the increase in residents they experienced over the following decade. U.S. Census Bureau, "1970 Census of Population and Housing: Census Tracts, Philadelphia, Pa.–N.J. Standard Metropolitan Statistical Area," General Characteristics of the Population Table P-1, *Index of United States Census Bureau*, https://www2.census.gov/library/publications/decennial/1970/phc-1/39204513p16ch05.pdf; U.S. Census Bureau, "1980 Census of Population and Housing: Census Tracts, Philadelphia, Pa.–N.J. Standard Metropolitan Statistical Area," Race and Spanish Origin Table P-7, *Index of United States Census Bureau*, https://archive.org/stream/1980censusofpo8022831unse; U.S. Census Bureau, "1990 Census of Population and Housing: Population and Housing Characteristics for

Census Tracts and Block Numbering Areas, Philadelphia, PA–NJ PMSA, Section 1," Race and Hispanic Origin Table 8, *Index of United States Census Bureau*, https://archive .org/stream/1990censusofpopu32591unse.

13. Philadelphia Department of Public Health, "Acquired Immune Deficiency Syndrome (AIDS) Cases in Philadelphia and Philadelphia Primary Metropolitan Statistical Area (PMSA) Monthly Report," August 3, 1984, box 4, folder "AIDS in Phila," SWP. Here I define Center City as bounded by I-676, South Street, and the Schuylkill and Delaware Rivers, which included census tracts 1 through 12. By this definition, Center City was around 90 percent white in 1970 and 1980 and 85 percent white in 1990. Racial discrimination was not unique to Philadelphia's gay community and hampered AIDS outreach efforts in other cities as well. See Bost, "At the Club"; Brier, *Infectious Ideas*; and Inrig, *North Carolina and the Problem of AIDS*.

14. "Lavender Health," n.d., box 4, folder "Lavender Health," SWP; "News and Views of the Institute for Social Medicine and Community Health," September 1982, box 4, folder "Lavender Health," SWP; Pat McKeown, "No AIDS Cure, so 'Buddies' Offer Comfort," *Philadelphia Daily News*, August 10, 1983, 8. Batza describes the development of gay health services such as Lavender Health during the 1970s in *Before AIDS*.

15. Stein, *City of Sisterly and Brotherly Loves*; de Marco interview.

16. Tommi Avicolli, "AIDS Outreach Aimed at Blacks," *Philadelphia Gay News*, July 15, 1983, ONE. Avicolli reported that 46 percent of Philadelphians were Black, but surveillance reports quoted a lower proportion—38 percent—which suggested a wider racial disparity in the city's AIDS epidemic. Philadelphia Department of Public Health, "Acquired Immune Deficiency Syndrome (AIDS) Cases."

17. Evelyn Dickerson, "Blacks Fall Victim to AIDS, Too," *Philadelphia Tribune*, July 31, 1984, 13; "Apathy Slows AIDS Fight," *Philadelphia Tribune*, July 31, 1984.

18. Smith interview.

19. As a younger man, de Marco identified as gay but now identifies himself as queer, which he sees as "more of a political statement than anything else." De Marco interview.

20. De Marco interview. Bay describes a similar inversion of racial stereotypes by Black intellectuals in *White Image in the Black Mind*. ABilly S. Jones-Hennin, a longtime activist and Black bisexual man, recalled in 2007 that in the early days of the epidemic, "There was a great deal of denial. There was a belief, due to lack of information, that this was a gay white disease. African Americans were not the only ones with that belief. In fact, there were some whites who suddenly found blacks sexually more appealing." Will O'Bryan, "Past and Present," *Metro Weekly* (blog), October 17, 2007, https://www .metroweekly.com/2007/10/past-and-present/.

21. Dickerson, "Blacks Fall Victim to AIDS, Too"; Burnette interview; Smith interview; de Marco interview.

22. Fawn Vrazo, "From Philly, a Rap Record about AIDS, for Black Men," *Chicago Tribune*, July 18, 1985, 10D; Vanessa Williams, "Among Black People, AIDS Is Taking a Heavier Toll," *Philadelphia Inquirer*, March 11, 1986; "Respect Yourself Rap Record Now on Sale," *Au Courant*, May 26, 1986, 6, JJWA; "Respect Yourself!" lyrics quoted in Bordowitz, *The AIDS Crisis Is Ridiculous*, 36; David Fair to Thomas Livers, November 24, 1986, box 4, folder "David Fair—various controversies," SWP. "Respect Yourself!" was later used by the New York AIDS activist video collective Testing the Limits in its work.

23. Cei Bell, "Racism Charges at Phila. AIDS Task Force Unfounded," *Philadelphia*

*Gay News*, April 4, 1986, 1, JJWA; Cei Bell, "Task Force Committed to Black Outreach, Says Ifft," *Philadelphia Gay News*, April 11–17, 1986, 26, JJWA.

24. Darlene Garner, IMPACT potluck dinner invitation, July 1, 1986, box 4, folder "David Fair—various controversies," SWP; "PCHA Elects New Board," *Au Courant*, May 19, 1986, 15, JJWA; Abdul-Khabeer interview; Fair interview; Anderson interview.

25. Smith interview.

26. David Fair, interview with Dan Daniels on *Gaydreams*, air date March 3, 1985, WXPN-FM, Philadelphia, box 4, folder "AIDS in Phila 1984–87," SWP.

27. Sign-in sheets dated April 6 and June 8, 1986, held by the Black LGBT Archivists Society of Philadelphia, in the possession of Kevin Trimell Jones. The sheets are not marked as such but according to Jones are from BEBASHI meetings. "BEBASHI Moves into 1199C Office Space," *Au Courant*, June 23, 1986, 17; Abdul-Khabeer interview; Wadlington interview.

28. Bell, "Racism Charges at Phila. AIDS Task Force Unfounded." According to Bell, *Philadelphia Gay News* editors altered the original headline, "Racism Charges at Phila. AIDS Task Force Unsubstantiated," due to space concerns. Although this did subtly change its meaning, she points out, "This wasn't an attempt on PGN's part to change the meaning of my article." Cei Bell, email message to author, February 27, 2018. Bell was also among those who attended the BEBASHI meetings mentioned above.

29. Bell, "Racism Charges at Phila. AIDS Task Force Unfounded"; Abdul-Khabeer interview.

30. Bell, "Racism Charges at Phila. AIDS Task Force Unfounded."

31. Although the 1964 Civil Rights Act predated the widespread use of federal block grants to fund local and state programs, the Department of Justice's Office of Legal Counsel determined in a 1982 legal opinion that federal block grants fell within the "literal terms" of the 1964 law. "Applicability of Certain Cross-Cutting Statutes to Block Grants under the Omnibus Budget Reconciliation Act of 1981," quoted in Bill Lann Lee to Executive Agency Civil Rights Directors, United States Department of Justice Civil Rights Division, January 28, 1999, https://www.justice.gov/crt/block-grant-memo; Cei Bell, "Task Force Committed to Black Outreach, Says Ifft," *Philadelphia Gay News*, April 11–17, 1986; David Fair, "Don't We Die Too?," 1986, Black LGBT Archivists Society of Philadelphia. Although Fair's name does not appear on the leaflet, he claimed authorship of it in an email to the author, January 2, 2019. View a digitized copy of "Don't We Die Too?" at the African American AIDS History Project, http://afamaidshist.fiu.edu/omeka-s/s/african-american-aids-history-project/item/1946.

32. David Wentroble, "PATF Is Attuned to Black Gays with AIDS," *Au Courant*, April 28, 1986, 8.

33. Wentroble, 8.

34. Tommi Avicolli, "Over 2000 Participate in AIDS Walk & Rally," *Philadelphia Gay News*, October 3–10, 1986, 1; Abdul-Khabeer interview.

35. AIDS vigil video recording, September 25, 1986, Rashidah Abdul-Khabeer personal collection. View the speech at the African American AIDS History Project at http://afamaidshist.fiu.edu/omeka-s/s/african-american-aids-history-project/item/762.

36. Abdul-Khabeer interview. Abdul-Khabeer gave a similar account of her "Malcolm X speech" to journalist Pat Loeb, recalling that she said, "You're willing to bend them over and screw them, but you won't take care of them." See Pat Loeb, "After

Tipping Point of Stonewall, AIDS Forged a New Kind of LGBT Activism," KYW News-radio, June 24, 2019, https://kywnewsradio.radio.com/articles/news/after-tipping-point-stonewall-aids-forged-new-kind-lgbt-activism. AIDS vigil video recording; Hinson interview.

37. Abdul-Khabeer interview.

38. Bill Whiting, "Divisive Events Hurt Everyone," *Philadelphia Gay News*, October 3–10, 1986, 9, JJWA. Whiting's influence in the Philadelphia gay community is hard to discern, but, perhaps tellingly, the *Philadelphia Gay News* paired his letter not with a defense of Hassan but with another editorial criticizing the vigil's "heavily religious program." Charlie O'Donnell, a resident of Lehighton, Pennsylvania, also criticized the march route for not going down Spruce Street and questioned the commitment of women to the fight against AIDS in a letter to the editor printed before the walk and vigil. See Charlie O'Donnell, "Divisiveness Is a Real Shame," letter to the editor, *Au Courant*, September 22, 1986, JJWA. On the planning of the candlelight walk, see Ryan Hall, "AIDS Candlelight March to City Hall Planned," *Au Courant*, July 28, 1986, 3, JJWA.

39. Whiting, "Divisive Events Hurt Everyone," 9.

40. Whiting, 30.

41. Whiting, 30.

42. Tommi Avicolli, "Goode's Hatchet Again Falls on Minority Necks," *Philadelphia Gay News*, May 9, 1986, 1; Tommi Avicolli, "New Minority Coordinator Honored at Local Reception," *Philadelphia Gay News*, October 10, 1986, 3, both in JJWA.

43. Kadaba, "Black Warning"; Tyree Johnson, "Unequal Treatment?," *Philadelphia Daily News*, February 26, 1987, 15, box 4, folder "David Fair—various controversies," SWP. Terence Young also reports interpersonal difficulties with Stoffa, leading to Young's demotion and eventual departure from the AIDS Task Force in 1988. In 1994, financial troubles at the agency led to Stoffa's resignation and a criminal investigation from the district attorney. The following year Stoffa was charged with stealing money from the AIDS Task Force; after a long trial he entered a plea of no contest the following year and was sentenced to four years' probation. See Young interview. Huntly Collins, "Head of AIDS Task Force Quits amid Criminal Probe," *Philadelphia Inquirer*, April 12, 1994, A1; Linda Loyd, "Stoffa Ordered to Stand Trial," *Philadelphia Inquirer*, September 29, 1995, B1; Linda Loyd, "AIDS Group's Ex-Boss Enters No-Contest Plea," *Philadelphia Inquirer*, November 7, 1996, B1.

44. Barbara Faggins, "AIDS Activists Angry, but Not Surprised at Firing," *Philadelphia Tribune*, March 3, 1987, 1A.

45. Anderson interview.

46. An introductory letter, signed by Hassan and Wadlington and attached to the copy of the report that is available in the Scott Wilds Papers, suggests that they at least contributed to the document. BEBASHI, "AIDS and Minorities: A Crisis Ignored," 1986, box 4, folder "AIDS in Phila 1984–87," SWP.

47. BEBASHI, "AIDS and Minorities" (emphasis in original). The terms *men who have sex with men* and *MSM* were adopted in the context of HIV research to account for sexual behaviors that do not align with gay or bisexual male identities. However, the terms—along with *women who have sex with women* or *WSW*—have been criticized in public health literature "because they obscure social dimensions of sexuality; undermine the self-labeling of lesbian, gay, and bisexual people; and do not sufficiently

describe variations in sexual behavior." Young and Meyer, "Trouble With 'MSM' and 'WSW'" (emphasis in original).

48. To say that the difference between manifestations of same-sex desire in white America versus Black America arises mainly from the homophobic attitudes of Black communities oversimplifies the complex lived reality of African American MSM. Such attitudes exist within Black communities, as they do in American society more generally, but using the congruity between Black men's sexual activities and their public identities to measure Black community attitudes reduces sexual and progressive politics alike to a single criterion of normatively white sexual expression. Mark Haile writes that "there is a construction of sexuality far more elaborate than mere 'straight' or 'gay,' especially in the black community. When coupled with the racism that is the history of this nation, that affects every aspect of life, the end result is a field of sexual identities for black lesbians and gay men that is identical to neither the white gay and lesbian community in America, nor the framework of sexual orientation as had been studied on the African continent." Mark Haile, "It Can Happen to Anybody. Even Me, Magic Johnson," *BLK* 3, no. 9 (1991): 20–25, quoted in Román, *Acts of Intervention*, 162. For a variety of perspectives on this issue, see Constantine-Simms, *Greatest Taboo*.

49. Wadlington interview.

50. Wadlington interview.

51. Smith interview.

52. BEBASHI, "AIDS and Minorities."

53. *BEBASHI News*, October 1989 and July 1990, BOF.

54. *BEBASHI News*, November 1989; *Hot, Horny & Healthy!* flyer, May 1989 and November 1990, all in BOF.

55. Alexis Moore, "Fighting AIDS in Phila.: A Mission to Inform Blacks," *Philadelphia Inquirer*, September 25, 1988, J1; Kadaba, "Black Warning"; "Interview with Rashidah Hassan and Richard Jennings," *Fresh Air*, NPR, January 28, 1992, http://39ea54ff11b298f9bcaa-1b99eba380497722926169d6da8b098e.r2.cf5.rackcdn.com/1992/FA19920128.mp3.

56. BEBASHI, "Training Manual," July 1986, box 6, folder "Bebashi 1986–1987 1990," AIDS Library (Philadelphia) Records, Temple University Special Collections Research Center.

57. BEBASHI, *Anybody Can Get AIDS* (brochure), n.d., box 4, folder "AIDS in Phila 1984–87," SWP. This brochure was likely produced in early 1987, to promote a radiothon benefit on the local station WDAS. See "Radiothon to Benefit BEBASHI," *Au Courant*, February 23, 1987, 14, JJWA; and BEBASHI, *You Don't Have to Be White or Gay to Get AIDS*, n.d., BOF. This brochure was produced sometime during BEBASHI's first few years, when its offices were inside the 1199C headquarters at 1319 Locust Street. BEBASHI, *BEBASHI [We Need You . . .* ], n.d., BOF. This brochure was produced while BEBASHI was located at 1528 Walnut Street.

The presentation of Black bodies has long been wrapped up with ideas about class within Black communities, in ways that mark light skin and straight hair as more respectable, and darker skin and Afro-textured hair as less respectable. Evelyn Brooks Higginbotham coined the term "politics of respectability" to describe the work of African American women in the National Baptist Convention in her book *Righteous Discontent*. For more on the historical context for Black women thinkers' appeals to respectability, see Cooper, *Beyond Respectability*. For more on the ways that concerns for respectability shaped Black women's activism against sexual assault, see McGuire, *At the Dark End of the Street*. For more on the ways that Black women challenged notions of respectability with regard to hair and clothing, see Ford, *Liberated Threads*.

58. The idea that children had to be protected from AIDS inspired protests by parents to prevent the admission of children with the disease to public schools, most famously in Kokomo, Indiana, where local parents organized for two years to prevent Ryan White from attending school. In Arcadia, Florida, the Ray family saw their home burned to the ground by an arsonist while they fought to enroll their three HIV-positive sons in DeSoto County public schools. Finally, the New York City Board of Education's decision to admit children with AIDS to public schools brought Black and white parents in Queens together in a cross-racial alliance to keep children with AIDS out of the classroom. See "Family in AIDS Case Quits Florida Town after House Burns," *New York Times*, August 30, 1987, A1; and Brier, "'Save Our Kids.'"

59. "BEBASHI Benefits from Record Promotion, 'Birthday Parties,'" *Au Courant*, July 13, 1987, 13, JJWA.

60. Kadaba, "Black Warning"; "BEBASHI News," February 1990, BOF.

61. Wadlington interview.

62. Professor Lazare Kaptue to Curtis Wadlington, August 28, 1989, Curtis Wadlington Collection, African American AIDS History Project; Wadlington interview. View a digitized copy of Kaptue's letter at the African American AIDS History Project at http://afamaidshist.fiu.edu/omeka-s/s/african-american-aids-history-project/item/2595.

63. Alexis Moore, "Fighting AIDS in Phila.: Programa Esfuerzo Reaches Out to Latinos," *Philadelphia Inquirer*, September 25, 1988, J1; Kadaba, "Black Warning"; Abdul-Khabeer interview.

64. "Editorial Viewpoints: Business as Usual," *Philadelphia Gay News*, August 19–25, 1988, box 4, folder "David Fair—various controversies," SWP; Kadaba, "Black Warning," 12.

65. Kadaba, "Black Warning," 27.

66. Kadaba, 12.

67. Kadaba, 12.

68. Huntly Collins and Marc Kaufman, "The Rise and Fall of a Pioneering AIDS Agency," *Philadelphia Inquirer*, October 6, 1993.

69. Collins and Kaufman.

70. Collins and Kaufman.

71. Shilpa Mehta, "BEBASHI Accused of Homophobia," *Au Courant*, November 8, 1993, 23, Clippings File, Black LGBT Archivists Society Collection, in possession of Kevin Trimell Jones.

72. Collins and Kaufman, "Rise and Fall of a Pioneering AIDS Agency."

73. Collins and Kaufman. On the origins of the "welfare queen" stereotype, see Levin, *Queen*.

74. Abdul-Khabeer interview.

75. Wadlington interview.

76. Marc Kaufman and Huntly Collins, "Pioneer AIDS Organization Leaves Bankruptcy, Plans to Raise Funds," *Philadelphia Inquirer*, December 22, 1994; Huntly Collins, "AIDS Agency Making Comeback," *Philadelphia Inquirer*, May 2, 1996; "Our Leadership and Staff," Bebashi: Transition to Hope, accessed April 18, 2019, https://www.bebashi.org/our-staff/.

## Chapter 2

1. "1950s—Cincinnati," Reggie Williams 1951–1999, accessed August 7, 2018, https://sites.google.com/site/reggiewilliamsexhibit/50s; Reggie Williams, "Complete Testimony to CDC Oversight Committee," July 2, 1992, box 28, DTP (at the time of archival research the Duncan Teague Papers were unprocessed; box numbers correspond to those of the collection in its unprocessed form); U.S. Department of Housing and Urban Development, "Environmental Assessment Determinations and Compliance Findings for HUD-Assisted Projects 24 CFR Part 50," HUD Exchange, October 5, 2017, https://www.hudexchange.info/resource/reportmanagement/published/ERR_900000010039103_Demolition-and-Disposition-of-Washington-Terrace-Apts_Cincinnati_OH_EA_AN_10052018_1507216200308.docx.

2. "1960s—Cincinnati," Reggie Williams 1951–1999, accessed August 7, 2018, https://sites.google.com/site/reggiewilliamsexhibit/60s; "1970s—Los Angeles," Reggie Williams 1951–1999, accessed August 7, 2018, https://sites.google.com/site/reggiewilliamsexhibit/70s. For more on gay and lesbian politics in San Francisco during the 1980s, see Hobson, *Lavender and Red*. For more on the Black history of the San Francisco Bay Area, see Broussard, *Black San Francisco*; Crowe, *Prophets of Rage*; Murch, *Living for the City*; and Self, *American Babylon*.

3. U.S. Census Bureau, "1980 Census of Population and Housing: Census Tracts, San Francisco, Oakland, Calif. Standard Metropolitan Statistical Area," Population Characteristics Table P-7, Internet Archive, https://archive.org/details/1980censusofpop802321unse. For more on BWMT see Gregory Conerly, "Black and White Men Together (BWMT)," in Stein, *Encyclopedia of Lesbian, Gay, Bisexual, and Transgender History in America*, 146–47. Records for the NABWMT are held at the ONE National Gay and Lesbian Archives at the University of Southern California, while records for local chapters are held at the San Francisco GLBT Historical Society, Cornell University, the Wisconsin Historical Society, the Atlanta History Center, and elsewhere.

4. Reggie Williams biography, n.d., box 4, folder 68; Reggie Williams to Roz Abrams, August 8, 1985, box 1, folder 27; "KWIC-FAN Mission Statement," [1986], box 4, folder 76, all in NTFAP-UCSF. For more on the Third World AIDS Advisory Task Force and the racial politics of AIDS prevention in San Francisco, see Brier, *Infectious Ideas*, 45–77.

5. "A Discussion with Reggie Williams," *Washington Blade*, [1989], box 4, folder 7, NTFAP-UCSF. "AIDS-related complex" was a diagnosis used in the early years of the epidemic for those who were beginning to show signs of HIV disease, such as weight loss and enlarged lymph nodes, but who had not yet developed opportunistic infections such as Kaposi's sarcoma or pneumocystic pneumonia. It has since fallen out of use.

6. Arthur Lazere, "AIDS Professionals—Taking Education to the People," *Outlines*, April 1989; and Lou Chibbaro Jr., "BWMT Gets $207,000 Grant to Educate Black Gays," *Washington Blade*, September 30, 1988, both in box 4, folder 7, NTFAP-UCSF; Centers for Disease Control and Prevention, "On the Front Lines : Fighting HIV/AIDS in African-American Communities," CDC Stacks, August 1999, https://stacks.cdc.gov/view/cdc/42659.

7. "NTFAP Notes," August 1993, box 31, DTP; Reggie Williams, "AIDS Groups Denounce State's Three Years of AIDS Neglect," 1991, box 1, folder 20, NTFAP-UCSF.

8. Frank Broderick, "BEBASHI Offers Help to Hispanic Community in AIDS

Education," *Au Courant*, February 16, 1987, JJWA; Alexis Moore, "Fighting AIDS in Phila.: Programa Esfuerzo Reaches Out to Latinos," *Philadelphia Inquirer*, September 25, 1988, J1; *GMAD Calendar*, March 1988, box 5, folder 1, GMAD-SC; *GMAD Calendar*, March 1992, box 5, folder 5, GMAD-SC; George Bellinger résumé and biographical sketch, n.d., box 3, folder 14, GMAD-SC; NTFAP, "Ujima Project Description," November 1995, box 14, DTP.

9. Avery F. Gordon and Christopher Newfield, "Introduction," in Gordon and Newfield, *Mapping Multiculturalism*, 5; Abdul-Khabeer interview. For an overview of historical scholarship on multicultural grassroots organizing, see Behnken, "Comparative Civil Rights"; and responses in *Journal of Civil and Human Rights* 3, no. 1 (Spring/ Summer 2017). For some examples of this scholarship, see Behnken, *Civil Rights and Beyond*; Brilliant, *Color of America Has Changed*; Kurashige, *Shifting Grounds of Race*; and Lee, *Building a Latino Civil Rights Movement*.

10. *Black and White Men Together/San Francisco* 6, no. 5, May 1985, box 1, folder 43, QRC. See also Brier, *Infectious Ideas*.

11. Diana Carpenter-Madoshi, "AIDS: The Black Community Fights Back," *San Francisco Bay Guardian*, October 4, 1989, box 4, folder 45, NTFAP-UCSF. Other groups included the Kapuna West Inner-City Child/Family AIDS Network (KWIC-FAN), founded by Dr. Calu Lester in 1986; the MidCity Consortium to Combat AIDS; AIDS Indigent Direct Services; and the AIDS Project of the East Bay in Oakland. Glide United Memorial Methodist Church also conducted outreach in San Francisco's Tenderloin neighborhood, where shared needles made for a common pathway for HIV transmission. In addition to the NTFAP records at UCSF, holdings for KWIC-FAN exist in the John Teamer Papers at the GLBT Historical Society of San Francisco, the AIDS Office of the San Francisco Department of Public Health Records at San Francisco Public Library, and the Hank Tavera Papers at the Ethnic Studies Library at UC Berkeley.

12. Reggie Williams and Larry Burnett to Jim Geary, December 12, 1985, box 1, folder 27.

13. Robert Henderson to Reggie Williams, January 7, 1986, box 1, folder 11; BWMT AIDS Task Force to Paul Volberding, n.d., box 1, folder 29; BWMT/SF AIDS Task Force to Paul Volberding, October 11, 1985, box 1, folder 27, all in NTFAP-UCSF.

14. Richard Stevenson to Lee, January 22, 1988, box 1, folder 15, NTFAP-UCSF. BWMT/ San Francisco, which around 1988 changed its name to BWMT/San Francisco Bay Area, reportedly had a "significant" Asian membership. See NTFAP, "Program Narrative," n.d., National Task Force on AIDS Prevention Records, box 1, folder 2, NTFAP-UCSF.

15. "Community Forum on Strategies for Survival of Black Gay Men," January 14, 1990, box 4, folder 36, NTFAP-UCSF.

16. Jim Marks, "Fractious Family," *Southern Voice*, August 2, 1990, box 28, DTP; Cleo Manago, "B.M.X., Filling the Deadly Cracks of AIDS among Black Men Who Love Men," *Real Read*, n.d., box 1, folder 22, NTFAP-UCSF. Manago was a controversial figure within Bay Area activist circles and found himself in the middle of a major labor dispute soon after taking over as executive director of the AIDS Project of the East Bay. Writing for the Black gay magazine *BLK*, L. Lloyd Jordan argued that the disputes arose from Manago's "lack of managerial experience in combination with his political naïveté." Jordan also noted that Manago had a long-running dispute with Phill Wilson and BWMT/Los Angeles going back to 1987, the result of Manago's "political and philosophic

discomfort with what he regards as bourgeois, conformist organizations." Apparently Manago was "convinced" that the AIDS Project of the East Bay "staff members were poisoned against him . . . by Wilson allies." See L. Lloyd Jordan, "Brouhaha by the Bay," *BLK*, February 1990, 17–22, https://archive.org/details/blk_15. For a first-person account of the politics surrounding Black gay men's groups in Oakland, see LaGrone, "Day the Unspeakable Screamed Its Name."

17. Reggie Williams to Perry Lang, November 20, 1985, box 1, folder 27; and NTFAP, "Statement of Purpose," n.d., box 1, folder 10, both in NTFAP-UCSF. For more on the BWMT/Philadelphia rap record, see chapter 1.

18. Chris Bull, "Black and White Men Together to Launch AIDS Education Program," *Gay Community News*, October 2, 1988, box 4, folder 7, NTFAP-UCSF; National Council of La Raza to Reggie Williams, December 6, 1988, box 1, folder 15, NTFAP-UCSF; Feeback interview. As Brier has shown, while socially conservative members of the Reagan administration and congressional Republicans opposed any response to AIDS that appeared to validate homosexuality, others pushed for a more realistic and compassionate approach. See *Infectious Ideas*, 78–121.

19. Steve Feeback, BWMT National Task Force on AIDS Prevention grant report, 1989, box 28, DTP; "First Task Force Meeting," August 13–14, 1988, box 28, DTP; Wilson interview; NTFAP, *Mutual Support*, no. 1, September 1988, box 2, folder 17, NTFAP-UCSF.

20. Credle interview; James Credle, "CDC and Its AIDS Conference," *Black/Out*, Fall 1988, Serial Collections, HSC.

21. NTFAP, *Hot, Horny & Healthy!* flyer, 1990, box 4, folder 6, NTFAP-UCSF; Luis Palacios-Jimenez and Michael Shernoff, "Facilitator's Guide to 'Hot, Horny & Healthy': Eroticizing Safer Sex," 1986, David Lourea Papers, box 2, folder 55, San Francisco Public Library; Phill Wilson and Health Education Committee of BWMT/Los Angeles, "Hot, Horny and Healthy! Facilitator's Manual," box 29, DTP.

22. NTFAP, "Second Quarterly Report—Budget Period 04," 1991, box 2, folder 4, NTFAP-UCSF; Lee Y. Woo to Louis Ashley, March 26, 1990, box 1, folder 32, NTFAP-UCSF; Bay Area HIV Support and Education Services, *Hot, Horny and Healthy!* flyer, 1990, box 1, folder 19, NTFAP-UCSF. For more on the "train the trainer" public health educational model, see Orfaly et al., "Train-the-Trainer as an Educational Model."

23. Eric Perez, "Safely Is Safety," 1989, box 4, folder 66, NTFAP-UCSF.

24. NTFAP, "HIV Prevention Services for African American Men with Men," 1990, box 3, folder 14, NTFAP-UCSF.

25. Perez, "Safely Is Safety." Woubshet describes the role of "compounding loss" in Black gay AIDS activism in *Calendar of Loss*.

26. Gus Arechavala, "CURAS Outreach Plan," December 1, 1990, box 2, folder 41; Phill Wilson, "'¡Caliente, con Ganas Y Saludable!' Manual Del Facilitador," trans. Martín Ornelas, n.d., box 2, folder 45; Steve Feeback and Douglas Yaranon, "R2T2 Final Report," September 5, 1991, box 2, folder 41, all in NTFAP-UCSF.

27. GMOCC, "Minority Community Health Coalition Demonstration Grant 4th Quarter/Budget Year 1 Report," 1992, box 2, folder 35, NTFAP-UCSF; "NTFAP Notes for Chapters," June 1991, box 27, DTP. In a report to the Bayview Hunter's Point Foundation, the Black Gay Men's Task Force, which included Wendell Carmichael of GMOCC, noted that "in Shanti's Multicultural Plan (1990), there seems to be no sensitivity to the fact that 'people of color' are not a monolithic group and that the nature and spread of

the disease in the Black community is not identical to that of other groups." Kenneth Monteiro, "A Framework for AIDS Services for Black Gay/Bisexual Men," February 1991, box 4, folder 73, NTFAP-UCSF.

28. GMOCC, "Minority Community Health Coalition Demonstration Grant 4th Quarter/Budget Year 1 Report."

29. In addition to the Third World AIDS Advisory Task Force, the five-month student strike led by the Third World Liberation Front at San Francisco State University in late 1968 and early 1969 was instrumental in establishing the university's College of Ethnic Studies. "Campus Commemorates 1968 Student-Led Strike," *SF State News*, September 22, 2008, https://www.sfsu.edu/~news/2008/fall/8.html; GMOCC, "Minority Community Health Coalition Demonstration Grant 4th Quarter/Budget Year 1 Report."

30. "First Task Force Meeting," August 13, 1988; "Second Task Force Meeting Minutes," January 1989, both in box 28, DTP.

31. Other similar studies were undertaken in San Francisco around the same time. A survey of Black San Francisco residents in 1988 and 1989 found that although many respondents knew about AIDS and could recall specific public health messages about HIV, they underestimated their own risk for contracting the virus. Around the same time, John L. Peterson, a Black gay psychologist at the UCSF Center for AIDS Prevention Studies, was also conducting research on sexual behavior and AIDS risk reduction among gay and bisexual Black men in San Francisco, Berkeley, and Oakland. Peterson, along with Gerardo Marín of the University of San Francisco, had also published "Issues in the Prevention of AIDS among Black and Hispanic Men." See "Many San Francisco Blacks Remain at High Risk for AIDS," n.d., box 2, folder 21; Tim Isbell to Thomas Coates and John Peterson, August 22, 1988, box 1, folder 30; John L. Peterson to Reggie Williams, May 25, 1989, box 1, folder 16; and John L. Peterson to Reggie Williams, October 4, 1991, box 1, folder 21, all in NTFAP-UCSF.

32. Feeback, BWMT National Task Force on AIDS Prevention grant report; Minns interview; Reggie Williams to Survey Interviewers, May 31, 1989, box 1, folder 31, NTFAP-UCSF; NTFAP, "Interviewer Instructions," n.d., box 28, DTP.

33. Reggie Williams, Steven Feeback, and Daniel R. Minns, "A Descriptive Analysis of AIDS Knowledge, Attitudes, and Risk Behaviors for HIV Infection among Black Males Who Have Sex with Other Men," 1990, box 1, folder 27, NTFAP-GLBT.

34. Williams, Feeback, and Minns, "Descriptive Analysis."

35. Williams, Feeback, and Minns, "Descriptive Analysis."

36. Boykin, *Beyond the Down Low*; Snorton, *Nobody Is Supposed to Know*.

37. Ron Goldberg, "Conference Call: When PWAs First Sat at the High Table," *POZ*, July 1998, https://www.poz.com/article/Conference-Call-7188-4737; NTFAP, "Second Quarterly Report—Budget Period 03," 1990, box 2, folder 4, NTFAP-UCSF.

38. Duncan Osborne, "GMHC Joins AIDS Confab Boycott," *OutWeek*, May 30, 1990; France, *How to Survive a Plague* (book), 418–19; Phyllida Brown, "The AIDS Debate Moves to the Streets," *New Scientist*, accessed July 27, 2018, https://www.newscientist.com/article/mg12617231-400-the-aids-debate-moves-to-the-streets-the-sixth international-conference-on-aids-held-in-san-francisco-last-week/; Dean Lance, "Letter to the Village Voice," ACT UP/New York, accessed July 27, 2018, http://www.actupny.org/%20othanniversary/voicelet.html. For more on DIVA TV and alternative video as a medium for AIDS activism, see Juhasz, *AIDS TV*.

39. Rex Wockner, "Seen but Not Heard," *OutWeek*, July 11, 1990; Elaine Herscher and Lori Olszewski, "ACT UP Drowns Out Louis Sullivan's Speech," *San Francisco Chronicle*, June 25, 1990, A1; Scott Shepard, "Irate Sullivan Brands Speech Protesters," *Palm Beach Post*, June 26, 1990, 3A.

40. Paul Feldman, "Chris Brownlie; Crusader for AIDS Care, Hospices," *Los Angeles Times*, November 29, 1989, http://articles.latimes.com/1989-11-29/news/mn-54_1 _chris-brownlie-hospice; Phill Wilson to Louis Sullivan, July 1, 1990, box 1, folder 19, NTFAP-UCSF.

41. NTFAP, "Second Quarterly Report—Budget Period 03," 1990, box 2, folder 4; Gay Men of Color AIDS Institute flyer, 1990, box 3, folder 21, both in NTFAP-UCSF.

42. *Safer Sex Comix*, no. 8, https://www.nlm.nih.gov/exhibition/survivingandthriving /digitalgallery/detail-safersexcomix.html; Jesse Helms, "S.Amdt.963 to H.R.3058— 100th Congress (1987–1988)," legislation, October 14, 1987, https://www.congress.gov /amendment/100th-congress/senate-amendment/963.

43. NTFAP, *Prevention Begins at Home* 1, no. 1, September 1988, box 28, DTP; NTFAP, *Mutual Support*, no. 1, September 1988, box 2, folder 17, NTFAP-UCSF.

44. Cal Thomas, "Taxes Pay for 'Horny & Hot' Workshops," *Milwaukee Journal*, November 4, 1990.

45. Thomas, "Taxes Pay for 'Horny & Hot' Workshops"; "Lawrence Welk Encore," *New York Times*, March 27, 1991, https://www.nytimes.com/1991/03/27/opinion/topics-of-the -times-lawrence-welk-encore.html.

46. Reggie Williams, "Text of Statement to the U.S. Congressional Black Caucus," draft, July 16, 1991, box 4, folder 18, NTFAP-UCSF.

47. Al Cunningham to Richard Sacks, June 11, 1991, box 4, folder 69, NTFAP-UCSF.

48. NTFAP, *Notes for Chapters*, no. 4, July 1991, box 28, DTP.

49. "That's Outrageous!," *Reader's Digest*, September 1991, 112–13.

50. "That's Outrageous!" On the origins of the "welfare queen" stereotype, see Levin, *Queen*.

51. NTFAP, "National Task Force on AIDS Prevention Disputes 'Outrageous' Reader's Digest Reprint," 1991, box 4, folder 69, NTFAP-UCSF.

52. Reggie Williams to William Roper, September 27, 1991; and Reggie Williams and Steve Feeback to Mario Solis-Marich et al., November 23, 1991, both in box 1, folder 33, NTFAP-UCSF. NTFAP, *Notes for Chapters*, no. 13, April 1992, box 28, DTP.

53. Reggie Williams to Members of the National Commission on AIDS, January 9, 1992, box 1, folder 34, NTFAP-UCSF.

54. Reggie Williams to Tom Horan, October 26, 1988, box 1, folder 30; John Teamer and Michael Warner to NABWMT Board of Directors, August 1989, box 1, folder 30; Reggie Williams to NABWMT Board of Directors/NTFAP Project Monitoring Committee, July 26, 1990, box 1, folder 19; Ronald L. Trosper to Reggie Williams, November 1, 1991, box 1, folder 21, all in NTFAP-UCSF; Feeback interview.

55. Feeback interview.

56. NTFAP, "Second Quarterly Report—Budget Period 04"; Feeback interview.

57. Reggie Williams to Fred Silverman and Dede Hapner, April 1, 1991, box 2, folder 42, NTFAP-UCSF.

58. NTFAP, AmFAR Public Policy Grants Program letter of intent, December 11, 1991,

box 2, folder 52, NTFAP-UCSF; "A Campaign for Fairness! A Call to Action!," n.d., box 28, DTP; "NTFAP Notes for Chapters," January 1992, box 17, DTP; Carole Midgen to James Curran, June 9, 1992, box 28, DTP; "NTFAP Notes for Chapters," December 1991, box 28, DTP; Barney Frank et al. to William Roper, June 8, 1992, box 28, DTP; Nancy Pelosi to Reggie Williams, January 7, 1993, box 1, folder 24, NTFAP-UCSF.

59. NTFAP, programs chart, 1992, box 4, folder 29, NTFAP-UCSF; Reggie Williams, "Complete Testimony to CDC Oversight Committee," July 2, 1992, box 28, DTP.

60. Nancy Pelosi to Reggie Williams, January 7, 1993, box 1, folder 24; and NTFAP, "Northern California Grantmakers AIDS Task Force Policy Initiative Grant Application 1994–95," September 1994, box 5, folder 7, both in NTFAP-UCSF. Box 14 of the Duncan Teague Papers also contains printed computer slides from a CDC presentation on HIV prevention community planning, which lists "PELOSI Legislation" as an "important antecedent" to the CDC's guidance. For more on HIV prevention community planning, see Valdisseri, Aultman, and Curran, "Community Planning."

61. *NTFAP Notes*, November/December 1993, box 2, folder 14, NTFAP-UCSF; Steve Lew, Campaign for Fairness meeting minutes, October 20, 1994, box 13, DTP. For more on the challenges of HIV prevention community planning, see Dearing et al., "Local Reinvention."

62. Office of the White House Press Secretary, "President Clinton Signs Executive Order for Creation of the Presidential Advisory Council on HIV/AIDS and Announces Twenty-Three Members of the Council," Clinton Presidential Materials Project, June 15, 1995, https://clintonwhitehouse6.archives.gov/1995/06/1995-06-15-president-names-23-to-hiv-aids-advisory-council.html; Morrow-Hall interview.

63. NTFAP, "Office of Minority Health Grant 2nd Quarter/Budget Year 2 Report," 1993, box 2, folder 37, NTFAP-UCSF. BAHSES appears to have suffered from a number of internal problems, including the unresolved nature of its relationship to BWMT and a tense relationship between the group's executive director, Lee Woo, and its board. See meeting minutes in box 1, folder 15, Bay Area HIV Support and Education Services Records, UCSF Special Collections.

64. San Francisco Department of Public Health, "CURAS Audit Report," October 1992, box 2, folder 49; CURAS Board of Directors, "CURAS Work Plan," October 1992, box 2, folder 49; "Notes for Discussion: Proyecto ContraSIDA—P/V," 1993, box 1, folder 35; "Fact Sheet: Proyecto ContraSIDA por Vida," n.d., box 3, folder 17, all in NTFAP-UCSF.

65. Bang Nguyen, "Gay Men of Color Consortium on AIDS Educational Models for Community Change (EMC2) Evaluation Report," December 20, 1993, box 3, folder 17, NTFAP-UCSF.

66. Wolfgang Schreiber, "Reggie Williams Exhibit," Reggie Williams 1951–1999, accessed September 11, 2016, https://sites.google.com/site/reggiewilliamsexhibit/.

67. Alan McCord, "AIDS Community Honors Activist Reggie Williams," December 10, 1993, National Task Force on AIDS Prevention Records, box 3, folder 16, UCSF Special Collections.

68. Randy Miller to NTFAP Board Finance Committee, March 5, 1994, box 3, folder 17, NTFAP-UCSF; Reggie Williams to Deborah Wallace, November 3, 1993, box 1, folder 25, NTFAP-UCSF; NTFAP, "Ujima Project Description," November 1995, box 14, DTP; *Strategem*, Summer 1997, box 14, DTP; Morrow-Hall interview. Part of Project Fire's history is

documented in the James Credle Papers, available at the African American AIDS History Project, http://afamaidshist.fiu.edu/omeka-s/s/african-american-aids-history-project/item-set/731.

69. Morrow-Hall interview; Wolfgang Schreiber, "Reggie Williams Exhibit."

## Chapter 3

1. Joseph Beam, "Caring for Each Other," *Philadelphia Gay News*, May 16–22, 1986, 9, box 7, folder 16, Joseph F. Beam Papers, SC.

2. Bost, *Evidence of Being*. The phrase "Black gay renaissance" may have been coined by Alden Reimonenq. See Steward, "Saint's Progeny."

3. Robinson quoted in Cohen, *Boundaries of Blackness*, 100; Bost, *Evidence of Being*; Phill Wilson, "Deciding Moment: Together We Are Greater Than AIDS," in Black AIDS Institute, *Back of the Line*, 5–6.

4. Phill Wilson, "Outreach to Black Gay/Bisexual Men," n.d., box 29, DTP. Here Wilson explicitly drew on the work of Black psychiatrist Alvin Poussaint, who argued (in Wilson's words) that "the legacy of centuries of forced servitude, social segregation and color discrimination has had a physically and psychologically brutalizing effect on many (if not all) Black people and our psyches. This brutalization can result in a generalized sense of powerlessness, and in a broad based self-perpetuating cultural lack of self-esteem."

5. In *Boundaries of Blackness* Cathy Cohen outlines "the three stages of response to AIDS in African-American communities." The first stage, "the emergence of AIDS and a visible Black gay identity," and the third, "the AIDS bureaucracy in African-American communities," are germane to this story. The former involves responses to AIDS from the artists and organizations that made up the Black gay renaissance, while the latter finds that "many organizations servicing people of color with AIDS pursue agendas structured around service provision and education, with little effort devoted to politics." While Cohen also writes in the same section that groups like GMAD had an "organizational vision and mission . . . broader than those of most AIDS service organizations," the process that Joe Pressley and Kevin McGruder describe in oral history interviews toward the end of this chapter point to GMAD becoming more like those professionalized and depoliticized AIDS service organizations. See Cohen, *Boundaries of Blackness*, 91–118.

6. Beam, "Making Ourselves from Scratch," 261; Beam, "Introduction," 13–14; Beam, "Brother to Brother," 231. In "Brother to Brother" Beam emphasized that "Black men loving Black men" is "the revolutionary act of the eighties," "an autonomous agenda for the eighties," and "a call to action, an acknowledgment of responsibility." Fred Carl, who founded the Blackheart Collective, tells a similar story about working at the Oscar Wilde Bookshop in New York City in McGruder, "To Be Heard in Print."

7. *BWMT/LA Newsletter*, no. 16, February 1982, Periodicals, BWMT Newsletters, BWMT–Los Angeles 1980–1982, ONE; Branner, "Blackberri."

8. Cliff, *Claiming an Identity They Taught Me to Despise*. Beam would also become friends and interlocutors with several notable Third World feminist thinkers. See Barbara Smith and Steven G. Fullwood, "On Joseph Beam: A Conversation," in Fullwood and Stephens, *Black Gay Genius*, 19–37.

9. According to Beam, the phrase "in the life" has overtones of both criminality and

sexuality, "used to describe 'street life' (the lifestyle of pimps, prostitutes, hustlers, and drug dealers) [and] also . . . to describe the 'gay life' (the lives of Black homosexual men and women)." Beam, *In the Life*, 12; Jacqueline Trescott, "Anthology of a Mother's Grief," *Washington Post*, August 17, 1991. For examples of reader responses to *In the Life*, see Chuck Tarver to Joseph Beam, n.d., box 4, folder 3, Joseph F. Beam Papers, SC; and Penn, "Hide, Seek, Arrive *In the Life*."

10. Bost, *Evidence of Being*, 59.

11. Both the NTFAP and GMAD hosted benefit screenings of the film. "'Paris Is Burning' Director, Star to Appear at Gala Premiere," 1991, box 4, folder 6; Jennie Livingston, "Making 'Paris Is Burning,'" box 4, folder 30, both in NTFAP-UCSF. For an overview of the ongoing *Paris Is Burning* controversy, see Ashley Clark, "Burning Down the House: Why the Debate over *Paris Is Burning* Rages On," *The Guardian*, June 24, 2015, https://www.theguardian.com/film/2015/jun/24/burning-down-the-house-debate-paris-is-burning.

12. Smith and Fullwood, "On Joseph Beam"; Black Gay and Lesbian Leadership Forum, "California Community Foundation Proposal," n.d., box 4, folder 13, NTFAP-UCSF. Kevin J. Mumford argues that Philadelphia Black Gays (PBG) members were instrumental to the passing of a local gay and lesbian nondiscrimination ordinance in 1982, whereas in his contribution to *In the Life* James Charles Roberts charged that many PBG members had been unwilling to take principled political positions and insisted that "PBG was all but dormant" when the ordinance passed. See Mumford, "Trouble with Gay Rights"; and Roberts, "Light That Failed." The first issue of *Black/Out* listed active black gay and lesbian groups. *Black/Out* 1, no. 1 (Summer 1986), Serial Collections, HSC.

13. See the shift from using "Third World" to "people of color" in the Third World Lesbian/Gay Conference advertised by the National Coalition of Black Gays in 1981 versus the Third World/People of Color Conference that the group advertised in late 1983. *Habari-Habari* 3, no. 2 (1981); *Habari-Daftari*, December 1983/January 1984, both in box 5, folder 21, QRC.

14. "David: 0 vs Goliath: 1," and Gil Gerald, "Reagan Must Go!" in *Habari-Daftari*, undated; Charles Stewart, "Minority Participation in the Gay/Lesbian Community" in *Habari-Daftari*, no. 4 (1984); "Chapter Happenings," in *Habari-Habari* 3, no. 2 (1981); Juana Maria Paz, "Lonnie M. Woods #14217: 'Just Cause I'm an Inmate Do I Have to Die?,'" in *Habari-Daftari*, December 1983/January 1984, all in box 5, folder 21, QRC. The National Coalition of Black Gays also provided copies of *Habari-Daftari* for free to incarcerated people. The National Coalition of Black Lesbians and Gays (having been renamed) printed pen pal requests from incarcerated people in *Black/Out*. See *Black/Out* 2, no. 1 (Fall 1988): 59, Serial Collections, HSC. The Blackheart Collective dedicated the second issue of its journal to "Black gay men who are, or have been, incarcerated." For more on concern for the plight of the incarcerated as part of the project of gay liberation, see Downs, *Stand by Me*, 143–67. The continued focus on prison issues within the Black gay and lesbian movement complicates Downs's declension narrative, which posits that gay prison activism "[fell] by the wayside" as "many gay people became more obsessed with themselves than with others or with their community."

15. Duberman, *Hold Tight Gently*, 113; Bost, *Evidence of Being*, 136, 140.

16. Colin Robinson, preliminary sketch by GMAD Statement of Purpose Committee, August 6, 1986; and "Men of Afrikan Descent (GMAD) Minutes," August 20, 1986, both in box 1, folder 1, GMAD-SC.

17. *GMAD Calendars*, March, July, September, October, December 1988, box 5, folder 1, GMAD-SC. Although Kimberlé Crenshaw ("Demarginalizing") coined the term "intersectionality" in 1989, well after GMAD was founded, I reference the concept here because it accurately describes the group's work. Crenshaw also traces the origins of the concept through a long line of black feminist thinkers, putting her in the same intellectual lineage as the artists, writers, and activists of the Black gay renaissance.

18. *Moja*, no. 3, April 3, 1979, QRC; J. R. Roberts, *Black Lesbians*; Craig G. Harris, "The NCBLG Family Gathers," *Black/Out* 1, no. 1 (Summer 1986), Serial Collection, HSC; "The Lesbian Herstory Archives: History and Mission," accessed March 18, 2019, http://www.lesbianherstoryarchives.org/history.html; Craig G. Harris, "Black Gay/Lesbian History: A Seldom-Told Tale," *Au Courant*, February 24, 1986, JJWA. Jim Downs has written about the emergence of gay history as a disciplinary subfield in the 1970s with African American history as its model. The development of a self-conscious Black gay history extends and complicates that story. See Downs, *Stand by Me*, 89–112.

19. Charles Michael Smith, "Bruce Nugent: Bohemian of the Harlem Renaissance," in Beam, *In the Life*, 209–20; Essex Hemphill, "Looking for Langston: An Interview with Isaac Julien" and "Undressing Icons" in Hemphill, *Brother to Brother*, 175–77, 181.

20. "US Conference of Mayors Collaborative HIV/AIDS Prevention Grant Monthly Update Report," February 1995, box 24, folder 4, GMAD-SC.

21. "African Americans Are Vocal about Gay Pride," *City Sun* (Brooklyn), July 28, 1995, box 22, folder 4, GMAD-SC. Other Countries also included an interview with Rustin in its first published collection. Redvers Jeanmarie, "An Interview with Bayard Rustin," in *Other Countries*, 3–16.

22. Cleaver quoted in Mumford, "Trouble with Gay Rights," 54; Welsing quoted in McBride, "Can the Queen Speak?" 369; Asante quoted in Carbado, *Black Men on Race, Gender, and Sexuality*, 284; Riggs, "Black Macho Revisited," 257. For a challenge to Black sexual essentialism from an Africanist perspective, see Murray and Roscoe, *Boy-Wives and Female Husbands*.

23. *GMAD Calendar*, July 1988, box 5, folder 1, GMAD-SC; Arit John, "Confusing a Country for a Continent: How We Talk About Africa," *Atlantic*, August 29, 2013, https://www.theatlantic.com/international/archive/2013/08/confusing-country-continent-how-we-talk-about-africa/311621/.

24. *GMAD Calendar*, May 1994, box 5, folder 7, GMAD-SC. The Egyptian focus of this program reflects a shift in orientation from West Africa to Egypt as the supposed cradle of a durable Black civilization. See Austin, *Achieving Blackness*. For a longer view on white American attitudes toward Africa as a backward and timeless place, see Bederman, *Manliness and Civilization*.

25. *Habari-Habari* 3, no. 2 (1981); *Habari-Daftari*, December 1983/January 1984, both in box 5, folder 21, QRC.

26. Beasley's article on ritual performance in Adodi, which draws on oral history sources, misstates the year of the group's founding as 1983. Beasley, "'Tribute to the Ancestors.'"

27. Adodi New York Habari Gani e-Newsletter Archive Homepage, accessed November 10, 2012, http://archive.constantcontact.com/fs065/1101859413381/archive/1102432339232.html. Also quoted from www.adodiintl.org in Beasley, "'Tribute to the Ancestors.'"

28. Michael Oatis, "A Voice in Our Wilderness," *Black/Out* 1, no. 3/4 (1987), Serial

Collections, HSC. Yemaya is also known as Yemoja, a water goddess in the Yoruba religion, whose worship in the Caribbean and the Americas is rooted in the history of the Atlantic slave trade. The Blackheart Collective also titled the first volume of its journal *Yemonja*, another variation on her name. Bost, *Evidence of Being*, 68.

29. Oatis, "A Voice in Our Wilderness"; Frank Broderick, "Adodi Black Gay Support Group to Hold Retreat," *Au Courant*, October 26, 1987, 13, JJWA; Adodi interview quoted in Beasley, "'Tribute to the Ancestors,'" 435; *GMAD Calendar*, May 1989, box 5, folder 2, GMAD-SC; *GMAD Calendar*, October/November 1990, August 1991, and September 1991, box 5, folder 4, GMAD-SC.

30. *GMAD Calendar*, June 1989; and "Ukwangela" in *GMAD Calendar*, July 1989, both in box 5, folder 2, GMAD-SC. The definition of *ukwangela* used here is a direct quote from Davidson, *The Africans*. "Palaver" came to English from the Portuguese *palavra*, which early traders in West Africa used to describe their interactions with the native population. See *Oxford Dictionary of Word Origins*, ed. Julia Cresswell, 2012 online edition, accessed via Oxford Reference electronic database.

31. *GMAD Calendar*, September 1991, box 5, folder 4; and *GMAD Calendar*, January/February 1992, box 5, folder 5, both in GMAD-SC.

32. In this way GMAD fit into the 1990s turn toward Afrocentrism. See Austin, *Achieving Blackness*. *GMAD Calendar*, June, September, and October 1993, box 5, folder 6; *GMAD Calendar*, July 1994, box 5, folder 7, all in GMAD-SC.

33. Austin criticizes Black gay and lesbian activists for grounding claims to gay legitimacy in African tradition rather than in "any abstract principle of justice or equality," but this interpretation misses the other purposes that a usable Black gay past served. See *Achieving Blackness*, 160.

34. Riggs, *Tongues Untied*.

35. Riggs, "Black Macho Revisited."

36. Woubshet describes this feeling as one of "compounding loss" in *Calendar of Loss*.

37. Ron Simmons, "Tongues Untied: An Interview with Marlon Riggs," in Hemphill, *Brother to Brother*, 193.

38. *Tongues Untied* won awards at the Berlin Film Festival and from the Los Angeles Film Critics Association, among others. "Tongues Untied," IMDB, accessed March 21, 2019, http://www.imdb.com/title/tt0103099/awards. Writing for the *Washington Post*, David Mills praised *Tongues Untied*, whereas his colleague Courtland Milloy criticized it for "ignor[ing] the heterosexual audience" and thus "miss[ing] a chance to contribute to changing the hostile climate that keeps black homosexuals in their closets." David Mills, "Cry of 'Tongues Untied,'" *Washington Post*, July 19, 1991, B1; Courtland Milloy, "Film on Black Gays Is Bold, but Ignores the Big Picture," *Washington Post*, July 18, 1991, C3; Dubin, *Arresting Images*; Bullert, *Public Television*; Mintcheva, "'Some Objects in This Exhibit May Be Disturbing to Certain Viewers.'"

39. "Motown Tongues Still Tied," June 1991, box 1, folder 33, NTFAP-UCSF; Out Fund for Lesbian and Gay Liberation, "Out with Our First Grants," 1991, box 1, folder 20, NTFAP-UCSF.

40. Bost, *Evidence of Being*; Colin Robinson and Robert Reid-Pharr to PBS, n.d., box 3, folder 8, GMAD-SC.

41. Everett, *I Shall Not Be Removed*.

42. *GMAD Calendar*, November 1989, box 5, folder 2, GMAD-SC. The "Uniéndonos"

program included Anthony Knight-Dewey, a Black gay man born in Queens; Aurelio Font, who sang in the gay a cappella group the Flirtations; Manuel Ramos Otero, a gay Puerto Rican writer; and Carlos Segura, a member of Other Countries Collective. "Our Founder," Baton Foundation, accessed March 20, 2019, https://thebatonfoundation.org /our-founder; Duberman, *Hold Tight Gently*; "Rare Book & Manuscript Library Acquires Archive of Puerto Rican Author Manuel Ramos Otero," Columbia University Libraries, March 12, 2014, https://library.columbia.edu/news/libraries/2014/2014-3-12 _RBML_Acquires_Ramos_Otero_Archive.html; Bost, *Evidence of Being*. GMAD *Calendar*, June 1989, box 5, folder 2, box 5; the October/November 1990 *GMAD Calendar* dropped "Latino" from program Friday Night Forum descriptions, while the June and August 1991 calendars referred to inclusion of Arab men, box 5, folder 4; *GMAD Calendar*, March 1992, box 5, folder 5, all in GMAD-SC.

43. *GMAD Calendar*, May 1989, box 5, folder 2; *GMAD Calendar*, September 1991, box 5, folder 4, both in GMAD-SC.

44. *GMAD Calendar*, March and June 1992, box 5, folder 5, GMAD-SC. The group did not publish a calendar for May 1992 due to financial and technical difficulties, so Anthony's letter and Jones's response may have originally been slated for the unpublished issue.

45. Pressley interview.

46. *GMAD Calendar*, June 1992.

47. *GMAD Calendar*, June 1992.

48. Having been founded in 1987 at a meeting called by the New York Urban League of over sixty of "New York City's highest ranking leaders," the BLCA advocated for public policy around AIDS among African Americans, developed programs, and provided technical assistance and financial advice to community-based groups. "Black Leadership Commission on AIDS Booklet," n.d., box 8, folder 21, GMAD-SC.

49. Black Leadership Commission on AIDS, "Clinicians' Teaching Guide for the Lifestyles Genesis Learning Series Program," n.d., box 8, folder 22; Black Leadership Commission on AIDS, "Lifestyles Genesis Planning Retreat Program," July 1990, box 9, folder 1, both in GMAD-SC.

50. Reggie Williams, Steven Feeback, and Daniel R. Minns, "A Descriptive Analysis of AIDS Knowledge, Attitudes, and Risk Behaviors for HIV Infection among Black Males Who Have Sex with Other Men," 1990, box 1, folder 27, NTFAP-GLBT.

51. GMAD Board of Directors meeting minutes, May 9, May 19, and June 20, 1991, all in box 4, folder 14, GMAD-SC; Colin Robinson to GMAD Brothers, April 5, 1991, box 3, folder 8, GMAD-SC; Fullwood, *Gay Men of African Descent, Inc. Records* [finding aid]. According to a version of the GMAD records finding aid furnished to the author by Fullwood (who was a GMAD member) in 2012, Elbert Gates served as GMAD's first executive director, following the group's incorporation in 1989. This information is not included in the version of the GMAD finding aid that is accessible online through the New York Public Library website. In contrast, Darius Bost writes in *Evidence of Being* that Colin Robinson was the group's first executive director. Although Robinson did serve as executive director of GMAD during the middle 1990s, none of the documents consulted for this book suggest that he held this position at an earlier point.

52. Gary Paul Wright, "VOCAL—Minutes for 21 August 1990," box 6, folder 38, Robert Garcia Papers, Cornell University Library Rare and Manuscript Collections, Ithaca;

Black Leadership Commission on AIDS, Lifestyles Genesis Draft Curriculum, n.d., box 8, folder 21, GMAD-SC.

53. GMAD leaders were present at larger events that included *Hot, Horny and Healthy!* trainings, and the group hosted the playshop twice in 1989. NTFAP, *Prevention Begins at Home*, October 1988, box 2, folder 17, NTFAP-UCSF; NTFAP, "Schedule of Workshops and Trainings," 1989, box 17, DTP; *GMAD Calendar*, June 1989, box 5, folder 2, GMAD-SC.

54. The "zap" was a direct-action protest tactic used in the 1970s by gay liberation and other activist groups such as the Gay Activists Alliance, the Gay Liberation Front, and Women's International Terrorist Conspiracy from Hell (or WITCH). Zaps disrupt the normal flow of activity in a target location, using noisemakers, banners, or activists' bodies to take up space and attract attention. Since 1987, ACT UP chapters have used zaps to influence decision makers and draw public attention to issues concerning people living with or at risk for HIV and AIDS. As part of their zaps, ACT UP members have staged theatrical "die-ins," unfurled banners at the New York Stock Exchange, and flooded the phone banks of pharmaceutical companies, elected representatives, and public health officials. ACT UP Phone Zaps page, accessed November 28, 2012, http://www.actupny.org/documents/PZ.html. Chapter 6 describes some of the zaps that ACT UP Philadelphia staged during campaigns against Medicaid privatization and to secure affordable AIDS drugs for African countries.

55. Black Leadership Commission on AIDS, Lifestyles Genesis Draft Curriculum.

56. GMAD Board of Directors meeting minutes, May 19, 1991; GMAD Board HIV Program Initiatives Committee to NY AIDS Institute, October 10, 1991, box 8, folder 19, GMAD-SC.

57. Colin Robinson to Board of Directors, February 27, 1994, box 2, folder 9, GMAD-SC; Pressley interview.

58. Other productions by AIDSFILMS also used a "behavior-modeling" approach. See Alexandra Juhasz, "So Many Alternatives: The Alternative AIDS Video Movement," *Cinéaste* 21, no. 1/2 (1995): 37–39. Colin Robinson to Fran Barrett, June 17, 1991, box 2, folder 7; Valyrie Laedlin and Denice Williams to Colin Robinson, July 5, 1991, box 2, folder 7; "GMAD News," March 1, 1993, box 7, folder 5; "AIDSFILM/GMAD Steering Committee for African American Gay Men's Film Meeting Minutes," May 5, 1992, box 10, folder 1, all in GMAD-SC. The memorial service arranged by Woods's family, which erased his sexuality and the true cause of his death, inspired an outburst from Woods's friend and fellow Black gay writer Assotto Saint and other gay friends, who then staged their own alternate service. The incident inspired Thomas Glave's short story "The Final Inning." See Bost, *Evidence of Being*; and Woubshet, *Calendar of Loss*.

59. *Party* script, 1992, box 10, folder 9, GMAD-SC. All references to dialogue and action in *Party* are taken from this script.

60. The language of "relapse" with respect to condom use was prevalent in AIDS research and advocacy during the 1990s. See, for example, Stall et al., "Relapse from Safer Sex"; and "A Call for a New Generation of AIDS Prevention for Gay and Bisexual Men in San Francisco," August 1993, box 4, folder 16, NTFAP-UCSF.

61. Here "burn" means to have or give a sexually transmitted infection.

62. Colin Robinson to Board of Directors, February 27, 1994; Colin Robinson to Board of Directors, March 12, 1994, both in box 2, folder 9, GMAD-SC.

63. "Proposal to the Paul Rapoport Foundation," June 1, 1995, box 2, folder 8, GMAD-SC. Italics in original.

64. Beam, "Brother to Brother," 231, and Riggs, "Black Macho Revisited," 254, quoted in GMAD, "USCM Collaborative HIV Prevention Grants Proposal," December 1993, box 24, folder 2, GMAD-SC.

65. Colin Robinson to Board of Directors, August 4, 1995, box 2, folder 10, GMAD-SC.

66. Lawrence DeWyatt Abrams, "Report of the Managing Director," December 14, 1995, box 1, folder 5; "Executive Committee Report," November 14, 1995, box 1, folder 5; Fullwood, *Gay Men of African Descent, Inc. Records* [finding aid]; GMAD Board of Directors Meeting Minutes, July 30, 1996, box 4, folder 18; GMAD Board of Directors Meeting Minutes," March 8, 1997, box 4, folder 19; C. Ralph Wilson to Stephen Williams, March 6, 1996, box 3, folder 13; Robert E. Penn to Board of Directors, June 11, 1997, box 4, folder 23; "GMAD Board of Directors Meeting Minutes," July 10, 1997, box 4, folder 19; Colin Robinson to Fran Barrett, June 17, 1991, box 2, folder 7; GMAD Board HIV Program Initiatives Committee to NY AIDS Institute, October 10, 1991, box 8, folder 19, all except finding aid in GMAD-SC.

67. Levenson, *Secret Epidemic*; Regina Aragón and Jennifer Kates, "HIV/AIDS Policy Brief: The Minority AIDS Initiative," Henry J. Kaiser Family Foundation, 2004, https://kaiserfamilyfoundation.files.wordpress.com/2013/01/minority-aids-initiative-policy-brief.pdf; McGruder interview.

68. McGruder interview.

69. McGruder interview; Pressley interview.

70. McGruder interview.

71. K. Woodward, "GMAD as Hell," City Limits, May 10, 2004, https://citylimits.org/2004/05/10/gmad-as-hell/; McGruder interview; Pressley interview.

72. The point about AIDS being the impetus for the first government funding for Black gay men's work was made during a panel discussion of *Black Gay Genius: Answering Joseph Beam's Call*, edited by Steven Fullwood and Charles Stephens. The discussion was hosted by the P.A.G.E.S. Men's Book Club in Philadelphia and included Carlos Carter, Steven Fullwood, andre m. carrington, Darius Omar Williams, Guy Weston, Arleen Olshan, and Ron Simmons.

73. McGruder interview; Pressley interview.

## Chapter 4

1. "War on AIDS," *Weekly Review*, December 15, 1989, box 10, folder "Africa-Health-AIDS-Kemron," Leroy T. Walker Africa News Service Archive, David M. Rubinstein Rare Book and Manuscript Library, Duke University, Durham. Koech gives his own account of the Kemron episode, along with much of the rest of his personal and professional life, in Elliott, *Reimagining Science*.

2. "Kenyan Researchers Announce Success with New AIDS Drug," *Reuter News Reports*, February 7, 1990; Abid Aslam and Patrick Logan, "African AIDS Drug Catches U.S. Unawares," *Inter Press Service*, March 16, 1990; "Tanzania Seeks Kenyan AIDS Drug Kemron," *Reuter News Service*, March 28, 1990; "International Testing for Kemron," *Weekly Review*, May 4, 1990, all in box 10, folder "Africa-Health-AIDS-Kemron," Leroy T. Walker Africa News Service Archive. Africans who traveled to Nairobi seeking

treatment were often met with disappointment and exploitation. Nelson Ocheng, a Ugandan man with AIDS, sold his house to cover the cost of travel to Nairobi after hearing about Kemron on the radio. Upon arrival he discovered that the drug was unavailable and instead paid a local healer for an ineffective herbal treatment. Having spent most of his money only to see his condition get progressively worse, Ocheng returned home to Uganda to die. Loretta Tofani, "A Man's Long Journey for a Sliver of Hope," *Philadelphia Inquirer*, March 28, 1991, 1A, box 38, folder 10, KKP.

3. Lawrence K. Altman, "New AIDS Experiments Stir Hope and Wariness," *New York Times*, April 4, 1990, A22; Charles Nguigi, "War of Words over Kemron," *The Standard* (Kenya), May 4, 1990, reprinted in *New York Native*, May 28, 1990, 6, box 38, folder 10, KKP. The first coverage of Kemron in the *Native* appears to be in April 1990, shortly after *Biotechnology Newswatch* reported Koech's results. Neenyah Ostrom, "Oral Alpha-Interferon: A Special Report," *New York Native*, April 16, 1990, 8. Ostrom believed that AIDS was related to chronic fatigue and immune dysfunction syndrome (CFIDS), questioned the link between HIV and AIDS, and saw Kemron as a potential remedy for CFIDS. She later appeared on *Tony Brown's Journal* to promote her book *America's Biggest Cover-Up: 50 More Things Everyone Should Know about the Chronic Fatigue Syndrome Epidemic and Its Link to AIDS*. See *Tony Brown's Journal*, "Disease: America's New Frontier," aired April 24, 1994, on PBS, tape 45306, NPAC. Others also saw Kemron and other forms of low-dose oral alpha interferon as a promising remedy for CFIDS. See Neenyah Ostrom, "'AIDS' Treatment Breakthrough: Oral Alpha Interferon," *New York Native*, April 16, 1990, 8; and "Low Dose Oral Alpha Interferon, a Promising Treatment for CFIDS," n.d., both in box 38, folder 10, KKP. Writing for the Gay Men's Health Crisis newsletter *Treatment Issues* in October 1990, Dave Roche pointed out all of the times that his and other newsletters had reported on Kemron. However, critics who charged that the Kemron story had been "ignored" were largely talking about the mainstream news media, not AIDS activist publications. *Treatment Issues*, October 12, 1990, box 38, folder 10, KKP.

4. Neil Henry, "Kenya Unveils Drug That Is Reputed to Alleviate the Impact of AIDS," *Washington Post*, July 28, 1990, A14.

5. Lawrence K. Altman, "New AIDS Experiments Stir Hope and Wariness," *New York Times*, April 4, 1990, A22.

6. Henry, "Kenya Unveils Drug." John James gave a thorough accounting of the questionable aspects of Koech's study in *AIDS Treatment News*, April 20, 1990, box 38, folder 10, KKP.

7. Cohen, *Boundaries of Blackness*; Burkett, *Gravest Show on Earth*, 169.

8. Some white scholars also pointed out the racist overtones of the African origin theory. See Sontag, *Illness as Metaphor*, 139; Farmer, *AIDS and Accusation*, 3; and Patton, *Inventing AIDS*, 80. The mapping of genetic differences among strains of the virus has since shown that HIV crossed into the human population from chimpanzees somewhere around Cameroon near the beginning of the twentieth century, possibly through a hunter who cut himself while butchering a monkey. From there, colonialism, urbanization, civil war, the global trade in blood products, sex tourism, and efforts to eradicate epidemic disease transformed a single initial infection into a worldwide pandemic. Pepin, *Origins of AIDS*.

9. Dalton, "AIDS in Blackface," 212.

10. Karen Grigsby Bates, "Is It Genocide?," *Essence*, September 1990, 76; Kalichman, *Denying AIDS*; Heller, "Rumors and Realities."

11. Herek and Capitanio, "Conspiracies, Contagion, and Compassion"; Klonoff and Landrine, "Do Blacks Believe That HIV/AIDS Is a Government Conspiracy against Them?"; Bogart and Thorburn, "Relationship of African Americans' Sociodemographic Characteristics"; Sallar, Williams, and Omishakin, "Are HIV/AIDS Conspiracy Beliefs Barriers?"; Seele interview.

12. Whorton, *Nature Cures*. In November 2012, Duesberg was a guest on *The Joe Rogan Experience*, a popular podcast. Rogan, an actor, frequently gives a platform to guests who espouse racist, misogynistic, and Islamophobic views. As of this writing, Rogan's YouTube channel has almost 7.5 million subscribers. "Joe Rogan Experience #282—Dr. Peter Duesberg & Bryan Callen," YouTube, January 19, 2013, https://www.youtube.com/watch?v=k1jjomUYJ_g; Caroline Haskins, "From Joe Rogan to the Far Right: Inside YouTube's Alt-Media Ecosystem," *Vice* (blog), September 26, 2018, https://www.vice.com/en_us/article/59ade5/inside-youtubes-alt-media-ecosystem.

13. Thomas and Quinn, "Tuskegee Syphilis Study"; David L. Kirp, "Blood, Sweat, and Tears: The Tuskegee Experiment and the Era of AIDS," *Tikkun*, March 1995; Freimuth, "African Americans' Views"; Reverby, *Examining Tuskegee*; Reverby, "'Normal Exposure' and Inoculation Syphilis."

14. Nicholas M. Horrock, "Senate Intelligence Panel Told of F.B.I. Attempt to Discredit Dr. King in 1964," *New York Times*, November 19, 1975, 16; John Kifner, "F.B.I. Sought Doom of Panther Party," *New York Times*, May 9, 1976, 1.

15. Ojanuga, "Medical Ethics of the 'Father of Gynaecology'"; P. Turner, *I Heard It through the Grapevine*, xvii; Skloot, *Immortal Life of Henrietta Lacks*.

16. Love, *One Blood*, 262.

17. John Roberts, "African American Belief Narratives"; Kelley, "Kickin' Reality"; Kelley, *Yo' Mama's DisFunktional!*

18. In *AIDS Conspiracy Theories*, David Gilbert, a prison AIDS educator who is serving a seventy-five-year sentence for his role in the Weather Underground's 1981 robbery of a Brink's armored truck, addressed the prevalence of conspiracy theories among Black inmates and the difficulty they presented to his HIV prevention efforts. Bogart and Thorburn, "Exploring the Relationship of Conspiracy Beliefs"; Bogart et al., "Conspiracy Beliefs about HIV"; Bogart et al., "Medical Mistrust"; McGregor, *Khabzela*; LeRoy Whitfield, "Marathon Man," *POZ*, May 2002, https://www.poz.com/article/Marathon-Man-853-6184. Whitfield wrote about AIDS conspiracy theories among African Americans, as well as the continued use of Kemron, in the December 2000 issue of *POZ*. See "The Secret Plot to Destroy African Americans," *POZ*, December 2000, https://www.poz.com/article/The-Secret-Plot-to-Destroy-African-Americans-7602-7053. According to Phill Wilson, Whitfield was "not an AIDS dissident," but his decision to forgo antiretrovirals was born of the suspicion that "doctors and AIDS service providers pushed people to start taking the demanding meds too quickly." "Remembering LeRoy Whitfield," blackaids.org, September 18, 2010, https://web.archive.org/web/20100918103805/http://www.blackaids.org/index.php?option=com_content&view=article&id=159:remembering-leroy-whitfield&catid=58:news-2005-older&Itemid=129.

19. Nattrass, "Understanding the Origins and Prevalence of AIDS Conspiracy Beliefs."

20. Cohen examines some of the same *Final Call* articles in *Boundaries of Blackness*, 244–47.

21. "A.I.D.S: A Killer behind Bars," *Final Call* 4, no. 1 (1984), Periodicals Collection, Schomburg Center. (All subsequent *Final Call* citations are from this collection.) Sex between men behind bars seems a likely route of transmission, and scientists would later discover that the virus can have a long latency phase, during which a person with HIV shows no symptoms. Hence men in prison could have been infected through sex or shared needles years earlier, and others either might not have recognized their own risk as non-gay-identified MSM or might have hidden their own sexual history.

22. Abdul Alim Muhammad, "A.I.D.S.: Widespread Death," *Final Call*, February 14, 1985; "AIDS Can Kill Us All," *Final Call*, May 15, 1987.

23. "1987 in Perspective: An Interview with Minister Louis Farrakhan," *Final Call*, January 22, 1988; Hassan Omowale, "AIDS Virus Attacks Victim's Body with Deception," *Final Call*, August 22, 1989. Omowale had been incarcerated since the 1970s and published *Book of the Living Dead: Essays for African-American Awareness* from prison. He devoted an entire chapter in his book to an endorsement of AIDS conspiracy theories. See Fred Richardson, "Preparing to Organize Again!," *Big Red News*, March 20, 1992. Meanwhile, Segal's claim was part of a Soviet misinformation campaign that spread rumors that the United States had developed AIDS as a biological weapon. Boghardt, "Operation INFEKTION."

24. Omowale, "AIDS Virus Attacks Victim's Body with Deception"; Sovella X Perry, "AIDS Is Quickly Killing Blacks," *Final Call*, August 30, 1986.

25. *Tony Brown's Journal*, "AIDS and Blacks," directed by Bob Morris, aired on PBS, available through Alexander Street. This episode is dated by Alexander Street as 1984, but the closing titles say 1985, and news sources suggest that it aired in 1985. See "Brown Discusses the Pros and Cons of Black Men and AIDS," *Philadelphia Tribune*, September 6, 1985. Around the same time, Brown also had Dr. Wayne Greaves of Howard University on as a guest to talk about opportunistic infections among African Americans with AIDS. Tony Brown, "AIDS Problem among Blacks," *Washington Informer*, August 28, 1985, 13.

26. *Tony Brown's Journal*, "AIDS and Blacks."

27. *Tony Brown's Journal*, "AIDS: Everybody's Problem," directed by Bob Morris, aired 1986 on PBS, available through Alexander Street.

28. Tony Brown, "AIDS Facts That Are Not True," *Tri-State Defender*, November 9, 1988, 8A. The following episodes of *Tony Brown's Journal* can be found in NPAC: "A Message to Arthur Ashe and Magic Johnson," aired January 24, 1993, on PBS, tape 38996; "AIDS and Health," aired July 25, 1993, on PBS, tape 41393; "A Man with His Own AIDS Treatment," aired April 3, 1994, on PBS, tape 45023; "The First AIDS Whistleblower," aired May 7, 1989, on PBS, tape 23087; "What Causes AIDS?," aired October 1, 1989, on PBS, tape 25486.

29. *Tony Brown's Journal*, "Hunting the Virus Hunter," directed by Bob Morris, aired May 19, 1991, on PBS, tape 31800, NPAC.

30. *Tony Brown's Journal*, "Has the Medical Establishment Failed Us?," aired May 21, 1989, on PBS, tape 23297, NPAC, also available through Alexander Street.

31. *Tony Brown's Journal*, "The People vs. Western Medicine," aired June 4, 1989, on PBS, tape 23539, NPAC, also available through Alexander Street.

32. Brown, *Black Lies, White Lies*, xviii, 145, 198.

33. *Tony Brown's Journal*, "AIDS: Everybody's Problem"; *Tony Brown's Journal*, "How Women Get AIDS," directed by Bob Morris, aired 1987, on PBS, available through Alexander Street.

34. Vinette K. Pryce, "Hopes High for Reported Cure for AIDS in Kenya," *New York Amsterdam News*, July 28, 1990, 1; "'Racist Media' Silent on Miracle Cure for AIDS," *New York Amsterdam News*, July 28, 1990, 10.

35. *New York Amsterdam News* editorial quoted in Mark Lowery and Laurie Garrett, "Sandiford in Africa for Controversial AIDS Treatment," *Newsday*, August 17, 1990; "CEMOTAP Observes Its 30th Anniversary of Media Activism," *New York Amsterdam News*, March 20, 2017, http://amsterdamnews.com/news/2017/mar/30/cemotap-observes-its-30th-anniversary-media-activi/. For an account of the trip to Kenya and the fight over Kemron from the perspective of a woman whose mother was treated with Kemron, see Rose, *In Search of Serenity*. Rose begins the book by claiming that "in all likelihood, HIV is not the cause of AIDS." She goes on to describe her experience of attending "a six-hour session of information by Gary Null," cites AIDS denialists such as Duesberg along with anti-gay Afrocentrists such as Frances Cress Welsing and Haki Madhubuti, and recommends both the Nation of Islam and Dr. Sebi's Usha Herbal Research Institute for their "support services."

36. J. Zamgba Browne, "AIDS Victim Blames Squabble over Kemron Cure on Profits," *New York Amsterdam News*, December 22, 1990, 4.

37. Vinette K. Pryce, "Two Call Kenya's Kemron a Miracle," *New York Amsterdam News*, October 6, 1990, 1; Browne, "AIDS Victim Blames Squabble over Kemron Cure on Profits."

38. Jane Perlez, "In Kenya, a New AIDS Drug Gets Mired in Politics and Financial Disputes," *New York Times*, October 3, 1990, A20; Laurie Garrett, "A Heavy Dose of Animosity Debate over AIDS Drug's Value, Origin," *Newsday*, August 19, 1990; Project Inform, *PI Perspective*, May 1990, box 1, folder 4, NTFAP-GLBT.

39. Perlez, "In Kenya, a New AIDS Drug Gets Mired in Politics and Financial Disputes"; Hutchinson and Cummins, "Low-Dose Oral Interferon in Patient with AIDS"; Garrett, "Heavy Dose of Animosity Debate over AIDS Drug's Value, Origin"; Amy Goldstein, "Some Dismiss Interferon, Others Praise It," *Washington Post*, September 27, 1993, A10.

40. Perlez, "In Kenya, a New AIDS Drug Gets Mired in Politics and Financial Disputes"; Koech et al., "Low Dose Oral Alpha-Interferon Therapy."

41. Obel and Koech, "Outcome of Intervention"; Koech and Obel, "Treatment of HIV Infections and AIDS." Both articles were reprinted in the August 13, 1990, issue of the *New York Native*, found in box 38, folder 10, KKP; "'AIDS' Drug Mired in Corruption and Controversy," *New York Native*, December 3, 1990, 6, box 38, folder 10, KKP. Kiyoshi Kuromiya's Critical Path AIDS Project later repeated the placebo claim in an article that was critical of the Kemron project, and especially of Drs. Muhammad and Justice. *Critical Path AIDS Project* (newsletter), April 1992, box 38, folder 10, KKP. Several years later, in 1996, Obel was back to promote another reported HIV cure, which he called "Pearl Omega." The "unapologetic, defiant, and brutal" doctor followed that with at least one other drug, called "Iconaire," in 2019. Elliott, *Reimagining*

*Science*; Mercy Adhiambo, "Prof Obel on HIV Drug, His Love for Cars and Women," *The Standard*, January 27, 2019, https://www.standardmedia.co.ke/article/2001310944 /prof-obel-on-hiv-drug-his-love-for-cars-and-women.

42. Bruce Lambert, "Medical and Racial Debate Follow a Drug Hailed as an AIDS Cure," *New York Times*, September 2, 1990, 42; Charles Ortleb, "New York PWA Health Group Disputes Oral Alpha-Interferon Findings in Kenya and Florida," *New York Native*, August 13, 1990, 6, box 38, folder 10, KKP; Garrett, "Heavy Dose of Animosity Debate over AIDS Drug's Value, Origin"; Project Inform, *PI Perspective*, October 1990, box 396, folder 35, Resource Center LGBT Collection, Special Collections, University of North Texas, Denton.

43. Larry Tate and Martin Delaney, "Hope, Folly, or Fraud?," *PI Perspective*, April 1992, 11–13, box 396, folder 35, Resource Center LGBT Collection, Special Collections, University of North Texas, Denton.

44. "Oh Captain, My Captain," *Los Angeles Sentinel*, November 20, 1991, 6A; William Reed, "Blue Smoke and Mirrors," *Michigan Citizen* (Detroit), January 19, 1991, 8; Ron Sturrup, "AIDS Sufferers Get New Lease on Life," *Atlanta Inquirer*, November 2, 1991, 1.

45. It is impossible to say how widely copies of the packet circulated. However, the fact that one ended up in the possession of Kiyoshi Kuromiya, an Asian American AIDS treatment activist and member of ACT UP Philadelphia, suggests a wide reach. In the late 1980s and early 1990s fax machines would have also made it possible to send the packet, or others like it, to activists around the country. Although the copy in Kuromiya's papers does not appear to have been transmitted via fax, the ubiquity of faxed materials across AIDS activist archives points to the widespread use of the technology. See "Out of Africa: AIDS Cure Is Found," 1990, box 38, folder 10, KKP.

The false story of Carter's population commission was reported by other conspiracy-minded outlets, such as Lyndon LaRouche's *Executive Intelligence Review*, which warned that "genocidalists" had "take[n] over U.S. policy." In reality Carter had in 1977 directed a handful of federal agencies "to make a one-year study of the probable changes in the world's population, natural resources, and environment through the end of the century." In the resulting report, *Global 2000: The Report to the President: Entering the Twenty-First Century*, author Gerald Barney warned, "If present trends continue, the world in 2000 will be more crowded, more polluted, less stable ecologically, and more vulnerable to disruption than the world we live in now" (1). It did not, however, propose genocide as a solution to these problems.

Through his Prevent AIDS Now Initiative Committee (PANIC) and alongside Republican representative William Dannemeyer, LaRouche, a constant fixture of the American political fringe during the late twentieth and early twenty-first century, sponsored Proposition 64, a 1986 California ballot measure that would have allowed for the quarantine of people with HIV. It was defeated by a wide margin. David L. Kirp, "LaRouche Turns to AIDS Politics," *New York Times*, September 11, 1986, A27; Jay Mathews, "LaRouche's Call to Quarantine AIDS Victims Trails in California," *Washington Post*, October 26, 1986. The records of the No on 64 campaign are held at the ONE National Gay and Lesbian Archives in Los Angeles; see https://oac.cdlib.org/findaid/ark:/13030 /c8qco1ww/entire_text/.

46. Quotations regarding Wallace Fard's teachings are drawn from R. Turner, *Islam*

*in the African-American Experience*, 148–51. The brief history of the Nation of Islam also draws from Gibson, *History of the Nation of Islam*; and Gardell, *In the Name of Elijah Muhammad*.

47. Lincoln, *Black Muslims in America*, xxiii.

48. Gibson, *History of the Nation of Islam*.

49. Gibson, *History of the Nation of Islam*.

50. Gardell, *In the Name of Elijah Muhammad*.

51. A. Nelson, "Black Mass as Black Gothic"; Pinn, *African American Religious Experience in America*, 112. Although the Yakub myth may have been deemphasized as part of the NOI cosmology under Farrakhan's leadership, the *Final Call* still occasionally mentioned Yakub, suggesting that readers were familiar with the story. See "The Filth That Produces the Filth," *Final Call*, June 3, 1991.

52. Ivan Van Sertima, "The Lost Sciences of Africa: Part I," *Final Call*, January 15, 1987, 29. In his best-selling book *They Came before Columbus*, Van Sertima also claimed that African explorers crossed the Atlantic centuries before the Christian era and exerted significant influence on Mesoamerica. With respect to this and other work, Van Sertima has been criticized for selectively using historical and archaeological evidence to piece together a view of Olmec, Aztec, and Mayan history that is no less patronizing than colonialist narratives of the African past. Haslip-Viera, Ortiz de Montellano, and Barbour, "Robbing Native American Cultures."

53. Gibson, *A History of the Nation of Islam*; *NOI POWER Proclamation*, 1985, quoted in Gardell, *In the Name of Elijah Muhammad*, 319. Gardell also discusses Farrakhan's economic program, 317–22. Reporters at the *Chicago Tribune* later found that the NOI's business ventures did more to enrich Farrakhan and his family than to spread wealth within Black communities. Rogers Worthington, "Farrakhan Stand Bad for Business," *Chicago Tribune*, October 28, 1985; David Jackson and William Gaines, "The Power and the Money: Farrakhan Prospers as Ventures Flounder," *Chicago Tribune*, March 12, 1995.

54. R. Turner, *Islam in the African-American Experience*, 149; Pinn, *African American Religious Experience in America*, 102; Louis Farrakhan, "Weighing Properly Mentally and Physically," *Final Call*, October 7, 1991, 20; Elijah Muhammad, "Reduce Doctor Bills," *Final Call*, October 7, 1991, 26; Elijah Muhammad, "Many Ailments Can Be Cured," *Final Call*, June 8, 1994, 28; "Meat Is against Life," *Final Call*, April 1, 1997, 28. Gardell describes Farrakhan's war on obesity in *In the Name of Elijah Muhammad*, 328–29.

55. Sturrup, "AIDS Sufferers Get New Lease on Life."

56. Abdul Wali Muhammad, "'Miracle' Drugs Relieve AIDS Symptoms," *Final Call*, October 7, 1991, 32.

57. "Dr. Koech Leading the Way in AIDS Research," *Final Call*, October 7, 1991, 6.

58. "D.C. Activist Travels to Kenya for Treatment," *Final Call*, October 7, 1991, 32. This article, along with the Koech interview, was quoted liberally in Sturrup, "AIDS Sufferers Get New Lease on Life."

59. According to a profile in the *Washington Post* published just before her 1991 trip, Evans "said she had no AIDS symptoms now." Five years later, in 1996, she told a different story to Gwen Gilmore of the *Afro-American Red Star*: "When I went to Africa in the summer of 1991 my T-cell count was below 300, and I was exhibiting symptoms of the disease such as weight loss, poor appetite, and pain in my joints so much that I was walking with a cane or crutches." Saundra Torry, "A D.C. Woman's Desperate Search

for Hope," *Washington Post*, July 20, 1991, A9; Gwen Gilmore, "Kemron Helped Lashaun Evans," *Afro-American Red Star*, May 11, 1996.

60. Joseph P. Fried, "Cedric Sandiford, 41, a Victim of 1986 Howard Beach Attack," *New York Times*, November 21, 1991; William Egyir, "Harlem Physician Plans to Meet Needs of Blacks," *New York Amsterdam News*, June 1, 1996, 16; Jean Griffith-Sandiford quoted in Burkett, *Gravest Show on Earth*, 174.

61. "Speaker Says Drugs Available for AIDS Cure," *Sacramento Observer*, April 22, 1992, B2; "AIDS Activists Briefed on Treatment from Africa," *Final Call*, October 28, 1991.

62. Ovie H. Mitchell, "African Treatment of AIDS Deliberately Overlooked," *Call and Post* (Cincinnati), May 28, 1992, 1A; Sturrup, "AIDS Sufferers Get New Lease on Life."

63. Lisa Ely, "AIDS Treatment Drug Reports 90% Success Rate," *Chicago Citizen*, April 12, 1992, 16; Sherry Stone, "Kenyan Researchers Find Possible AIDS Cure," *Philadelphia Tribune*, November 5, 1991, 5A.

64. BEBASHI, "AIDS Treatment Found in Africa," 1991, box 38, folder 10, KKP; Mitchell, "African Treatment of AIDS Deliberately Overlooked." It's not entirely clear that Alim Muhammad used the phrase "crude powder" in his presentation, but it seems likely from the following: "He [Koech] developed a crude powder, according to Muhammad, that he administered to a Kenyan diplomat who was dying from full-blown AIDS." Stone, "Kenyan Researchers Find Possible AIDS Cure."

65. DC Coalition of Black Lesbians and Gay Men, *The Fire This Time*, Fall 1991, box 27, DTP.

66. LeRoy Whitfield, "Bite the Bullet," *POZ*, July 2000, https://www.poz.com/articl /Bite-The-Bullet-10295-4551; Ely, "AIDS Treatment Drug Reports 90% Success Rate"; Stone, "Kenyan Researchers Find Possible AIDS Cure."

67. David Fair to Barbara Justice (draft), October 30, 1991, box 38, folder 10, KKP.

68. David Fair to Barbara Justice (draft), October 30, 1991.

69. "Kemron Not Discovered in Kenya," *Inter Press Service*, November 14, 1990, box 10, folder "Africa-Health-AIDS-Kemron," Leroy T. Walker Africa News Service Archive, David M. Rubinstein Rare Book and Manuscript Library, Duke University, Durham.

70. Pfeiffer, "Oral Alpha-Interferon Craze"; Sally Squires, "NIH Reverses Controversial AIDS Drug," *Washington Post*, November 3, 1992, 6.

71. "NOI Gets Exclusive Rights to Immunex," *Call and Post*, March 26, 1992, 1A.

72. "We Must Depend on Allah and Ourselves" and "Unity: The Key to Black Economic Success in the 90s," *Final Call*, January 25, 1993, 31; "White Brutality Must Force Black Self-Determination," *Final Call*, June 29, 1992, 24. NOI had notably "cleaned up" Mayfair in the late 1980s through patrols by Fruit of Islam, the group's security wing, to keep drug dealers out of the neighborhood. Patrice Gaines-Carter, "The Nation of Islam a Close-Knit Society," *Washington Post*, September 18, 1988.

73. AIDS Research Advisory Committee, "Executive Summary [Low-Dose Oral Alpha Interferon Report]," box 38, folder 9, KKP; "Speaker Says Drugs Available for AIDS Cure," *Sacramento Observer*, April 22, 1992, B2; James Bolden, "War on AIDS: Nation of Islam Draws Battle Lines on Deadly AIDS Virus," *Los Angeles Sentinel*, August 20, 1992, A4; Patricia Anstett, "African AIDS Drug Rejected in US to Be Reevaluated," *Boston Globe*, August 24, 1992; Leslie A. Murdock, "AIDS Group Pushes for Kemron Testing," *Bay State Banner* (Boston), September 17, 1992, 19.

74. Malik Shabazz, "NMA to Hear Need for Drugs," *Afro-American Red Star*, October 24, 1992, A1; Warren E. Leary, "U.S. Will Sponsor AIDS-Drug Trials," *New York Times*, October 29, 1992, B12; Squires, "NIH Reverses Controversial AIDS Drug," 6.

75. Squires, "NIH Reverses Controversial AIDS Drug"; Malik Shabazz, "NIH, NMA Agree on AIDS Trial," *Afro-American Red Star*, October 31, 1992, A1; Amy Goldstein, "A D.C. Clinic's Controversial Rx for AIDS," *Washington Post*, September 27, 1993, A1.

76. Shabazz, "NIH, NMA Agree on AIDS Trial"; Denise Clay, "FDA to Test AIDS Drug Introduced by Nation of Islam," *Philadelphia Tribune*, May 4, 1993, 1A.

77. Clay, "FDA to Test AIDS Drug Introduced by Nation of Islam"; Benjamin Dudley, "New AIDS Medicine to Be Called Immuviron," *Afro-American Red Star*, April 3, 1993, A1.

78. Brenda Lein, "Immune-Based Therapies: New Emphasis in AIDS Research," *Project Inform Briefing Paper*, no. 3 (July 1993): 8–9, box 396, folder 34, Resource Center LGBT Collection, Special Collections, University of North Texas.

79. Gwen Gilmore, "Dr. Muhammad: 'Treatment Works,'" *Afro-American Red Star*, September 11, 1993, A1.

80. Goldstein, "A D.C. Clinic's Controversial Rx for AIDS."

81. Gardell, *In the Name of Elijah Muhammad*, 328.

82. Debra Freeman, "ADL and the Gay Lobby Are Playing Politics with D.C.'s AIDS Epidemic [interview with Dr. Abdul Alim Muhammad]," *Executive Intelligence Review*, April 1, 1994, 61–67.

83. Amy Goldstein, "Black Gays in New D.C. AIDS Coalition Wary about Muslim Doctor's Role," *Washington Post*, September 29, 1993. For more on Robinson's role in the National Task Force on AIDS Prevention, see the NTFAP Records at UCSF, especially box 3, folders 14 and 16.

84. Muhammad, "A.I.D.S.: Widespread Death."

85. National Black Gay and Lesbian Leadership Forum, "A Call to Action: The Role of Black Gay Men and Lesbians in the Million Man March," September 24, 1995, box 36, DTP. Around the same time, GMAD hosted "a town meeting on the [Million Man March] and the role that Black Gay men should play in it." The group invited a representative from the Nation of Islam to the meeting, although it is not clear that one attended. "AIDS Institute Peer Initiative Monthly Report," October 1995, box 22, folder 6, GMAD-SC.

86. Julie Wakefield, "Trial and Error," *Washington City Paper*, April 11, 1997, http://www.washingtoncitypaper.com/news/article/13012836/trial-and-error.

87. Gwen Gilmore, "Kemron Trials Delayed Again," *Afro-American Red Star*, August 6, 1994, A1; William Egyir, "Harlem Physician Plans to Meet Needs of Blacks," *New York Amsterdam News*, June 1, 1996, 16.

88. Gwen Gilmore, "560 Sought for Kemron Trials: HIV Positive?," *Afro-American Red Star*, April 27, 1996, A13; Desiree Allen Graves, "IRS Stifles Abundant Life Clinic," *Afro-American Red Star*, September 7, 1996, A1; Gwen Gilmore, "Kemron Trials Ended," *Afro-American Red Star*, June 28, 1997, A1.

89. Gilmore, "Kemron Trials Ended"; "Expanded Access and Patient Assistance Programs for Other Experimental Drugs from Their Manufacturers: Alpha Interferon (Kemron, Low Dose, Oral)," *Critical Path AIDS Project*, no. 32 (1997): 46–47.

90. Despite a significant increase in access to antiretroviral therapy in recent years,

just over 60 percent of people with HIV worldwide were accessing such treatments as of 2018. "Global Statistics," HIV.gov, July 31, 2019, https://www.hiv.gov/hiv-basics /overview/data-and-trends/global-statistics.

## Chapter 5

1. Seele interview.

2. Seele interview; Laurie Goodstein, "Harlem Effort against AIDS Opens with Prayer," *Washington Post*, September 11, 1989, A12. For other work on The Balm in Gilead, see Harris, *AIDS, Sexuality, and the Black Church*; Harris, "AIDS Promotion within the Black Church"; and Harris, "Panic at the Church."

Although I refer to "the Black church" throughout this chapter, we should recognize that Black Christians in the United States are far from monolithic in their expressions of faith or experiences of worship. They come from a wide range of denominations and from congregations big and small, and some belong to churches that are not predominantly Black. However, Black churches *have* played a singular role in the long struggle for Black freedom in America, and that history is important context for the work of The Balm in Gilead. Following the lead of other scholars, I use the phrase "the Black church" when discussing the institution in the abstract, and "Black churches" when referring to The Balm in Gilead's work with specific congregations.

3. Seele interview; Hannah Alani, "Lincolnville, SC, Recognized 151 Years after It Was Founded by Freed Blacks Following Civil War," *Post and Courier* (Charleston, S.C.), accessed November 29, 2018, https://www.postandcourier.com/news/lincolnville-sc -recognized-years-after-it-was-founded-by-freed/article_a73c3ca4-cb30–11e8-ad01 –8fccbd6856bd.html.

4. Seele interview.

5. Seele interview; Goodstein, "Harlem Effort against AIDS Opens with Prayer."

6. *Harvard AIDS Letter*, December 1992, box 75, folder 5, Gay Men's Health Crisis Records, New York Public Library; Seele interview; Goodstein, "Harlem Effort against AIDS Opens with Prayer."

7. Seele interview; Jeremiah 8:22. The title of this book is drawn from the same spiritual.

8. Aisha Satterwhite, "Nigeria," Balm in Gilead, December 6, 2002, cached by Wayback Machine, February 18, 2004, http://web.archive.org/web/20040218031628/http:// www.balmingilead.org/special_feature/journey/nigeria_1.asp. The Wayback Machine is a "bot" that periodically stores ("caches") versions of websites on the Internet Archive's server, making them easily accessible for the future. Using the Wayback Machine, historians can view cached versions of a page, tracking changes to it over time, or view pages that have since disappeared. The Wayback Machine main page can be viewed at http:// archive.org/web/web.php.

9. E. Franklin Frazier, *Negro Church in America*.

10. Higginbotham, *Righteous Discontent*; Fullilove and Fullilove, "Stigma as an Obstacle to AIDS Action," 1118. For a critique of heterosexism and homophobia in the Black church, see Douglas, *Sexuality and the Black Church*. In *Between Sundays*, Frederick finds that women in the contemporary Black church are not entirely silent on sexual issues, as some make it a point to talk about sex with younger women and girls to keep

them from suffering the kinds of sexual abuse or trauma that they themselves experienced. In *Righteous Content*, Wiggins similarly found that women in the Black church were unlikely to discuss stories of sexual trauma with their pastors but created their own informal structures and networks for counseling one another.

11. Raboteau, *Slave Religion*; Lincoln and Mamiya, *Black Church in the African American Experience*; Wimbush, *Bible and African Americans*, 4.

12. Higginbotham, *Righteous Discontent*, 187; Griffin, *Their Own Receive Them Not*, 18; L. Harris, "From Abolitionist Amalgamators to 'Rulers of the Five Points'"; Dew, *Apostles of Disunion*; Gaines, *Uplifting the Race*; Griffin, *Their Own Receive Them Not*.

13. Russell, "Color of Discipline"; Retzloff, "'Seer or Queer?'" 288.

14. According to Retzloff, Powell also attacked Prophet Jones in a 1951 article for *Ebony* with a thinly reference to Jones's "unnatural relationship" with his male assistant. Adam Clayton Powell Jr., "Sex in the Church," *Ebony*, November 1951, 27–34 quoted in Retzloff, 271. Wilkins quoted in D'Emilio, *Lost Prophet*, 338. In another example of the ethic of respectability, teenager Claudette Colvin was arrested for refusing to give up her seat on a Montgomery bus in March 1955, nine months before the arrest of Rosa Parks sparked a boycott to end segregation and racist abuse on the city's bus lines. Colvin might have become the face of the boycott, but she was dark-skinned, came from a poor family on the wrong side of town, and within months of her arrest had become pregnant. Local civil rights leaders, who were already organizing to challenge segregation on Montgomery buses, decided that they could not organize a boycott with Colvin at the center. E. D. Nixon, Alabama state president of the NAACP, remarked, "She's just not the kind we can win a case with." Nixon quoted in McGuire, *At the Dark End of the Street*, 91.

15. Downs, *Stand By Me*; Mumford, *Not Straight, Not White*; Tinney, "Why a Black Gay Church?," 76. According to Donald Burch III, Tinney "was told that his grandmother was part black . . . [and] that he could call himself black if he wanted to, although his family didn't consider themselves black." In *Queer Capital*, Beemyn refers to Tinney as a "black-identified" white gay man (214). Donald Burch III, June 22, 1999, quoted in Beemyn, *Queer Capital*, 231n111.

16. Griffin, *Their Own Receive Them Not*, 194–98; "Founder," Minority AIDS Project, accessed September 27, 2019, http://minorityaidsproject.org/founder/. The mainstream Church of God in Christ does not ordain women, but Flunder found a leadership role as assistant pastor at Love Center Ministries, an open-minded Bay Area offshoot of the denomination. From there, she split off to form Ark of Refuge and received a doctor of ministry degree from San Francisco Theological Seminary. Flunder interview; Garner interview.

17. In this vein, the Black gay writer James Baldwin compared the pastor at the church where he became a teenage preacher to the "pimps and racketeers on the Avenue." James Baldwin, "Letter from a Region in My Mind," *New Yorker*, November 10, 1962; McCoy quoted in Tinney, "Why a Black Gay Church?," 73; Fullilove and Fullilove, "Stigma as an Obstacle to AIDS Action."

18. C. Harris, "Cut Off from among Their People," 65–67.

19. Thomas Glave quoted in Woubshet, *Calendar of Loss*, 15; Nero, "Fixing Ceremonies," xiii; Hemphill, "Tomb of Sorrow," 76; Chuck Tarver, "Take Care of Your Blessings," *The Blackstripe*, January 8, 1996, http://www.qrd.org/qrd/www/culture/black/essex/blessings.html.

20. Woodyard, Peterson, and Stokes, "'Let Us Go into the House of the Lord,'" 459. Note that John L. Peterson, a Black gay psychologist who had worked at UCSF's Center for AIDS Prevention Studies, was involved in this research as well. For more on religious responses to AIDS, see Petro, *After the Wrath of God*.

21. Seele interview.

22. Seele interview.

23. Seele interview; Pernessa Seele, "AIDS, Spirituality and the African American Church: A Call for a Greater Response," Balm in Gilead, cached by Wayback Machine, August 18, 2000, http://web.archive.org/web/20000818174053/http://www.balmingilead.org/resources/spirituality.htm.

24. Seele was not alone in describing her work concerning AIDS as the result of a higher calling. Pastors and lay leaders who later replicated the Harlem Week of Prayer for the Healing of AIDS in other cities reported being "led by the spirit" and "called to this task as part of being a Christian." See Norris, "Black Church Week of Prayer for the Healing of AIDS," 82–85.

25. Creel, *Peculiar People* and "Slave Women of the Sea Islands of the South." Thanks to Hilary Jones for this insight.

26. Seele interview.

27. Balm in Gilead, "The Black Church Comprehensive HIV/AIDS Education Kit Funding Proposal," and Pernessa Seele CV, grant 0950-0543, reel 7637, FFG, italics in original.

28. Seele had also worked at Sloan Kettering Cancer Center and Rockefeller University before landing at Harlem Hospital. Seele interview; Balm in Gilead, "CDC National Partnerships for HIV Prevention Funding Proposal," August 7, 1998, Balm in Gilead Office Files, in possession of Balm in Gilead, Inc., Richmond, Va.

29. The cities were Atlanta, Macon (Ga.), Cleveland, Kansas City (Mo.), Raleigh-Durham, and Nashville. See Norris, "Black Church Week of Prayer for the Healing of AIDS"; and CDC, "Guidelines for Health Education and Risk Reduction Activities," wonder.cdc.gov, April 1, 1995, http://wonder.cdc.gov/wonder/prevguid/p0000389/p0000389.asp. Janet Wise reported findings from her study of attitudes among Black church leaders, conducted at the Revival of the African American Faith Community for the Protection and Healing of AIDS in Statesville, North Carolina, an event modeled on the Black Church Week of Prayer. Wise did not indicate whether organizers of the revival attended the Emory workshop, nor did she name the other cities represented there. Elsewhere, Pernessa Seele mentioned that the Black Church Week of Prayer model had been replicated in Boston, Birmingham, and Albuquerque, but whether organizers from these cities attended the Emory training is also unclear. See Wise, "Changing Clergy and Lay Leader Attitudes about HIV/AIDS"; and Balm in Gilead, "About The Balm in Gilead, Inc.," grant 0950-0543, reel 7637, FFG.

30. W. Steve Lee to Alexis Herman et al., February 23, 1994, Clinton Digital Library, http://www.clintonlibrary.gov/assets/storage/Research%20-%20Digital%20Library/rascosubject/Box%20003/r_612956-aids-1994-3.pdf; "The African American Clergy's Declaration of War on HIV/AIDS," February 28, 1994, box 75, folder 5, Gay Men's Health Crisis Records.

31. Wilson, "A Message to Black Clergy," 31–32.

32. Wilson, 33.

33. Brownlie quoted in Wilson, 35.

34. Wilson describes Brownlie's passing in "I'm Not Done Yet." Reprinted online at TheBody.com, http://www.thebody.com/content/art2485.html.

35. Gary Paul Wright to Robert Penn, January 10, 1994, box 1, folder 1, Robert E. Penn Papers, Schomburg Center, New York.

36. Balm in Gilead, *Who Will Break the Silence?* (1995), 12.

37. GMAD, "AIDS Institute Peer Initiative Monthly Report," October 1995, box 22, folder 6, GMAD-SC.

38. The Prayer Group's exegetical conversations were included in the original 1995 edition of *Who Will Break the Silence?* but disappeared from the 2010 edition. Otherwise, the prayers and liturgies in the two versions are almost identical. The 2010 edition also lists the members of the Prayer Group: Jay Hines, Jacqueline Holland, Joseph Long, Julia Mayo-Quinlan, Donna M. Prince, Janine Quinlan, William J. Vila, and Judith Hoch Wray. Balm in Gilead, *Who Will Break the Silence?* (1995), 13; Balm in Gilead, *Who Will Break the Silence?* (2010), 6.

39. Balm in Gilead (1995), 3, 86–87.

40. Balm in Gilead (1995), 13, 69.

41. Balm in Gilead (2010), 11.

42. Balm in Gilead (1995), 70–71; (2010), 13.

43. Balm in Gilead (1995), 28. This prayer became "Prayer of a Gay Christian" in the 2010 edition. Balm in Gilead (2010), 17.

44. Balm in Gilead (1995), 82–84.

45. Clara "Mother" Hale founded the Hale House Center, a home for abandoned and orphaned babies, including those born with HIV and/or addicted to drugs. Bruce Lambert, "Clara Hale, Founder of Home for Addicts' Babies, Dies at 87," *New York Times*, December 19, 1992, A1; Balm in Gilead, *Who Will Break the Silence?* (2010), 18, 27.

46. Balm in Gilead, *Who Will Break the Silence?* (1995), 12–13; (2010), 54.

47. Cary Goodman, Balm in Gilead executive administrator, email to author, August 12, 2013.

48. Balm in Gilead, "Final Report: Cooperative Agreement #U62/CCU220997-03-3," September 2005, Balm in Gilead Office Files.

49. Seele, "Church's Role in HIV/AIDS Prevention."

50. Balm in Gilead, "Programmatic Three Year Strategic Plan, 1998–2000," grant 09601141, reel 8074, FFG.

51. Sandy Thurman, "Report on the Presidential Mission on Children Orphaned by AIDS in Sub-Saharan Africa: Findings and Plan of Action," July 19, 1999, Clinton Digital Library, http://www.clintonlibrary.gov/assets/storage/Research-Digital Library/Reed -Subject/98/647386-aids-policy-1.pdf.

52. Daniels quoted in Stanford, *Homophobia in the Black Church*, 31; Balm in Gilead, "Final Report."

53. Balm in Gilead, "Final Report."

54. Balm in Gilead, "Final Report."

55. Balm in Gilead, "Final Report."

56. Aisha Satterwhite, "Together Let's Fight against AIDS [Côte d'Ivoire]," Balm in Gilead, cached by Wayback Machine, December 6, 2002, http://web.archive.org/web

/20021206150915/http://www.balmingilead.org/special_feature/journey/journey_1.asp; Aisha Satterwhite LinkedIn profile, accessed September 29, 2019, https://www.linkedin .com/in/aishasatterwhite/.

57. Although Igbo and Ibo refer to the same ethnic group, the language they speak is called Igbo.

58. Aisha Satterwhite, "We Cannot Fold Our Hands [Nigeria]," Balm in Gilead, cached by Wayback Machine, December 6, 2002, http://web.archive.org/web/20040218031628 /http://www.balmingilead.org/special_feature/journey/nigeria_1.asp.

59. Satterwhite, "We Cannot Fold Our Hands."

60. Satterwhite, "Making a Way Out of No Way [Zimbabwe]," *Balm in Gilead*, cached by Wayback Machine, December 6, 2002, https://web.archive.org/web/20021206112824 /http://www.balmingilead.org/special_feature/journey/zimbabwe_1.asp.

61. Satterwhite, "Together Let's Fight against AIDS [Côte d'Ivoire]," italics added. Public health data on HIV transmission, which relies on reported behavior, also likely underrepresents the extent of homosexual transmission in Africa because of the stigma against homosexuality. For critiques of scientific knowledge and discourse about patterns of HIV transmission in Africa, see Patton, *Inventing AIDS* and *Globalizing AIDS*.

62. The International HIV/AIDS Faith Advisory Board of The Balm in Gilead, "A Theological Call to Action," Balm in Gilead, cached by Wayback Machine, September 5, 2004, http://www.balmingilead.org/programs/africa2004/images/white_paper_english .pdf.

63. Map International and The Balm in Gilead, *Helpers for a Healing Community*, 13. The 1994 and 2004 editions of *Helpers for a Healing Community* are significantly different from one another. Much of what is described here is unique to the 2004 edition.

64. Map International and The Balm in Gilead, 17, 20.

65. Map International and The Balm in Gilead, 23–24.

66. Map International and The Balm in Gilead, 12, 16, 31, 56; Dortzbach and Kiiti, *Helpers for a Healing Community*, 28.

67. Balm in Gilead, "Final Report."

68. Black, Koopman, and Ryden, *Of Little Faith*; Seele interview; Teresa Lyles Holmes, "In State of the Union, President Bush Pledges to Work with African American Churches to Address HIV/AIDS," Balm in Gilead press release, February 1, 2006, cached by Wayback Machine, February 7, 2006, http://web.archive.org/web/2006 0207225735/http://www.balmingilead.org/press/releases/release_state_union. asp. The Supreme Court of the United States struck down some of PEPFAR's more controversial requirements in 2013 with a 6–2 decision in *Agency for International Development v. Alliance for Open Society International*. Elias Groll, "The Public Health Trends behind the Supreme Court's PEPFAR Decision," *Foreign Policy Blogs*, June 20, 2013, http://blog.foreignpolicy.com/posts/2013/06/20/the_public_health_trends_behind _the_supreme_court_pepfar_decision.

69. Seele interview; Patterson, *Politics of AIDS in Africa*. As Hartman recounts in *Lose Your Mother*, the romantic notions that some African Americans hold about their connection to the African continent are not always shared by the people who live there.

## Chapter 6

1. ACT UP/New York, "Candidate Gore Zaps," ACT UP/New York, accessed March 27, 2013, http://www.actupny.org/actions/gorezaps.html; ACT UP Philadelphia, Barshefsky protest photo, October 6, 1999, box 2, JDP; Gus Cairns, "America's New Activism," *Positive Nation* (UK), June 2002, box 1, JDP. The title of this chapter is taken from a sign carried by a member of ACT UP Philadelphia at a demonstration in June 2001 in Washington, D.C. Lance Lattig, "Acting Up Again," *Village Voice*, June 19, 2001, http://www.villagevoice.com/2001-06-19/news/acting-up-again/.

2. Petty, "Divine Interventions," 105–6.

3. France, *How to Survive a Plague*; Hubbard, *United in Anger*; Gould, *Moving Politics*; Siplon, *AIDS and the Policy Struggle in the United States*; Smith and Siplon, *Drugs into Bodies*.

4. Brier, *Infectious Ideas*. The Global Fund and PEPFAR emerged in a complex policy environment; in focusing on ACT UP Philadelphia I do not mean to discount the work of other actors. For other views, see Smith and Siplon, *Drugs into Bodies*; Kidder, *Mountains beyond Mountains*; and D'Adesky, *Moving Mountains*.

5. Smith and Siplon, *Drugs into Bodies*; Siplon, *AIDS and the Policy Struggle in the United States*; Gould, *Moving Politics*; Lawrence Altman, "Scientists Display Substantial Gains in AIDS Treatment," *New York Times*, July 12, 1996, A1; Crimp, *AIDS Demo Graphics*.

6. Around the same time that ACT UP Philadelphia was fighting for global treatment access, some former ACT UPers began to ask whether funding from the pharmaceutical industry had compromised some of the larger AIDS advocacy groups. See Stephen Gendin, "Last Word," *POZ*, October 2000, http://www.poz.com/article/Last-Word-7782-7059; and Larry Kramer, "Be Very Afraid," *POZ*, October 2000, http://www.poz.com/article/Be-Very-Afraid-1384-2823.

ACT UP Philadelphia also benefited (at least indirectly) from drug companies' largesse: Glaxo Wellcome awarded a $25,000 grant to Project TEACH in 1998. That did not stop ACT UP Philadelphia from criticizing the company. After Glaxo tried to stop the sale of a generic version of its drug Combivir in Ghana, ACT UP Philadelphia and Health GAP issued an action alert titled "Glaxo SmithKline Delivers Killer Greed—in Time for the Holidays." (Glaxo Wellcome merged with SmithKline Beecham in 2000.) ACT UP Philadelphia provided supporters with a sample letter of protest to send to Glaxo SmithKline executives, and Asia Russell, JD Davids, and others sent their own detailed letter of protest as well. Project TEACH, "Glaxo Wellcome, Inc—Final Grantee Report," 2000, box 1, JDP; Mark Schoofs, "Glaxo Enters Fight in Ghana on AIDS Drug," *Wall Street Journal*, December 1, 2000; ACT UP Philadelphia and Health GAP Coalition, "Glaxo SmithKline Delivers Killer Greed—in Time for the Holidays," December 2000, box 1, JDP; ACT UP Philadelphia and Health GAP Coalition, "Sample Letter to Robert Ingram," December 2000, box 1, JDP; Asia Russell et al. to Sir Richard Sykes, Jean-Pierre Garnier, and Robert Ingram, February 5, 2001, box 1, JDP; Gould, *Moving Politics*; Brier, *Infectious Ideas*; Pierre Thomas, "FBI Accused of Spying on AIDS Activists," *Washington Post*, May 16, 1995, A6; Davids interview.

7. Huntly Collins, "AIDS: Death Drop Bypassed Blacks," *Philadelphia Inquirer*, March 11, 1997, B1.

8. Davids interview; Lawrence Goodman, "Send Bohos, Nuts, and Addicts," *Phila-

*delphia Magazine*, November 2001, cached by Wayback Machine, June 16, 2002, http://web.archive.org/web/20020616161122/http://www.phillymag.com/Archives/2001Nov/actup_1.html; Krauss interview; *Housing Works AIDS Issues Update*, April 4, 2008, http://www.hwupdate.org/update/2008/04/global_gogetters.html; ACT UP Philadelphia, Philadelphia Foundation grant report, March 12, 1998, box 1, JDP. JD Davids has a former name that he prefers not to be used.

9. Driscoll interview.

10. Philadelphia FIGHT, Peer-Based Advocacy Initiative proposal, 2000, box 1, JDP.

11. Sowell interview; "Project TEACH Instructors' Handbook," TheBody.com, November 2002, http://www.thebody.com/content/art13347.html; Stanya Kahn, "TEACH the People," *HIV Plus* 7, February 2000, www.aidsinfonyc.org, cached by Wayback Machine, September 20, 2000, http://web.archive.org/web/20000920005615/http://www.aidsinfonyc.org/hivplus/issue7/report/positive.html; "John Bell 1946–2012," Philadelphia FIGHT, accessed July 7, 2013, http://fight.org/about-fight/fights-history/john-bell/.

12. "About Prevention Point Philadelphia," Prevention Point, accessed June 10, 2014, http://ppponline.org/about; Petty, "Divine Interventions," 100–102.

13. Petty, "Divine Interventions," 100–102.

14. Petty, 100–102. It is unclear whether this was the same spine as the one used in the HealthChoices campaign, although it appears to have been specially constructed for the National Day of Reckoning. In any case, the demonstrators carrying the spine were arrested and the spine itself was confiscated; ACT UP Philadelphia, Philadelphia Foundation grant report, March 12, 1998, box 1, JDP.

15. Mark Fazlollah, "A Protest at AIDS Service; Condoms Taken to Archbishop," *Philadelphia Inquirer*, May 19, 1991, B1; ACT UP, "Protesters Demand U.S. Trade Representative Barshefsky Extend South African Trade Agreement on Medicines to All Nations," September 30, 1999, box 1, JDP; Bell interview.

16. ACT UP Philadelphia, "Projects," critpath.org/actup, cached by Wayback Machine, February 18, 1999, http://web.archive.org/web/19990218065238/http://www.critpath.org/actup/projects.html; Krauss interview; Hayes interview. In a feature-length piece on recovery houses for *Philadelphia City Paper*, Gwen Shaffer interviewed men and women who told her the programs had saved their lives by helping them to get clean. But she also noted that the houses could be coercive—even exploitative—places. The residents of one house worked at the manager's neighboring businesses for free, and others helped to staff voter registration drives and political rallies for local Democratic politicians. Gwen Shaffer, "Silent Treatment," *Philadelphia City Paper*, November 8, 2001, box 1, JDP, http://mycitypaper.com/articles/110801/cs.cover1.shtml.

17. "Lessons Learned from Recent Demonstrations, with Suggested Remedies," ACT UP Philadelphia Subject File, John J. Wilcox Jr. Archives, William Way Community Center, Philadelphia; Bell interview.

18. Maskovsky, "'Fighting for Our Lives,'" 118–19.

19. Bell interview.

20. Sowell interview; Shabazz-El interview; ACT UP Philadelphia, Bread and Roses funding proposal, 1998, box 1, JDP; Susan Phillips, "Tough Act to Follow," *Philadelphia Weekly*, August 1, 2001, box 2, JDP. Waheedah Shabazz-El would go on to be a founding member of Positive Women's Network-USA and deliver the closing keynote at the 2010 International AIDS Conference in Vienna. "No. 6 of 20 Most Amazing HIV-Positive

Women: Waheedah Shabazz-El," *Plus*, February 11, 2015, http://www.hivplusmag.com /people/2015/02/11/no-6–20-most-amazing-hiv-positive-women-waheedah-shabazz-el.

21. Gilbert M. Gaul, "Health Plan Is Greeted Coolly," *Philadelphia Inquirer*, May 25, 1993, C1; Walter F. Roche, "State Health Proposal Rejected," *Philadelphia Inquirer*, August 31, 1993, B1.

22. Walter F. Roche, "Now, Health Insurers Compete for Poor Clients," *Philadelphia Inquirer*, March 17, 1992, B1; Walter F. Roche, "Managed Care Approved for Phila. Needy," *Philadelphia Inquirer*, November 20, 1993, B1; Marc Meltzer, "Privatizing Health Care Firms Seek Needy Clients," *Philadelphia Daily News*, December 2, 1993; Monica Rhor, "As Medicaid Yields to HMOs, Clients Get Bruised," *Philadelphia Inquirer*, October 9, 1994, B1; Walter F. Roche, "Health-Care Profits Come under Fire," *Philadelphia Inquirer*, December 1, 1994, B1.

23. For a narrative that is more sympathetic to Clinton, see Wilentz, *Age of Reagan*.

24. Rodgers, *Age of Fracture*.

25. ACT UP Philadelphia, "Resisting HealthChoices: Two Years of Activism in Southeastern PA," ACT UP Philadelphia, April 1997, cached by Wayback Machine, July 7, 1997, http://web.archive.org/web/19970707132413/http://www.critpath.org/actup/hchoices .htm.

26. Mario Cattabiani and Megan O'Matz, "Governor Offers Lean Budget," *Morning Call* (Allentown, Pa.), February 7, 1996, A1; Megan O'Matz, "Spending Plan Would Cut Medical Benefits for Poor," *Morning Call*, February 7, 1996, A1.

27. Marie McCullough, "Planned Health Cuts Causing Winces," *Philadelphia Inquirer*, February 24, 1996, A1.

28. McCullough, "Planned Health Cuts Causing Winces."

29. Courtney Cairns, "New AIDS Drugs Available Free from State," *Morning Call*, August 6, 1996, B5; Megan O'Matz, "Pa. Budget Process Frustrates Some Democrats," *Morning Call*, June 30, 1996, A6; Mary Flannery, "Stricken from the Rolls," *Philadelphia Daily News*, August 12, 1996, 4; ACT UP Philadelphia, "Resisting HealthChoices."

30. ACT UP Philadelphia, "Resisting HealthChoices"; Julie Knipe Brown, "Activists Want Enormity to Strike Home," *Philadelphia Daily News*, December 2, 1996, 3; Mary Petty, "Art and Social Change: AIDS Activism in Philadelphia," University of Pennsylvania School of Social Work, February 1997, http://www.sp2.upenn.edu/siap/docs /culture_builds_community/art_and_social_change.pdf.

31. ACT UP Philadelphia, "Resisting HealthChoices"; Huntly Collins, "Plan's Options Unclear to AIDS Patients," *Philadelphia Inquirer*, February 6, 1997, B1; Karl Stark and Huntly Collins, "Busy Lines, Confusion, Protests," *Philadelphia Inquirer*, February 4, 1997, A1.

32. ACT UP Philadelphia, "Resisting HealthChoices"; Julie Davids, "Philly AIDS Protest, Wednesday at Noon," sci.med.aids, March 3, 1998, https://groups.google.com/forum /-!msg/sci.med.aids/Le7CjI1UgBo/xJLOG7rNqygJ; Huntly Collins, "AIDS Protesters Say State Falls Short on Medicine, Money," *Philadelphia Inquirer*, March 5, 1998, B3; Richard G. Barnes, "Protesters Take a Stand for Better AIDS Program," *Philadelphia Tribune*, March 6, 1998, 2A; Project TEACH, "Final Grantee Report: Peer-Based Advocacy Initiative," 2000, box 1, JDP.

33. ACT UP Philadelphia, "Resisting HealthChoices"; Terry Pristin, "Protesting Law on Prison Care," *New York Times*, March 1, 1996, New Jersey edition, B1; Chris Mondics

and Andrea Knox, "N.J. Will Privatize Prison Clinics," *Philadelphia Inquirer*, November 29, 1995, S1; Gregory Smith, "Prisoners with AIDS Are under Attack," ACT UP Philadelphia, June 1997, cached by Wayback Machine, December 24, 2002, http://web.archiv
.org/web/20021224223521/http://www.critpath.org/actup/Project 2.htm.

34. Maskovsky, "'Fighting for Our Lives'"; Davids interview; Petty, "Divine Interventions," 90–91. New Jersey ended its contract with CMS (now called Corizon) in 2008, five years after Smith's death in 2003. The company and other correctional HMOs have come under fire for the appallingly negligent care that they provide to those who reside out of sight and mind for many Americans. See the Prison Policy Initiative's list of related resources at www.prisonpolicy.org/cms.html, especially Wil S. Hylton, "Sick on the Inside," *Harper's Magazine*, August 2003, 43–54. For more on the end of New Jersey's contract with CMS, see Rick Hepp, "UMDNJ to Manage Health Care at State Prisons," nj.com, April 1, 2008, https://www.nj.com/news/2008/03/umdnj_to_take_over_health
_care.html. For more on Greg Smith's case and the political funeral that ACT UP Philadelphia staged for him in 2004, see Dan Royles, "Love and Rage," *Nursing Clio* (blog), March 9, 2017, http://nursingclio.org/2017/03/09/love-and-rage/.

35. De Marco interview; Susan Phillips, "Tough Act to Follow," *Philadelphia Weekly*, August 1, 2001, box 2, JDP.

36. Goodman, "Send Bohos, Nuts, and Addicts."

37. Siplon, *AIDS and the Policy Struggle in the United States*, 119; Lattig, "Acting Up Again"; Critical Path AIDS Project, "Our Name and Logo," Critical Path AIDS Project, cached by Wayback Machine, April 16, 2000, http://web.archive.org/web/2000
0416190529/http://www.critpath.org/docs/namelogo.htm; Douglas Martin, "Kiyoshi Kuromiya, 57, Fighter for the Rights of AIDS Patients," *New York Times*, May 28, 2000, 34.

38. Global Exchange, "Top Ten Reasons to Oppose the IMF," n.d., box 1, JDP. On the connection between World Bank and IMF lending practices and AIDS in Africa, see Bob Lederer and Joyce Millen, "Banking on Disaster," *POZ*, July 1998, https://www.poz.com
/article/Banking-on-Disaster-1641-6866.

39. Andrew Sullivan, "When Plagues End," *New York Times Magazine*, November 10, 1996; Eric Sawyer, "Remarks at the Opening Ceremony," ACT UP/New York, accessed March 8, 2013, http://www.actupny.org/Vancouver/sawyerspeech.html; Kiyoshi Kuromiya, "Vancouver: An Activist's Journal," *Critical Path AIDS Project* 31 (Fall 1996): 1, 22–23. For more on the "end" of AIDS, see Rofes, *Dry Bones Breathe*.

40. On the founding of Health GAP, see Mark Milano, Alan Berkman, and David Hoos, "Breaking the Silence: Activist Efforts to Improve Global Access to AIDS Medications," ACT UP/New York, July 6, 2000, http://www.actupny.org/reports/milano
.html; Smith and Siplon, *Drugs into Bodies*, 58–60; and Reverby, "Fielding H. Garrison Lecture."

41. U.S. State Department, "U.S. Government Efforts to Negotiate the Repeal, Termination or Withdrawal of Article 15(c) of the South African Medicines and Related Substances Act of 1965," Consumer Project on Technology, February 5, 1999, http://www
.cptech.org/ip/health/sa/stdept-feb51999.html; Huntly Collins, "AIDS Activists Target a Disparity of Care," *Philadelphia Inquirer*, March 5, 2001, A1; Treatment Action Campaign, "An Explanation of the Medicines Act and the Implications of the South African Court Victory," ACT UP/New York, April 24, 2001, https://actupny.org/reports/TAC
statement.html; Siplon, *AIDS and the Policy Struggle in the United States*.

42. Davids interview; UNAIDS and WHO, "Report on the Global HIV/AIDS Epidemic," data.unaids.org, June 1998, http://data.unaids.org/pub/Report/1998/19981125 _global_epidemic_report_en.pdf; ACT UP Philadelphia, "Fight AIDS in Sub-Saharan Africa!," critpath.org/actup, cached by Internet Archive, January 22, 2000, http://web. archive.org/web/20000122195100/http://www.critpath.org/actup/project3.html; JD Davids email to COMM-ORG electronic mailing list, comm-org.wisc.edu, April 13, 2000, http://comm-org.wisc.edu/pipermail/colist/2000-April/000644.html; ACT UP/New York, "Protesting Congressional African Trade Bill," ACT UP/New York, accessed April 7, 2013, https://actupny.org/actions/africaaction.html; Jesse Jackson Jr., "Keep HOPE Alive," POZ, July 1999, http://www.poz.com/articles/216_10387.shtml; "The Africa Bills, Intellectual Property, and HIV/AIDS," n.d., box 1, JDP.

43. ACT UP/New York, "Candidate Gore Zaps"; ACT UP Philadelphia, "Hundreds of African American, HIV Positive, and Gay and Lesbian Voters to Confront Gore at Fundraising Dinner," June 24, 1999, box 1, JDP; Robert Zausner, "Gore Coming to Phila. for Dinner and Dollars," Philadelphia Inquirer, June 28, 1999, A1; Huntly Collins, "S. Africa Dispute Hits Gore in Phila.," Philadelphia Inquirer, June 29, 1999, A8; Paul Davis, email to aidsact@critpath.org, treatment@critpath.org, and bob1@poz.com, June 29, 1999, http://lists.essential.org/pharm-policy/msg00151.html; Smith and Siplon, Drugs into Bodies, 66; Siplon, AIDS and the Policy Struggle in the United States.

44. ACT UP/New York, "Candidate Gore Zaps"; Steven Lee Myers, "South Africa and U.S. End Dispute over Drugs," New York Times, September 18, 1999, A8; ACT UP, "Gore Concedes to Life-Saving Compromise on SA Drug Policy," September 17, 1999, box 1, JDP. The zaps against Gore also drew media attention to his ties to pharmaceutical industry insiders and lobbyists. Karine Cunqueiro, "Health-Trade: Hostile AIDS Activists Target Gore," Inter Press Service, July 18, 1999, https://web.archive.org/web/20010306102645 /http://www.aegis.com/news/ips/1999/ip990703.html; John B. Judis, "K Street Gore," American Prospect, July/August 1999, 18–21.

45. ACT UP/New York, "Candidate Gore Zaps"; Ralph Nader, James Love, and Robert Weissman to Charlene Barshefsky, October 6, 1999, box 1, JDP; Barshefsky protest photo, October 6, 1999, box 2, JDP; Paul Davis, "ACT UP Demands Essential Medicines for All," Essentialdrugs.org, November 19, 1999, http://www.essentialdrugs.org/edrug /archive/199911/msg00101.php; Goodman, "Send Bohos, Nuts, and Addicts"; Milano interview; Kaiser Family Foundation, "AIDS Drugs: Activists March on White House over Compulsory Licensing," December 1, 1999, box 1, JDP.

46. Bill Clinton, "Remarks to the Ministers Attending the WTO Meetings," The White House, December 1, 1999, https://clintonwhitehouse3.archives.gov/WH/New/WTO-Conf -1999/remarks/19991201-1505.html; Sabin Russell, "Poor Nations Given Hope on AIDS Drugs," SFGate, December 3, 1999, https://www.sfgate.com/health/article/Poor-Nations -Given-Hope-on-AIDS-Drugs-New-2892857.php; ACT UP/New York, "Candidate Gore Zaps"; U.S. President, "Executive Order 13155 of May 10, 2000, Access to HIV/AIDS Pharmaceuticals and Medical Technologies," Federal Register 65, no. 93, May 12, 2000: 30521– 3, https://www.govinfo.gov/content/pkg/FR-2000-05-12/html/00-12177.htm. Clinton was under pressure not only from AIDS activists on December 1, 1999; his announcement came in the middle of the World Trade Organization ministerial in Seattle, where the status quo on trade policy came under attack from developing nations within the meeting as well as from those who protested outside of it.

47. Peter Lurie, "Statement before the Committee on Government Reform, Subcommittee on Criminal Justice, Drug Policy, and Human Resources, U.S. House of Representatives," July 22, 1999, box 1, JDP; Helene Cooper, Rachel Zimmerman, and Laurie McGinley, "AIDS Epidemic Traps Drug Firms in a Vise: Treatment vs. Profits," *Wall Street Journal*, March 2, 2001, A1. The African Growth and Opportunity Act amendment, proposed by Senator Dianne Feinstein of California, would have barred the trade representative from punishing African countries that pursued compulsory licensing and parallel imports. Following the president's announcement, Feinstein chastised her colleagues for bowing to pharmaceutical lobbyists. "Why . . . did my amendment meet such stiff opposition?" she asked, before concluding, "There can be only one answer to that question—profits and corporate greed." "Defiant Clinton Approves Cheaper AIDS Drugs for Africa," *SFGate*, May 11, 2000, http://www.sfgate.com/health/article /Defiant-Clinton-Approves-Cheaper-AIDS-Drugs-for-2760389.php.

48. Robert Naiman and Neil Watkins, "A Survey of the Impacts of IMF Structural Adjustment in Africa: Growth, Social Spending, and Debt Relief," Preamble Center, April 1999, https://web.archive.org/web/20000816025551/preamble.org/imfinafrica.htm; "Join ACT UP—Protest the World Bank and IMF Deadly Policies," September 2001, box 1, JDP.

49. *Breaking the Bank*; Angela Couloumbis, "Area Activists Plan to Make Their Voices Heard," *Philadelphia Inquirer*, April 16, 2000, A16; John H. Bell, "Speech at Demonstration against the IMF/WB," April 16, 2000, box 1, JDP; ACT UP Philadelphia, "ACT UP Shuts Down the IMF/World Bank" and "Fight the Global AIDS Crisis!," April 2000, ACT UP Philadelphia Subject File; Jonathan Peterson, "Clashes in the Capital," *Los Angeles Times*, April 17, 2000, A1.

50. Huntly Collins, "AIDS Activists Target a Disparity of Care"; ACT UP/New York, "Global March at the International AIDS Conference, Durban South Africa," ACT UP/New York, July 9, 2000, http://www.actupny.org/reports/durban-march.html; Winnie Madikizela-Mandela, "The Extent of the AIDS Disaster," speech, Treatment Action Campaign, July 9, 2000, http://www.tac.org.za/Documents/Speeches/wm000709 .txt.

51. ACT UP/New York, "ACT UP @ Republican National Convention, Philadelphia July/August 2000," ACT UP/New York, accessed March 21, 2013, http://www.actupny .org/reports/rnc-7-31-00.html; ACT UP/New York, "1000 AIDS Activists Demonstrate against G. W. Bush at Republican National HQ," ACT UP/New York, accessed April 7, 2013, http://www.actupny.org/reports/bushzap10-13-00.html.

52. Health GAP Coalition, "Action Alert: Failing the Test on Global AIDS," University of Pennsylvania—African Studies Center, May 10, 2001, http://www.africa.upenn.edu /Urgent_Action/apic-051001.html; David E. Sanger, "Bush Says US Will Give $200 Million to World AIDS Fund," *New York Times*, May 12, 2001, A4.

53. Lattig, "Acting Up Again"; Daryl Lindsey, "AIDS Activists Change Their Act," Salon, June 25, 2001, http://www.salon.com/2001/06/25/aids_11/; Esther Kaplan, "The Mighty ACT UP Has Fallen: The Philadelphia Story," *POZ*, November 2001, http://www .poz.com/articles/194_1278.shtml.

54. ACT UP Philadelphia, "Weathering the Storm," November 14, 2001, ACT UP Philadelphia Subject File. The Church of the Advocate has its own place in the history of Philadelphia's civil rights and Black Power movements. See "Civil Rights Period,"

Church of the Advocate, accessed September 5, 2019, http://www.churchoftheadvocate
.org/civil-rights-period.html.

55. World Trade Organization, "Declaration on the TRIPS Agreement and Public Health," World Health Organization, November 14, 2001, https://www.who.int/medicines /areas/policy/tripshealth.pdf?ua=1; Médecins Sans Frontières, "From Durban to Barcelona: Overcoming the Treatment Deficit," M S F | A I D S, July 2002, https://web.archive.org /web/20020803230918/https://www.msf.es/msf_aids/politica_eng.asp; Patterson, *Politics of AIDS in Africa*, 15.

56. "AIDS Activists, Danny Glover, Rep. Barbara Lee Rally at Capital against Global AIDS Disaster," ACT UP/New York, April 4, 2002, http://www.actupny.org/reports /gap4-10-02.html; ACT UP/New York, "November 26 World AIDS Day Mobilization," ACT UP/New York, November 26, 2002, http://www.actupny.org/reports/WAD02.html; ACT UP, "World AIDS Day NYC Flyer," STOP GLOBAL AIDS NOW, accessed June 30, 2014, http://web.archive.org/web/20030315091726/http://www.stopglobalaidsnow.org/112602 _WAD_flyer_nyc.pdf.

57. Stop Global AIDS Now, "Money for AIDS, Not for War," STOP GLOBAL AIDS NOW, November 22, 2002, http://web.archive.org/web/20021121193641/http://www.stopglobal aidsnow.org/; ACT UP/New York, "November 26 World AIDS Day Mobilization."

58. ACT UP/New York, "November 26 World AIDS Day Mobilization"; ACT UP/New York, "Bush's State of the Union Address 2003 (AIDS Excerpt)," ACT UP/New York, accessed July 10, 2014, http://www.actupny.org/reports/bushstate03.html; "Key Initiatives in the President's State of the Union Message," The White House, January 28, 2003, https://web.archive.org/web/20030412195133/http://www.whitehouse.gov/news/releases /2003/01/20030128-14.html.

59. ACT UP/New York, "Bush's State of the Union Address 2003 (AIDS Excerpt)."

60. Sheryl Gay Stolberg, "Politics of Abortion Delays $15 Billion to Fight AIDS," *New York Times*, March 6, 2003, A22; "Global AIDS Bill Hits Snag in Congress," Associated Press, April 1, 2003, http://www.foxnews.com/story/2003/04/01/global-aids-bill-hits -snag-in-congress; Sheryl Gay Stolberg, "$15 Billion AIDS Plan Wins Final Approval in Congress," *New York Times*, May 22, 2003, A30; "PEPFAR," avert.org, accessed July 2, 2014, http://www.avert.org/pepfar.htm.

61. Bendavid and Bhattacharya, "President's Emergency Plan"; Erika Check Hayden, "An Unlikely Champion," *Nature* 457 (January 2009): 254–56; Eugene Robinson, "Bush's Greatest Legacy," *Washington Post*, July 27, 2012, A21; "The U.S. President's Emergency Plan for AIDS Relief (PEPFAR)," *Henry J. Kaiser Family Foundation* (blog), August 2, 2019, https:// www.kff.org/global-health-policy/fact-sheet/the-u-s-presidents-emergency-plan-for/.

62. Jose de Marco et al., "Does the AIDS Movement Still Need ACT UP? Lessons from ACT UP Philadelphia on Changing Tactics for a Changing Epidemic," poster presentation, Nineteenth International AIDS Conference, Washington, D.C., July 22–27, 2012, http://pag.aids2012.org/EPosterHandler.axd?aid=7748; de Marco interview; Davids interview; Krauss interview; Sowell interview.

63. Sheryl Gay Stolberg and Richard W. Stevenson, "Bush AIDS Effort Surprises Many, but Advisers Call It Long Planned," *New York Times*, January 30, 2003, A1; Stolberg, "$15 Billion AIDS Plan Wins Final Approval in Congress"; Donnelly, "President's Emergency Plan for AIDS Relief."

64. Gleeson et al., "Trans Pacific Partnership Agreement." The Trans-Pacific Partner-

ship, a now-defunct 2016 regional trade agreement for countries on the Pacific Rim, included intellectual property provisions that favor pharmaceutical companies. President Donald Trump signed an executive order withdrawing from the Trans-Pacific Partnership soon after taking office in January 2017 as part of a larger program of economic protectionism. This does not mean that the Trump administration is any less friendly to drug companies than Clinton or Bush was. The appointment of Alex Azar, a former executive with Eli Lilly and Company, as secretary of Health and Human Services in late 2017 indicates an especially cozy relationship between his administration and the pharmaceutical industry. Peter Baker, "Trump Abandons Trans-Pacific Partnership, Obama's Signature Trade Deal," *New York Times*, January 20, 2018, https://www .nytimes.com/2017/01/23/us/politics/tpp-trump-trade-nafta.html; Robert Pear, "Senate Confirms Trump Nominee Alex Azar as Health Secretary," *New York Times*, December 10, 2018, https://www.nytimes.com/2018/01/24/us/politics/alex-azar-health-and-human-service -secretary-confirmed-senate.html.

## Chapter 7

1. Dázon Dixon Diallo in Hirshorn, *Nothing without Us.*
2. Corea, *Invisible Epidemic.*
3. Cohen, "Punks, Bulldaggers, and Welfare Queens."
4. Dixon Diallo interview by Ross.
5. B. Smith, "Press of Our Own."
6. Dixon Diallo, email to author, October 20, 2019.
7. Dixon Diallo interview by Ross.
8. *Political Environments* [newsletter of the Committee on Women, Population, and the Environment], no. 8 (Winter/Spring 2001), grant 0990-0619, reel 8830, FFG.
9. Dixon Diallo interview by Ross.
10. Dixon Diallo interview by Ross.
11. SisterLove, Inc., "An Evaluation of the Healthy Love Workshop Draft Proposal," January 2005, untitled manila folder, box 4, SLR; AID Atlanta, "P.S., I Love You," 1985, folder "P.S. I Love You—AID Atlanta," box 5, SLR; Maureen Downey, "Party Has Role in AIDS Prevention," *Atlanta Journal-Constitution*, February 16, 1987, B1.
12. Women's AIDS Prevention Project, "The Facilitator's Guide to the Safe Sex Party 'Party 'til You Drop Unsafe Sex Practices,'" 1988, box 1, unmarked gray folder, SLR; "Is Your Love Healthy? A Facilitator's Guide to the Healthy Love Party, and AIDS Workshop for Women," 1995, box 1, folder "1995 Healthy Love manual," SLR.
13. Dixon Diallo interview by Ross.
14. Dixon Diallo interview by Ross. As Jennifer Nelson argues in *More Than Medicine*, the Operation Rescue campaign was part of a larger effort to weaken abortion clinics financially, through direct action as well as costly regulation.
15. Dixon Diallo interview by Ross.
16. "SisterLove: Women's AIDS Project History," 1990, and Dázon Dixon, "Is Your Love Healthy? Facilitator's Guide to the Healthy Love Party, and AIDS Workshop for Women Only," October 1990, box 1, both in unmarked black folder, SLR.
17. "Is Your Love Healthy? A Facilitator's Guide to the Healthy Love Party, and AIDS Workshop for Women," 1995, box 1, folder "1995 Healthy Love manual," SLR.

18. American Foundation for AIDS Research, "Women United for Women at Risk Project Description," 1990, box 11, folder "WUWAR Proposal Copy," SLR.

19. Dázon Dixon, "Women United for Women at Risk Grant Summary," 1991, box 4, untitled purple folder, SLR.

20. McGovern, "S. P. v. Sullivan." The AIDS definition campaign and actions at the CDC and Health and Human Services offices are documented in Hubbard, *United in Anger*.

21. ACT UP/Network Women's Committee, "ACT UP Demands That the Centers for Disease Control Expand the AIDS Surveillance Definition!!," n.d., and ACT UP Network, "Background on the Centers for Disease Control," n.d., both in box 4, untitled purple folder, SLR; McGovern interview.

22. ACT UP, "Phyllis Sharpe," Jon Cohen AIDS Research Collection, University of Michigan Library, accessed December 11, 2018, http://name.umdl.umich.edu/5571095 .0422.008; Hubbard, *United in Anger*; "Katrina Haslip Dies; AIDS Worker Was 33," *New York Times*, December 3, 1992; "Katrina Haslip," *Nothing without Us* (blog), June 23, 2013, http://womanatthereel.com/katrina-haslip/; Levine interview.

23. Dázon Dixon, "ACT UP Speech," January 9, 1990, box 4, folder "CDC/ACT UP Speech 1/9/90," SLR. A slightly different version of this speech was also printed as "Facing Reality: AIDS Education and Women of Color" in the ACT UP/NY Women and AIDS Book Group, *Women, AIDS, and Activism*, 227–29.

24. SisterLove: Women's AIDS Project, "Revised Agenda: C.A.R.E. Fair 1990," October 1990, box 1, folder 4, ACT UP Chicago Records, Special Collections Research Center, University of Chicago; Wolfe interview.

25. Hubbard, *United in Anger*; Dixon Diallo interview by Ross.

26. See, for example, Risa Denenberg, "Pregnant Women and HIV," 159–64, and Marion Banzhaf, Tracy Morgan, and Karen Ramspacher, "Reproductive Rights and AIDS: The Connections," 199–209, in the ACT UP/NY Women and AIDS Book Group, *Women, AIDS, and Activism*.

27. Dixon Diallo interview by Ross.

28. Dixon Diallo interview by White.

29. Dixon Diallo interview by White.

30. "LoveHouse HOPWA Project Description," 1993, box 2, folder "HOPWA '93 Support Letter Faxes," SLR.

31. SisterLove, Inc., "Love House Program Description," n.d., folder "LoveWorks Day Activity Program," and Dázon Dixon, "Memo to Gail Watson," May 13, 1993, folder "LoveHouse," both in box 2, SLR; "SisterLove Women's AIDS Project: Programs and Projects," n.d., unfiled, box 4, SLR; "CityHelp," *Atlanta Journal-Constitution*, June 2, 1994, sec. Buckhead City Life supplement.

32. Dázon Dixon Diallo, "Letter to Erskine Hawkins," December 2, 2003, folder "misc grant files," and SisterLove, Inc.–South Africa, "Board of Directors Manual," 2003, untitled manila folder, both in box 3, SLR; SisterLove, Inc., "We Are Not Alone Project Proposal," n.d., box 4, untitled green folder, SLR.

33. "SisterLove Newsletter," April 1, 1992, SisterLove Records, box 3, untitled green folder, SLR.

34. Dixon Diallo interview by Ross; SisterLove, Inc., "OurTime Funding Proposal," 1993, box 3, folder "Proposal Stuff 9/93 MACF/Grant Accept," SLR.

35. *SisterLove Newsletter* 1, no. 1, April 1, 1992, untitled green folder, and SisterLove, Inc., OurTime brochure, 1993, untitled green folder, both in box 3, SLR; Oyotunji home page, accessed January 23, 2019, http://www.oyotunji.org/.

36. Smith, "Introduction," xxv; J. Nelson, *More Than Medicine.* See Brier's discussion of feminist perspectives on development in *Infectious Ideas*, 126–28. She cites, among others, Corrêa, *Population and Reproductive Rights*; Basu, *Challenge of Local Feminisms*; Jain, *Women, Development, and the UN*; and Antrobus, *Global Women's Movement.*

37. Dixon Diallo interview by Ross.

38. Dixon Diallo interview by Ross.

39. McIntosh and Finkle, "Cairo Conference"; United Nations, *Beijing Declaration and Platform for Action*, quoted in Rodriguez-Trias, "Topics for Our Times"; Dixon Diallo interview by Ross.

40. Jennifer Nelson devotes a chapter in *More Than Medicine* to Ross's story. Ross has also published several written accounts of her journey as an activist. The most recent is "Reproductive Justice as Intersectional Feminist Activism," which includes a list of the Black women who caucused together at the Illinois conference. See also *Political Environments* [newsletter of the Committee on Women, Population, and the Environment], no. 8 (Winter/Spring 2001), grant 0990-0619, reel 8830, FFG; and Ross interview.

41. Ross, "Reproductive Justice as Intersectional Feminist Activism"; Ross, "Understanding Reproductive Justice," SisterSong, May 2006, https://d3n8a8pro7vhmx.cloudfront .net/rrfp/pages/33/attachments/original/1456425809/Understanding_RJ_Sistersong .pdf?1456425809. In earlier accounts Ross placed the Illinois conference three months *after* the Cairo meeting but has most recently recounted the conference as taking place three months before. Given that the group, calling themselves "Women of African Descent for Reproductive Justice," took out an ad in the *Washington Post* outlining their demands for health care reform in August 1994, a month before the Cairo meeting, this revised time line makes more sense. The text of the ad is reproduced at Black Women for Reproductive Justice, accessed January 17, 2019, https://bwrj.wordpress.com/category /wadrj-on-health-care-reform.

42. SisterLove, Inc., "Training on Reproductive Tract Infections, Self-Help and Human Rights Education," n.d., grant 0985-1763, reel 8124, FFG.

43. Brier, *Infectious Ideas*; Ross interview.

44. SisterLove, Inc., "Anchor Concept Paper: SisterSong Women of Color Reproductive Health Project," 1998, grant 0990-0619, reel 8830, FFG.

45. Dixon Diallo discussed her impending departure in *LoveNotes*, Fall 1995, box 3, untitled green folder, SLR; Dázon Dixon, "Letter to Reena Marcelo," May 15, 1998, grant 0985-1763, reel 8124, FFG.

46. Ross interview.

47. SisterLove, Inc., "Report to Ford Foundation," December 31, 1999, and "SisterSong End of Year Report to the Ford Foundation," 2000, grant 0990-0619, reel 8830; Alliance of Black Women Organizations, World AIDS Day Meeting flyer, November 1999, grant 0990-0639, reel 8874, all in FFG.

48. Chukwudi Onwuachi Saunders, "Program Officer's Memo," 2002, box 823, folder "Reports 016095," Catalog Reports, Ford Foundation Records, Rockefeller Archive Center; Ross interview.

49. Saunders, "Program Officer's Memo."

50. SisterSong, SisterSong Women of Color Reproductive Health and Sexual Rights National Conference brochure, 2003, Women and Gender Printed Collection, Georgia State University Library Digital Collections, http://digitalcollections.library.gsu.edu /cdm/ref/collection/women_print/id/539; Ross interview.

51. SisterLove, "Women and AIDS Program Funding Proposal," April 1991, box 3, folder "Proposals/Writeups," SLR.

52. Dixon Diallo interview by Ross.

53. Other grantees included the National Latino/a Lesbian, Gay, Bisexual, and Trans-gender Organization, which partnered with Bienestar, a Los Angeles Latino/a AIDS service organization; La Clinica del Pueblo, a culturally competent community health clinic in Washington, D.C.; and two Central American groups: Organizacion de Apoyo a una Sexualidad Integral Frente al SIDA, in Guatemala, and Comunidad Gay Sam-pegrana, in Honduras. M. Bahati Kuumba, "A Transnational Partnership 'How-To': Recipes for HIV/AIDS Prevention Cross-Border Linkages," November 2003, unfiled, box 4, SLR.

54. Kuumba, "Transnational Partnership 'How-To.'"

55. Kuumba, "Transnational Partnership 'How-To'"; SisterLove, Inc., "Major Accom-plishment International Programs for Year 2002," box 10, folder "SLI International Pro-grams," SLR.

56. Cowie, *Capital Moves*; Elmore, *Citizen Coke*.

57. Kuumba, "Transnational Partnership 'How-To.'"

58. SisterLove, Inc., "SisterLove/GAP Organizational Capacity Building Initiative," 2001, box 11, folder "Funded Grant Program Plan GAP," SLR; SisterLove, Inc., "Sister-Love HIV/AIDS Capacity Building Project Year 01 Fourth Quarter Report," October 2002, box 2, untitled manila folder, SLR.

59. For more on AIDS and the discourse of globalization, see introduction, note 22.

60. Söderbaum and Taylor, "Transmission Belt?"

61. Two municipalities, Thembisile Hani and Dr JS Moroka, had populations that were over 99 percent black, according to the 1996 South African census. SisterLove, Inc., "SisterLove HIV/AIDS Capacity Building Project Year 01 Fourth Quarter Report"; "SisterLove, Incorporated-International Programs Capability Statement," n.d., box 10, folder "SLI International Programs," SLR. Wolpe is noted for his "cheap labor thesis" regarding the function of apartheid in reproducing cheap black labor as South Africa transitioned to a capitalist society. See Wolpe, "Capitalism and Cheap Labour-Power."

62. Bemnet Fantu, "SisterLove, South Africa Board Meeting Minutes," October 2003, box 10, folder "YR 02, Qq 04 Trip to SA," SLR; Busisiwe Baloyi, "SisterLove Staff Re-sponse," n.d., box 10, folder "Intern—Morgan Dooley," SLR.

63. SisterLove, Inc., "Year 02 Second Quarter Progress Report," 2003, folder "HCBP YR 2 2nd Quarter Rep.," and SisterLove, Inc., "Thembuhlelo HIV/AIDS Capacity Build-ing Project Year 03 Revised Plan of Action," August 6, 2003, folder "SLI International Programs," both in box 10, SLR.

64. Morgan Dooley, "HCBP Year 03 Data Collection—Catherine Molsepe," August 12, 2004, folder "Intern—Morgan Dooley," and Women's Health Project, "Final Report of the SisterLove Thembuhlelo HIV/AIDS Capacity Building (HCBP) Evaluation," n.d., folder "SLI International Programs," both in box 10, SLR.

65. Women's Health Project, "Final Report."

66. Bemnet Fantu, "CDC Post Assessment Debriefing Notes," September 22, 2003, box 10, folder "YR 02, Q 04 Trip to SA," SLR.

67. "Year 03 1st Quarter South Africa Visitation Risk Management Assessment Meeting Notes," January 29, 2004, SisterLove Records, unfiled, box 10, SLR.

68. SisterLove, Inc., "Thembuhlelo HIV Capacity Building Project Phase II: Greater Groblersdal and Greater Marble Hall Situational Analysis and Needs Assessment Report," March 2003, box 10, folder "HCBP, YR 02—GG/GM Situational Analysis and Needs Assessment Report," SLR; Fantu, "SisterLove, South Africa Board Meeting Minutes."

69. "SisterLove, Inc. South Africa HIV/AIDS Capacity Building Project for NGOs/CBOs Budget Period 01 Progress Report," 2002, box 2, untitled manila folder (SisterLove manual); Women's Health Project, "Final Report"; SisterLove, Inc., "Thembuhlelo HIV Capacity Building Project Phase II."

70. Dooley, "Catherine Molsepe"; Morgan Dooley, "HCBP Year 03 Data Collection—Sonto Mlangeni," August 11, 2004, box 10, manila folder "Intern–Morgan Dooley," SLR; SisterLove, Inc., "Thembuhlelo HIV/AIDS Capacity Building Project Year 02 Final Progress Report," October 2003, box 10, folder "SLI International Programs," SLR.

71. Seseni Nu, "SisterLove/GAP Capacity Building Initiative Project Year 01 Second Quarter Report," April 2002, box 10, folder "Quarterly Report for Year 01," SLR; Barron et al., "Eliminating Mother-to-Child HIV Transmission"; Women's Health Project, "Final Report."

72. South Africa National Office of the Department of Land Affairs, "Annual Report: 1 April 2006–31 March 2007," UNPAN, 2007, http://unpan1.un.org/intradoc/groups/public/documents/cpsi/unpan028127.pdf; Linda Villarosa, "The Lady with the Dildoes Has Plenty of Sister Love," TheBody.com, August 7, 2008, http://www.thebody.com/content/art48138.html.

73. John T. Edge, "The Hidden Radicalism of Southern Food," *New York Times*, May 6, 2017, https://www.nytimes.com/2017/05/06/opinion/sunday/the-hidden-radicalism-of-southern-food.html; Edge, *Potlikker Papers*; White, *Freedom Farmers*; J. Nelson, *More Than Medicine*; Dixon Diallo interview by Ross.

74. "Vice Presidential Candidates Debate," C-SPAN, October 5, 2004, https://www.c-span.org/video/?183584–1/vice-presidential-candidates-debate. Ifill's question appears at timestamp 01:04:04.

## Conclusion

1. Philip Bump, "It's True Trump Didn't Pledge Obamacare Repeal in 64 Days. He Pledged It in One," *Washington Post*, March 24, 2017, https://www.washingtonpost.com/news/politics/wp/2017/03/24/its-true-trump-didnt-pledge-obamacare-repeal-in-64-days-he-pledged-it-in-one; Algernon Austin, "Obamacare Reduces Racial Disparities in Health Coverage," Center for Global Policy Solutions, 2016, http://globalpolicysolutions.org/resources/obamacare-reduces-racial-disparities-in-health-coverage; "Exhibit A for Republican Obamacare Repeal Challenge: People with HIV," Reuters, January 5, 2017, http://www.reuters.com/article/us-usa-obamacare-hiv-analysis-idUSKBN14P228.

2. Aengenheyster et al., "Point of No Return"; Darryl Fears, "One Million Species

Face Extinction, U.N. Report Says. And Humans Will Suffer as a Result," *Washington Post*, May 6, 2019, https://www.washingtonpost.com/climate-environment/2019/05/06/one-million-species-face-extinction-un-panel-says-humans-will-suffer-result/.

3. "Climate Gentrification Could Exacerbate Housing Crisis in South Florida," Sierra Club, December 20, 2018, https://www.sierraclub.org/sierra/climate-gentrification-could-exacerbate-housing-crisis-south-florida; Carmin Chappell, "Climate Change in the US Will Hurt Poor People the Most, According to a Bombshell Federal Report," CNBC, November 26, 2018, https://www.cnbc.com/2018/11/26/climate-change-will-hurt-poor-people-the-most-federal-report.html; "Climate Change Will Affect Developing Countries More Than Rich Ones," *The Economist*, May 9, 2018, https://www.economist.com/graphic-detail/2018/05/09/climate-change-will-affect-developing-countries-more-than-rich-ones; Isabelle Gerretsen, "How Climate Change Is Fueling Extremism," CNN, March 10, 2019, https://www.cnn.com/2019/03/06/world/climate-change-terrorism-extremism-africa-middle-east-intl/index.html.

4. Tess Riley, "Just 100 Companies Responsible for 71% of Global Emissions, Study Says," *The Guardian*, July 10, 2017, https://www.theguardian.com/sustainable-business/2017/jul/10/100-fossil-fuel-companies-investors-responsible-71-global-emissions-cdp-study-climate-change; Vann R. II Newkirk, "Environmental Racism Is Real, According to Trump's EPA," *The Atlantic*, February 28, 2018, https://www.theatlantic.com/politics/archive/2018/02/the-trump-administration-finds-that-environmental-racism-is-real/554315/.

# BIBLIOGRAPHY

Because this book is a work of recent history, the lines between primary and secondary sources are quite blurry. For that reason, I have listed sources that readers may expect to find in university libraries as "Academic Sources." Some of those listed as "Printed Primary Sources" may be found in university libraries as well.

## Manuscript Collections

Atlanta, Ga.
   Auburn Avenue Research Library
      Duncan Teague Papers
Berkeley, Calif.
   University of California, Berkeley, Bancroft Library, University Archives
      Queer Resource Center Resource Files
Chicago, Ill.
   University of Chicago, Special Collections Research Center
      ACT UP Chicago Records
Denton, Tex.
   University of North Texas, Special Collections
      Resource Center LGBT Collection
Digital Collections
   ACT UP Oral History Project
   African American AIDS History Project
      Curtis Wadlington Collection
      James Credle Papers
      Rashidah Abdul-Khabeer Collection
   Clinton Digital Library
   Georgia State University Library Digital Collections
      Women and Gender Printed Collection
   LGBTQ Religious Archives Network Oral Histories
   University of Michigan Library
      Jon Cohen AIDS Research Collection
Durham, N.C.
   Duke University, David M. Rubinstein Rare Book and Manuscript Library
      Leroy T. Walker Africa News Service Archive
Fort Lauderdale, Fla.
   Stonewall National Museum and Archives

Ithaca, N.Y.
    Cornell University Library, Rare and Manuscript Collections
        Human Sexuality Collection
        Robert Garcia Papers
Los Angeles, Calif.
    University of California, Los Angeles, Film and Television Archive
        News and Public Affairs Collection
New York, N.Y.
    New York Public Library
        Gay Men's Health Crisis Records
    Schomburg Center
        Gay Men of African Descent Records
        Joseph F. Beam Papers
        Periodicals Collection
        Robert E. Penn Papers
Northampton, Mass.
    Smith College, Sophia Smith Collection
        SisterLove Records
        Voice of Feminism Oral History Project
Philadelphia, Pa.
    Temple University Special Collections Research Center
        AIDS Library (Philadelphia) Records
        Scott Wilds Papers
    William Way LGBT Community Center, John J. Wilcox Jr. Archives
        ACT UP Philadelphia Subject File
        BEBASHI Organizational Files
        JD Davids Papers
        Kiyoshi Kuromiya Papers
Privately Held
    The Balm in Gilead Office Files, in possession of the Balm in Gilead, Inc.,
        Richmond, Va.
    Black LGBT Archivists Society Collection, in possession of Kevin Trimell Jones
San Francisco, Calif.
    Gay, Lesbian, Bisexual, Transgender Historical Society
        National Task Force on AIDS Prevention Records
    San Francisco Public Library
        David Lourea Papers
    University of California, San Francisco, Archives and Special Collections
        Bay Area HIV Support and Education Services Records
        National Task Force on AIDS Prevention Records
Sleepy Hollow, N.Y.
    Rockefeller Archive Center
        Ford Foundation Grant Files
        Ford Foundation Records

## Published Primary Sources

The ACT UP/NY Women and AIDS Book Group. *Women, AIDS, and Activism.* Boston: South End Press, 1990.

The Balm in Gilead. *Though I Stand at the Door and Knock: Discussions on the Black Church Struggle with Homosexuality and AIDS.* New York: Balm in Gilead, 1997.

———. *Who Will Break the Silence? Liturgical Resources for the Healing of AIDS.* New York: Balm in Gilead, 1995.

———. *Who Will Break the Silence? Liturgical Resources for the Healing of AIDS.* New York: Balm in Gilead, 2010.

Barney, Gerald O. *Global 2000: The Report to the President: Entering the Twenty-First Century.* 1980. Revised version, Cabin John, Md.: Seven Locks Press, 1991. https://www.cartercenter.org/resources/pdfs/pdf-archive/global2000reporttothepresident--enteringthe21stcentury-01011991.pdf.

Beam, Joseph. "Brother to Brother: Words from the Heart." In *In the Life: A Black Gay Anthology*, edited by Joseph Beam, 230–42. Boston: Alyson Books, 1986.

———. "Introduction: Leaving the Shadows Behind." In *In the Life: A Black Gay Anthology*, edited by Joseph Beam, 13–18. Boston: Alyson Books, 1986.

———. "Making Ourselves from Scratch." In *Brother to Brother: New Writings by Black Gay Men*, edited by Essex Hemphill, 261–62. Boston: Alyson Publications, 1991.

———, ed. *In the Life: A Black Gay Anthology.* Boston: Alyson Books, 1986.

Black AIDS Institute. *Back of the Line: The State of AIDS among Black Gay Men in America.* Los Angeles: Black AIDS Institute, 2012.

*Blackheart 2: The Prison Issue.* New York: The Blackheart Collective, 1984. https://archive.org/details/blackheart_2.

Branner, Bernard. "Blackberri: Singing for Our Lives." In *In the Life: A Black Gay Anthology*, edited by Joseph Beam, 170–84. Boston: Alyson Books, 1986.

Brown, Tony. *Black Lies, White Lies.* New York: William Morrow, 1995.

Cliff, Michelle. *Claiming an Identity They Taught Me to Despise.* Watertown, Mass: Persephone Press, 1980.

Crimp, Douglas. *AIDS Demo Graphics.* Seattle: Bay Press, 1990.

DeMarco, Joe. "Gay Racism." In *Black Men/White Men: A Gay Anthology*, edited by Michael J. Smith, 109–18. San Francisco: Gay Sunshine Press, 1983.

Dortzbach, Karl, and Ndunge Kiiti, eds. *Helpers for a Healing Community: A Pastoral Counseling Manual for AIDS.* Nairobi, Kenya: Map International, 1994.

Fullwood, Steven G., and Charles Stephens, eds. *Black Gay Genius: Answering Joseph Beam's Call.* New York: Vintage Entity Press, 2014.

Gilbert, David. *AIDS Conspiracy Theories: Tracking the Real Genocide.* Montreal: Abraham Guillen Press, 2002.

Harris, Craig G. "Cut Off from among Their People." In *In the Life: A Black Gay Anthology*, edited by Joseph Beam, 63–67. Boston: Alyson Books, 1986.

Hemphill, Essex. *Ceremonies: Prose and Poetry.* 2nd ed. San Francisco: Cleis Press, 2000.

———. "The Tomb of Sorrow." In *Brother to Brother: New Writings by Black Gay Men*, edited by Essex Hemphill, 75–83. Boston: Alyson Publications, 1991.

———, ed. *Brother to Brother: New Writings by Black Gay Men*. Boston: Alyson Publications, 1991.

Hurston, Zora Neale. *Their Eyes Were Watching God*. Philadelphia: J. B. Lippincott, 1937. 1st HarperLuxe ed., New York: HarperCollins, 2008. Page numbers refer to 2008 edition.

Levy, Paul R. *Queen Village, the Eclipse of Community: A Case Study of Gentrification and Displacement in a South Philadelphia Neighborhood*. Philadelphia: Institute for the Study of Civic Values, 1978.

Map International and The Balm in Gilead. *Helpers for a Healing Community: A Pastoral Counseling Manual for HIV/AIDS*. 3rd ed. Nairobi, Kenya: Map International, 2004. Cached by WayBack Machine July 2, 2015, https://web.archive.org/web /20150702013522/http://www.balmingilead.org/downloads/resources/Helpers %20For%20A%20Healing%20Community%20-%20Pastoral%20Counseling%20 Manual%20-%20Intro%20-Table%20of%20Contents-Parts%201--2--34.pdf.

*Other Countries: Black Gay Voices—A First Volume*. New York: Other Countries, 1988.

Penn, Robert E. "Hide, Seek, Arrive *In the Life*." In *Black Gay Genius: Answering Joseph Beam's Call*, edited by Steven G. Fullwood and Charles Stephens. New York: Vintage Entity Press, 2014.

Riggs, Marlon T. "Black Macho Revisited: Reflections of a Snap! Queen." In *Brother to Brother: New Writings by Black Gay Men*, edited by Essex Hemphill, 253–57. Boston: Alyson Publications, 1991. Also printed in *Black American Literature Forum* 25, no. 2 (Summer 1991): 389–94. https://doi.org/10.2307/3041695.

Roberts, James Charles. "A Light That Failed." In *In the Life: A Black Gay Anthology*, edited by Joseph Beam, 87–92. Boston: Alyson Books, 1986.

Roberts, J. R. *Black Lesbians: An Annotated Bibliography*. Tallahassee, Fla.: Naiad Press, 1981.

Rose, Patti Renee. *In Search of Serenity: A Black Family's Struggle with the Threat of AIDS*. Chicago: Third World Press, 1993.

Smith, Barbara. "Introduction." In *Home Girls: A Black Feminist Anthology*, edited by Barbara Smith, xix–lvi. New York: Kitchen Table: Women of Color Press, 1983.

Tinney, James S. "Why a Black Gay Church?" In *In the Life: A Black Gay Anthology*, edited by Joseph Beam, 70–86. Boston: Alyson Books, 1986.

United Nations. *Beijing Declaration and Platform for Action*. 1995. http://www .unwomen.org/-/media/headquarters/attachments/sections/csw/pfa_e_final _web.pdf.

Wilson, Phill. "I'm Not Done Yet." In *Gay Widowers: Life after the Death of a Partner*, edited by Michael Shernoff, 125–36. New York: Routledge, 1997.

———. "A Message to Black Clergy." In *Though I Stand at the Door and Knock: Discussions on the Black Church Struggle with Homosexuality and AIDS*, by the Balm in Gilead, 31–35. New York: Balm in Gilead, 1997.

## Academic Sources

Adams, Carolyn, David Bartlelt, David Elesh, Ira Goldstein, Nancy Kleniewski, and William Yancey. *Philadelphia: Neighborhoods, Division, and Conflict in a Postindustrial City*. Philadelphia: Temple University Press, 1991.

Adimora, Adoara A., and Victor J. Schoenbach. "Social Context, Sexual Networks, and Racial Disparities in Rates of Sexually Transmitted Infections." *Journal of Infectious Diseases* 191, suppl. 1 (2005): S115–22.

Adimora, Adaora A., Victor J. Schoenbach, and Michelle A. Floris-Moore. "Ending the Epidemic of Heterosexual HIV Transmission among African Americans." *American Journal of Preventive Medicine* 37, no. 5 (November 2009): 468–71. https://doi .org/10.1016/j.amepre.2009.06.020.

Adimora, Adaora A., Victor J. Schoenbach, Francis E. A. Martinson, Tamera Coyne-Beasley, Irene Doherty, Tonya R. Stancil, and Robert E. Fullilove. "Heterosexually Transmitted HIV Infection among African Americans in North Carolina." *Journal of Acquired Immune Deficiency Syndromes* 41, no. 5 (April 2006): 616–23. https://doi .org/10.1097/01.qai.0000191382.62070.a5.

Adimora, Adaora A., Victor J. Schoenbach, Francis E. A. Martinson, Kathryn H. Donaldson, Robert E. Fullilove, and Sevgi O. Aral. "Social Context of Sexual Relationships among Rural African Americans." *Sexually Transmitted Diseases* 28, no. 2 (February 2001): 69–76. https://doi.org/10.1097/00007435-200102000-00002.

Adimora, Adaora A., Victor J. Schoenbach, Francis E. A. Martinson, Kathryn H. Donaldson, Tonya R. Stancil, and Robert E. Fullilove. "Concurrent Partnerships among Rural African Americans with Recently Reported Heterosexually Transmitted HIV Infection." *Journal of Acquired Immune Deficiency Syndromes* 34, no. 4 (December 2003): 423–29. https://doi.org/10.1097/00126334-200312010-00010.

Aengenheyster, Matthias, Qing Yi Feng, Frederick van der Ploeg, and Henk A. Dijkstra. "The Point of No Return for Climate Action: Effects of Climate Uncertainty and Risk Tolerance." *Earth System Dynamics* 9, no. 3 (August 2018): 1085–95. https://doi .org/10.5194/esd-9-1085-2018.

Altman, Dennis. "Globalization, Political Economy, and HIV/AIDS." *Theory and Society* 28, no. 4 (August 1999): 559–84.

Anderson, Carol. *Eyes off the Prize: The United Nations and the African American Struggle for Human Rights, 1944–1955.* New York: Cambridge University Press, 2003.

Anderson, Warwick. "The New York Needle Trial: The Politics of Public Health in the Age of AIDS." *American Journal of Public Health* 81, no. 11 (November 1991): 1506–17.

Austin, Algernon. *Achieving Blackness: Race, Black Nationalism, and Afrocentrism in the Twentieth Century.* New York: NYU Press, 2006.

Barron, Peter, Yogan Pillay, Tanya Doherty, Gayle Sherman, Debra Jackson, Sanjana Bhardwaj, Precious Robinson, and Ameena Goga. "Eliminating Mother-to-Child HIV Transmission in South Africa." *Bulletin of the World Health Organization* 91, no. 1 (January 2013): 70–74. https://doi.org/10.2471/BLT.12.106807.

Batiste, Stephanie Leigh. *Darkening Mirrors: Imperial Representation in Depression-Era African American Performance.* Durham: Duke University Press, 2012.

Batza, Katie. *Before AIDS: Gay Health Politics in the 1970s.* Philadelphia: University of Pennsylvania Press, 2018.

Bay, Mia. *The White Image in the Black Mind: African-American Ideas about White People, 1830–1925.* New York: Oxford University Press, 2000.

Beasley, Myron M. "'Tribute to the Ancestors': Ritual Performance and Same-Gender-Loving Men of African Descent." *Text and Performance Quarterly* 28, no. 4 (October 2008): 433–57. https://doi.org/10.1080/10462930802352045.

Bederman, Gail. *Manliness and Civilization: A Cultural History of Gender and Race in the United States, 1880–1917.* Chicago: University of Chicago Press, 1996.

Beemyn, Genny. *A Queer Capital: A History of Gay Life in Washington, D.C.* New York: Routledge, 2014.

Behnken, Brian D. "Comparative Civil Rights: Notes on the Field of Black-Brown Relations and Multiethnic Freedom Struggles." *Journal of Civil and Human Rights* 1, no. 2 (2015): 212–30.

———, ed. *Civil Rights and Beyond: African American and Latino/a Activism in the Twentieth-Century United States.* Athens: University of Georgia Press, 2016.

Bendavid, Eran, and Jayanta Bhattacharya. "The President's Emergency Plan for AIDS Relief in Africa: An Evaluation of Outcomes." *Annals of Internal Medicine* 150, no. 10 (May 2009): 688–95.

Bérubé, Allan. "How Gay Stays White and What Kind of White It Stays." In *The Making and Unmaking of Whiteness*, edited by Birgit Brander Rasmussen, Eric Klinenberg, Irene J. Nexica, and Matt Wray, 234–65. Durham: Duke University Press, 2001.

Black, Amy E., Douglas L. Koopman, and David K. Ryden. *Of Little Faith: The Politics of George W. Bush's Faith-Based Initiatives.* Washington, D.C.: Georgetown University Press, 2004.

Blain, Keisha. *Set the World on Fire: Black Nationalist Women and the Global Struggle for Freedom.* Philadelphia: University of Pennsylvania Press, 2018.

Bogart, Laura M., and Sheryl Thorburn. "Exploring the Relationship of Conspiracy Beliefs about HIV/AIDS to Sexual Behaviors and Attitudes among African-American Adults." *Journal of the National Medical Association* 95, no. 11 (November 2003): 1057–65.

———. "Relationship of African Americans' Sociodemographic Characteristics to Belief in Conspiracies about HIV/AIDS and Birth Control." *Journal of the National Medical Association* 98, no. 7 (July 2006): 1144–50.

Bogart, Laura M., Glenn Wagner, Frank H. Galvan, and Denedria Banks. "Conspiracy Beliefs about HIV Are Related to Antiretroviral Treatment Nonadherence among African American Men with HIV." *Journal of Acquired Immune Deficiency Syndromes* 53, no. 5 (April 2010): 648–55.

Bogart, Laura M., Glenn J. Wagner, Harold D. Green, Matt G. Mutchler, David J. Klein, Bryce McDavitt, Sean J. Lawrence, and Charles L. Hilliard. "Medical Mistrust among Social Network Members May Contribute to Antiretroviral Treatment Nonadherence in African Americans Living with HIV." *Social Science and Medicine* 164 (September 2016): 133–40. https://doi.org/10.1016/j.socscimed.2016.03.028.

Boghardt, Thomas. "Operation INFEKTION: Soviet Bloc Intelligence and Its AIDS Disinformation Campaign." *Studies in Intelligence* 53, no. 4 (December 2009): 1–24.

Bordowitz, Gregg. *The AIDS Crisis Is Ridiculous and Other Writings, 1986–2003.* Edited by James Meyer. Cambridge, Mass.: MIT Press, 2004.

Bost, Darius. "At the Club: Locating Early Black Gay AIDS Activism in Washington, D.C." *Occasion* 8 (August 31, 2015): 1–9. http://arcade.stanford.edu/occasion/club-locating-early-black-gay-aids-activism-washington-dc.

———. *Evidence of Being: The Black Gay Cultural Renaissance and the Politics of Violence.* Chicago: University of Chicago Press, 2018.

Boykin, Keith. *Beyond the Down Low: Sex, Lies, and Denial in Black America*. New York: Carroll and Graf, 2004.

Brier, Jennifer. *Infectious Ideas: U.S. Political Responses to the AIDS Crisis*. Chapel Hill: University of North Carolina Press, 2009.

———. "'Save Our Kids, Keep AIDS Out': Anti-AIDS Activism and the Legacy of Community Control in Queens, New York." *Journal of Social History* 39, no. 4 (2006): 965–87.

Brilliant, Mark. *The Color of America Has Changed: How Racial Diversity Shaped Civil Rights Reform in California, 1941–1978*. New York: Oxford University Press, 2010.

Broussard, Albert S. *Black San Francisco: The Struggle for Racial Equality in the West, 1900–1954*. Lawrence: University Press of Kansas, 1993.

Bullert, B. J. *Public Television: Politics and the Battle over Documentary Film*. New Brunswick: Rutgers University Press, 1997.

Burkett, Elinor. *The Gravest Show on Earth: America in the Age of AIDS*. Boston: Houghton Mifflin, 1995.

Burrows, Vanessa, and Barbara Berney. "Creating Equal Health Opportunity: How the Medical Civil Rights Movement and the Johnson Administration Desegregated U.S. Hospitals." *Journal of American History* 105, no. 4 (March 2019): 885–911. https://doi.org/10.1093/jahist/jaz004.

Carbado, Devon W. *Black Men on Race, Gender, and Sexuality: A Critical Reader*. New York: NYU Press, 1999.

Carroll, Tamar W. *Mobilizing New York: AIDS, Antipoverty, and Feminist Activism*. Chapel Hill: University of North Carolina Press, 2015.

Chambré, Susan M. *Fighting for Our Lives: New York's AIDS Community and the Politics of Disease*. New Brunswick: Rutgers University Press, 2006.

Cochrane, Michelle. *When AIDS Began: San Francisco and the Making of an Epidemic*. New York: Routledge, 2003.

Cohen, Cathy. *The Boundaries of Blackness: AIDS and the Breakdown of Black Politics*. Chicago: University of Chicago Press, 1999.

———. "Punks, Bulldaggers, and Welfare Queens: The Radical Potential of Queer Politics?" *GLQ: A Journal of Lesbian and Gay Studies* 3, no. 4 (May 1997): 437–65. https://doi.org/10.1215/10642684--3-4--437.

Constantine-Simms, Delroy, ed. *The Greatest Taboo: Homosexuality in Black Communities*. Los Angeles: Alyson Books, 2001.

Cooper, Brittney C. *Beyond Respectability: The Intellectual Thought of Race Women*. Urbana: University of Illinois Press, 2017.

Corbould, Clare. *Becoming African Americans: Black Public Life in Harlem, 1919–1939*. Cambridge, Mass.: Harvard University Press, 2009.

Corea, Gena. *The Invisible Epidemic: The Story of Women and AIDS*. New York: HarperPerennial, 1993.

Countryman, Matthew. *Up South: Civil Rights and Black Power in Philadelphia*. Philadelphia: University of Pennsylvania Press, 2006.

Cowie, Jefferson. *Capital Moves: RCA's 70-Year Quest for Cheap Labor*. Ithaca: Cornell University Press, 1999.

Crane, Johanna Tayloe. *Scrambling for Africa: AIDS, Expertise, and the Rise of American Global Health Science*. Ithaca: Cornell University Press, 2013.

Creel, Margaret Washington. *A Peculiar People: Slave Religion and Community Culture among the Gullah*. New York: NYU Press, 1988.

———. "Slave Women of the Sea Islands of the South." *Negro History Bulletin* 63, nos. 1–4 (2000): 8–16.

Crenshaw, Kimberle. "Demarginalizing the Intersection of Race and Sex: A Black Feminist Critique of Antidiscrimination Doctrine, Feminist Theory and Antiracist Politics." *University of Chicago Legal Forum* 1989 (1989): 139–68.

Crowe, Daniel E. *Prophets of Rage: The Black Freedom Struggle in San Francisco, 1945–1969*. New York: Garland, 2000.

D'Adesky, Anne-Christine. *Moving Mountains: The Race to Treat Global AIDS*. London: Verso, 2006.

Dalton, Harlon L. "AIDS in Blackface." *Daedalus* 118, no. 3 (Summer 1989): 205–27.

Davidson, Basil. *The Africans: An Entry to Cultural History*. London: Longmans, Green, 1969. http://archive.org/details/in.ernet.dli.2015.107751.

Dearing, James W., R. Sam Larson, Liisa M. Randall, and Randall S. Pope. "Local Reinvention of the CDC HIV Prevention Community Planning Initiative." *Journal of Community Health* 23, no. 2 (April 1998): 113–26.

D'Emilio, John. *Lost Prophet: The Life and Times of Bayard Rustin*. Chicago: University of Chicago Press, 2004.

Dew, Charles B. *Apostles of Disunion: Southern Secession Commissioners and the Causes of the Civil War*. Charlottesville: University Press of Virginia, 2001.

Donnelly, John. "The President's Emergency Plan for AIDS Relief: How George W. Bush and Aides Came to 'Think Big' on Battling HIV." *Health Affairs* 31, no. 7 (July 2012): 1389–96.

Douglas, Kelly Brown. *Sexuality and the Black Church: A Womanist Perspective*. Maryknoll, N.Y.: Orbis Books, 1999.

Downs, Jim. *Stand by Me: The Forgotten History of Gay Liberation*. New York: Basic Books, 2016.

Duberman, Martin. *Hold Tight Gently: Michael Callen, Essex Hemphill, and the Battlefield of AIDS*. New York: New Press, 2014.

Dubin, Steven C. *Arresting Images: Impolitic Art and Uncivil Actions*. London: Routledge, 1992.

Edge, John T. *The Potlikker Papers: A Food History of the Modern South*. New York: Penguin Press, 2017.

Edlin, Brian R., Kathleen L. Irwin, Sairus Faruque, Clyde B. McCoy, Carl Word, Yolanda Serrano, James A. Inciardi, Benjamin P. Bowser, Robert F. Schilling, and Scott D. Holmberg. "Intersecting Epidemics—Crack Cocaine Use and HIV Infection among Inner-City Young Adults." *New England Journal of Medicine* 331, no. 21 (November 1994): 1422–27.

Elliott, Denielle. *Reimagining Science and Statecraft in Postcolonial Kenya: Stories from an African Scientist*. New York: Routledge, 2018.

Elmore, Bartow J. *Citizen Coke: The Making of Coca-Cola Capitalism*. New York: W. W. Norton, 2015.

Epstein, Steven. *Impure Science: AIDS, Activism, and the Politics of Knowledge*. Berkeley: University of California Press, 1996.

Farmer, Paul. *AIDS and Accusation: Haiti and the Geography of Blame*. Berkeley: University of California Press, 1992.

Fee, Elizabeth, and Daniel M. Fox, eds. *AIDS: The Burdens of History*. Berkeley: University of California Press, 1988.

Ford, Tanisha C. *Liberated Threads: Black Women, Style, and the Global Politics of Soul*. Chapel Hill: University of North Carolina Press, 2015.

France, David. *How to Survive a Plague: The Inside Story of How Citizens and Science Tamed AIDS*. New York: Knopf, 2016.

Frazier, E. Franklin. *The Negro Church in America*. New York: Schocken, 1964.

Frazier, Robeson Taj. *The East Is Black: Cold War China in the Black Radical Imagination*. Durham: Duke University Press, 2014.

Frederick, Marla F. *Between Sundays: Black Women and Everyday Struggles of Faith*. Berkeley: University of California Press, 2003.

Freimuth, Vicki S. "African Americans' Views on Research and the Tuskegee Syphilis Study." *Social Science and Medicine* 52 (March 2001): 797–808.

Fullilove, Mindy Thompson, and Robert E. Fullilove. "Stigma as an Obstacle to AIDS Action." *American Behavioral Scientist* 42, no. 7 (April 1999): 1117–29.

Fullilove, Robert E., Mindy Thompson Fullilove, Benjamin P. Bowser, and Shirley A. Gross. "Risk of Sexually Transmitted Disease among Black Adolescent Crack Users in Oakland and San Francisco, Calif." *JAMA: Journal of the American Medical Association* 263, no. 6 (February 1990): 851–55. https://doi.org/10.1001/jama.1990.03440060097039.

Fullwood, Steven. *Gay Men of African Descent, Inc. Records* [finding aid]. The New York Public Library, Schomburg Center for Research in Black Culture, 2004. http://archives.nypl.org/scm/21213.

Gaines, Kevin K. *American Africans in Ghana: Black Expatriates and the Civil Rights Era*. Chapel Hill: University of North Carolina Press, 2006.

———. *Uplifting the Race: Black Leadership, Politics, and Culture in the Twentieth Century*. Chapel Hill: University of North Carolina Press, 1996.

Gamble, Vanessa Northington. *Making a Place for Ourselves: The Black Hospital Movement, 1920–1945*. New York: Oxford University Press, 1995.

Gardell, Mattias. *In the Name of Elijah Muhammad: Louis Farrakhan and the Nation of Islam*. Durham: Duke University Press, 1996.

Geary, Adam M. *Antiblack Racism and the AIDS Epidemic: State Intimacies*. New York: Palgrave Macmillan, 2014.

Gibson, Dawn-Marie. *A History of the Nation of Islam: Race, Islam, and the Quest for Freedom*. Santa Barbara, Calif.: Praeger, 2012.

Gleeson, Deborah, Joel Lexchin, Ruth Lopert, and Burcu Kilic. "The Trans Pacific Partnership Agreement, Intellectual Property and Medicines: Differential Outcomes for Developed and Developing Countries." *Global Social Policy* 18, no. 1 (April 2018): 7–27. https://doi.org/10.1177/1468018117734153.

Gordon, Avery F., and Christopher Newfield, eds. *Mapping Multiculturalism*. Minneapolis: University of Minnesota Press, 1996.

Gostin, Lawrence O., Zita Lazzarini, T. Stephen Jones, and Kathleen Flaherty.

"Prevention of HIV/AIDS and Other Blood-Borne Diseases among Injection Drug Users." *JAMA: Journal of the American Medical Association* 277, no. 1 (January 1997): 53–62. https://doi.org/10.1001/jama.1997.03540250061033.

Gould, Deborah B. *Moving Politics: Emotion and ACT UP's Fight against AIDS.* Chicago: University of Chicago Press, 2009.

Griffin, Horace L. *Their Own Receive Them Not: African American Lesbians and Gays in Black Churches.* Cleveland, Ohio: Pilgrim Press, 2006.

Hammett, Theodore M., and Abigail Drachman-Jones. "HIV/AIDS, Sexually Transmitted Diseases, and Incarceration among Women: National and Southern Perspectives." *Sexually Transmitted Diseases* 33 (July 2006): S17–22. https://doi.org/10.1097/01.olq.0000218852.83584.7f.

Harris, Angelique. "AIDS Promotion within the Black Church: Social Marketing in Action." *Social Marketing Quarterly* 16, no. 4 (December 1, 2010): 71–91. https://doi.org/10.1080/15245004.2010.522762.

———. *AIDS, Sexuality, and the Black Church: Making the Wounded Whole.* New York: Peter Lang, 2010.

———. "Panic at the Church: The Use of Frames, Social Problems, and Moral Panics in the Formation of an AIDS Social Movement Organization." *Western Journal of Black Studies* 34, no. 3 (Fall 2010): 337–46.

Harris, Leslie M. "From Abolitionist Amalgamators to 'Rulers of the Five Points': The Discourse of Interracial Sex and Reform in Antebellum New York City." In *Sex, Love, Race: Crossing Boundaries in North American History*, edited by Martha Hodes, 191–212. New York: NYU Press, 1999.

Hartman, Saidiya. *Lose Your Mother: A Journey along the Atlantic Slave Route.* New York: Farrar, Straus and Giroux, 2007.

Haslip-Viera, Gabriel, Bernard Ortiz de Montellano, and Warren Barbour. "Robbing Native American Cultures: Van Sertima's Afrocentricity and the Olmecs." *Current Anthropology* 38, no. 3 (June 1997): 419–41. https://doi.org/10.1086/ca.1997.38.issue-3.

Heller, Jacob. "Rumors and Realities: Making Sense of HIV/AIDS Conspiracy Narratives and Contemporary Legends." *American Journal of Public Health* 105, no. 1 (January 2015): e43–50. https://doi.org/10.2105/AJPH.

Herek, Gregory M., and John P. Capitanio. "Conspiracies, Contagion, and Compassion: Trust and Public Reactions to AIDS." *AIDS Education and Prevention* 6, no. 4 (August 1994): 365–75.

Higginbotham, Evelyn Brooks. *Righteous Discontent: The Women's Movement in the Black Baptist Church, 1880–1920.* Cambridge, Mass.: Harvard University Press, 1993.

Hobson, Emily K. *Lavender and Red: Liberation and Solidarity in the Gay and Lesbian Left.* Oakland: University of California Press, 2016.

Hutchinson, Val, and Joseph M. Cummins. "Low-Dose Oral Interferon in Patient with AIDS." *Lancet*, December 26, 1987, 1530–31.

Inrig, Stephen J. *North Carolina and the Problem of AIDS: Advocacy, Politics, and Race in the South.* Chapel Hill: University of North Carolina Press, 2011.

Juhasz, Alexandra. *AIDS TV: Identity, Community, and Alternative Video.* Durham: Duke University Press, 1995.

———. "So Many Alternatives: The Alternative AIDS Video Movement." *Cinéaste* 21, nos. 1/2 (1995): 37–39.

Kalichman, Seth. *Denying AIDS: Conspiracy Theories, Pseudoscience, and Human Tragedy*. New York: Springer, 2009.

Kelley, Robin D. G. "Kickin' Reality, Kickin' Ballistics: 'Gangsta Rap' and Postindustrial Los Angeles." In *Race Rebels: Culture, Politics, and the Black Working Class*, 183–227. New York: Free Press, 1994.

———. *Yo' Mama's DisFunktional! Fighting the Culture Wars in Urban America*. Boston: Beacon Press, 1997.

Khan, Maria R., Irene A. Doherty, Victor J. Schoenbach, Eboni M. Taylor, Matthew W. Epperson, and Adaora A. Adimora. "Incarceration and High-Risk Sex Partnerships among Men in the United States." *Journal of Urban Health* 86, no. 4 (July 2009): 584–601.

Khan, Maria R., David A. Wohl, Sharon S. Weir, Adaora A. Adimora, Caroline Moseley, Kathy Norcott, Jesse Duncan, Jay S. Kaufman, and William C. Miller. "Incarceration and Risky Sexual Partnerships in a Southern US City." *Journal of Urban Health* 85, no. 1 (January 2008): 100–113.

Kidder, Tracy. *Mountains beyond Mountains: The Quest of Dr. Paul Farmer, a Man Who Would Cure the World*. Reprint ed. New York: Random House, 2009.

Klonoff, Elizabeth A., and Hope Landrine. "Do Blacks Believe That HIV/AIDS Is a Government Conspiracy against Them?" *Preventive Medicine* 28, no. 5 (May 1999): 451–57. https://doi.org/10.1006/pmed.1999.0463.

Koech, Davy K., and Arthur O. Obel. "Treatment of HIV Infections and AIDS: New Horizons." *East African Medical Journal* 67, no. 7 (July 1990): 77–81.

Koech, Davy K., Arthur O. Obel, Jun Minowada, Val A. Hutchinson, and Joseph M. Cummins. "Low Dose Oral Alpha-Interferon Therapy for Patients Seropositive for Human Immunodeficiency Virus Type-1 (HIV-1)." *Molecular Biotherapy* 2, no. 2 (June 1990): 91–95.

Kurashige, Scott. *The Shifting Grounds of Race: Black and Japanese Americans in the Making of Multiethnic Los Angeles*. Princeton: Princeton University Press, 2008.

LaGrone, Kheven Lee. "The Day the Unspeakable Screamed Its Name: My Memories of a Black Gay Men's Movement in 1990s Oakland." *Journal of Civil and Human Rights* 2, no. 2 (2016): 186–206. https://doi.org/10.5406/jcivihumarigh.2.2.0186.

Lee, Sonia Song-Ha. *Building a Latino Civil Rights Movement: Puerto Ricans, African Americans, and the Pursuit of Racial Justice in New York City*. Chapel Hill: University of North Carolina Press, 2014.

Levenson, Jacob. *The Secret Epidemic: The Story of AIDS and Black America*. New York: Pantheon, 2004.

Levenstein, Lisa. *A Movement without Marches: African American Women and the Politics of Poverty in Postwar Philadelphia*. Chapel Hill: University of North Carolina Press, 2009.

Levin, Josh. *The Queen: The Forgotten Life behind an American Myth*. New York: Little, Brown, 2019.

Lincoln, C. Eric. *The Black Muslims in America*. New York: Kayaod, 1963.

Lincoln, C. Eric, and Lawrence H. Mamiya. *The Black Church in the African American Experience*. Durham: Duke University Press, 1990.

Love, Spencie. *One Blood: The Death and Resurrection of Charles R. Drew*. Chapel Hill: University of North Carolina Press, 1997.

Manhart, Lisa E., Sevgi O. Aral, King K. Holmes, and Betsy Foxman. "Sex Partner Concurrency: Measurement, Prevalence, and Correlates among Urban 18–39-Year-Olds." *Sexually Transmitted Diseases* 29, no. 3 (March 2002): 133–43.

Marable, Manning. *Race, Reform, and Rebellion: The Second Reconstruction in Black America*. Jackson: University Press of Mississippi, 1991.

McBride, David. *From TB to AIDS: Epidemics among Urban Blacks since 1900*. Albany: State University of New York Press, 1991.

McBride, Dwight A. "Can the Queen Speak? Racial Essentialism, Sexuality, and the Problem of Authority." *Callaloo* 21, no. 2 (Spring 1998): 363–79.

McGovern, Theresa M. "S. P. v. Sullivan: The Effort to Broaden the Social Security Administration's Definition of AIDS." *Fordham Urban Law Journal* 21, no. 4 (1994): 1083–96.

McGregor, Liz. *Khabzela: The Life and Times of a South African*. Johannesburg: Jacana, 2005.

McGruder, Kevin. "To Be Heard in Print: Black Gay Writers in 1980s New York." *Obsidian III: Literature in the African Diaspora* 6, no. 1 (Spring 2005): 49–65.

McGuire, Danielle L. *At the Dark End of the Street: Black Women, Rape, and Resistance—A New History of the Civil Rights Movement from Rosa Parks to the Rise of Black Power*. Reprint ed. New York: Vintage, 2011.

McIntosh, C. Alison, and Jason L. Finkle. "The Cairo Conference on Population and Development: A New Paradigm?" *Population and Development Review* 21, no. 2 (June 1995): 223–60. https://doi.org/10.2307/2137493.

McKay, Richard A. *Patient Zero and the Making of the AIDS Epidemic*. Chicago: University of Chicago Press, 2017.

Mealer, Bryan. *Muck City: Winning and Losing in Football's Forgotten Town*. New York: Crown Archetype, 2012.

Meriwether, James H. *Proudly We Can Be Africans: Black Americans and Africa, 1935–1961*. Chapel Hill: University of North Carolina Press, 2001.

Mintcheva, Svetlana. "'Some Objects in This Exhibit May Be Disturbing to Certain Viewers': Art Controversies and the Ascent of the Religious Right." In *Potentially Harmful: The Art of American Censorship*, edited by Cathy Byrd and Susan Richmond, 88–95. Atlanta: Georgia State University, Ernest G. Welch School of Art and Design Gallery, 2006.

Mumford, Kevin J. *Not Straight, Not White: Black Gay Men from the March on Washington to the AIDS Crisis*. Chapel Hill: University of North Carolina Press, 2016.

———. "The Trouble with Gay Rights: Race and the Politics of Sexual Orientation in Philadelphia, 1969–1982." *Journal of American History* 98, no. 1 (June 2011): 49–72.

Murch, Donna Jean. *Living for the City: Migration, Education, and the Rise of the Black Panther Party in Oakland, California*. Chapel Hill: University of North Carolina Press, 2010.

Murray, Ashley, Zaneta Gaul, Madeline Y. Sutton, and Jose Nanin. "'We Hide . . .': Perceptions of HIV Risk among Black and Latino MSM in New York City." *American Journal of Men's Health* 12, no. 2 (March 2018): 180–88. https://doi.org/10.1177/1557988317742231.

Murray, Stephen O., and Will Roscoe, eds. *Boy-Wives and Female Husbands: Studies of African Homosexualities*. New York: St. Martin's Press, 1998.

Nattrass, Nicoli. "Understanding the Origins and Prevalence of AIDS Conspiracy Beliefs in the United States and South Africa." *Sociology of Health and Illness* 35, no. 1 (2013): 113–29. https://doi.org/10.1111/j.1467–9566.2012.01480.x.

Nelson, Alondra. "A Black Mass as Black Gothic: Myth and Bioscience in Black Cultural Nationalism." In *New Thoughts on the Black Arts Movement*, edited by Lisa Gail Collins and Margo Natalie Crawford, 138–52. New Brunswick: Rutgers University Press, 2006.

——. *Body and Soul: The Black Panther Party and the Fight against Medical Discrimination.* Minneapolis: University of Minnesota Press, 2011.

Nelson, Jennifer. *More Than Medicine: A History of the Feminist Women's Health Movement.* New York: NYU Press, 2015.

Nero, Charles I. "Fixing Ceremonies: An Introduction." In *Ceremonies: Prose and Poetry,* by Essex Hemphill, xi–xxiii. 2nd ed. San Francisco: Cleis Press, 2000.

——. "Why Are Gay Ghettoes White?" In *Black Queer Studies: A Critical Anthology,* edited by E. Patrick Johnson and Mae Henderson, 228–45. Durham: Duke University Press, 2005.

Obel, Arthur O., and Davy K. Koech. "Outcome of Intervention with or without Low Dose Oral Interferon Alpha in Thirty-Two HIV-1 Seropositive Patients in a Referral Hospital." *East African Medical Journal* 67, no. 7 (July 1990): 71–76.

Ojanuga, D. "The Medical Ethics of the 'Father of Gynaecology,' Dr. J. Marion Sims." *Journal of Medical Ethics* 19, no. 1 (March 1993): 28–31. https://doi.org/10.1136/jme.19.1.28.

Oppenheimer, Gerald M. "In the Eye of the Storm: The Epidemiological Construction of AIDS." In *AIDS: The Burdens of History,* edited by Elizabeth Fee and Daniel M. Fox, 267–300. Berkeley: University of California Press, 1988.

Orfaly, Rebecca A., Joshua C. Frances, Paul Campbell, Becky Whittemore, Brenda Joly, and Howard Koh. "Train-the-Trainer as an Educational Model in Public Health Preparedness." *Journal of Public Health Management Practice,* November 2005, S123–27.

Patterson, Amy S. *The Politics of AIDS in Africa.* Boulder, Colo.: Lynne Rienner, 2006.

Patton, Cindy. *Globalizing AIDS.* Minneapolis: University of Minnesota Press, 2002.

——. *Inventing AIDS.* London: Routledge, 1990.

Pepin, Jacques. *The Origins of AIDS.* New York: Cambridge University Press, 2011.

Peterson, John L., Joseph A. Catania, M. Margaret Dolcini, and Bonnie Faigeles. "Multiple Sexual Partners among Blacks in High-Risk Cities." *Family Planning Perspectives* 25, no. 6 (November 1993): 263–67. https://doi.org/10.2307/2136143.

Peterson, John L., and Gerardo Marín. "Issues in the Prevention of AIDS Among Black and Hispanic Men." Psychology and AIDS. Special issue, *American Psychologist,* 43, no. 11 (November 1988): 871–77. https://doi.org/10.1037/0003-066X.43.11.871.

Petro, Anthony M. *After the Wrath of God: AIDS, Sexuality, and American Religion.* New York: Oxford University Press, 2015.

Pfeiffer, Naomi. "The Oral Alpha-Interferon Craze: Still an Experimental Drug." *AIDS Patient Care* 5, no. 1 (February 1991): 34–38. https://doi.org/10.1089/apc.1991.5.34.

Pinn, Anthony B. *The African American Religious Experience in America.* Westport, Conn.: Greenwood, 2005.

Raboteau, Albert J. *Slave Religion: The "Invisible Institution" in the Antebellum South.* Updated ed. New York: Oxford University Press, 2004.

Raimondo, Meredith. "'AIDS Capital of the World': Representing Race, Sex and Space in Belle Glade, Florida / La Capital de SIDA Del Mundo: Representaciones de Raza, Sexo, y Espacio En Belle Glade, Florida." *Gender, Place and Culture* 12, no. 1 (March 2005): 53–70. https://doi.org/10.1080/09663690500082950.

Retzloff, Tim. "'Seer or Queer?' Postwar Fascination with Detroit's Prophet Jones." *GLQ* 8, no. 3 (2002): 271–96.

Reverby, Susan M. *Examining Tuskegee: The Infamous Syphilis Study and Its Legacy.* Chapel Hill: University of North Carolina Press, 2009.

———. "The Fielding H. Garrison Lecture: Enemy of the People/Enemy of the State: Two Great(ly Infamous) Doctors, Passions, and the Judgment of History." *Bulletin of the History of Medicine* 88, no. 3 (October 2014): 403–30. https://doi.org/10.1353/bhm.2014.0062.

———. "'Normal Exposure' and Inoculation Syphilis: A PHS 'Tuskegee' Doctor in Guatemala, 1946–1948." *Journal of Policy History* 23, no. 1 (January 2011): 6–28. https://doi.org/10.1017/S0898030610000291.

Roberts, John. "African American Belief Narratives and the African Cultural Tradition." *Research in African Literatures* 40, no. 1 (Spring 2009): 112–26.

Robertson, Gil L., IV, ed. *Not in My Family: AIDS in the African-American Community.* Chicago: Agate, 2006.

Rodgers, Daniel T. *Age of Fracture.* Cambridge, Mass.: Belknap Press, 2011.

Rodriguez-Trias, Helen. "Topics for Our Times: From Cairio to Beijing—Women's Agenda for Equality." *American Journal of Public Health* 86, no. 3 (March 1996): 305–6. https://doi.org/10.2105/AJPH.86.3.305.

Rofes, Eric. *Dry Bones Breathe: Gay Men Creating Post-AIDS Identities and Cultures.* New York: Haworth Press, 1998.

Román, David. *Acts of Intervention: Performance, Gay Culture, and AIDS.* Bloomington: Indiana University Press, 1998.

Ross, Loretta J. "Reproductive Justice as Intersectional Feminist Activism." *Souls* 19, no. 3 (July 2017): 286–314. https://doi.org/10.1080/10999949.2017.1389634.

Russell, Thaddeus. "The Color of Discipline: Civil Rights and Black Sexuality." *American Quarterly* 60, no. 1 (2008): 101–28. https://doi.org/10.1353/aq.2008.0000.

Sallar, Anthony, Patrick Bassey Williams, and Ademola Omishakin. "Are HIV/AIDS Conspiracy Beliefs Barriers to HIV Prevention among African American Men Residing in Southern United States?" Presented at the XVI International AIDS Conference, Toronto, 2006. http://www.abstract-archive.org/Abstract/Share/59032.

Scarce, Michael. *Smearing the Queer: Medical Bias in the Healthcare of Gay Men.* New York: Haworth Press, 1999.

Seele, Pernessa. "The Church's Role in HIV/AIDS Prevention." *Anglican Theological Review* 77, no. 4 (1995): 550–51.

Self, Robert. *American Babylon: Race and the Struggle for Postwar Oakland.* Princeton: Princeton University Press, 2003.

Shilts, Randy. *And the Band Played On: Politics, People, and the AIDS Epidemic.* New York: St. Martin's Press, 1987.

Sidbury, James. *Becoming African in America: Race and Nation in the Early Black Atlantic*. New York: Oxford University Press, 2007.

Siplon, Patricia D. *AIDS and the Policy Struggle in the United States*. Washington, D.C.: Georgetown University Press, 2002.

Skloot, Rebecca. *The Immortal Life of Henrietta Lacks*. New York: Crown, 2010.

Smith, Barbara. "A Press of Our Own: Kitchen Table: Women of Color Press." *Frontiers: A Journal of Women Studies* 10, no. 3 (1989): 11–13. https://doi.org/10.2307/3346433.

Smith, Raymond A., and Patricia D. Siplon. *Drugs into Bodies: Global AIDS Treatment Activism*. Santa Barbara, Calif.: Praeger, 2006.

Smith, Susan. *Sick and Tired of Being Sick and Tired: Black Women's Health Activism in America, 1890–1950*. Philadelphia: University of Pennsylvania Press, 1995.

Snorton, C. Riley. *Nobody Is Supposed to Know: Black Sexuality on the Down Low*. Minneapolis: University of Minnesota Press, 2014.

Söderbaum, Fredrik, and Ian Taylor. "Transmission Belt for Transnational Capital or Facilitator for Development? Problematising the Role of the State in the Maputo Development Corridor." *Journal of Modern African Studies* 39, no. 4 (2001): 675–95.

Sontag, Susan. *Illness as Metaphor and AIDS and Its Metaphors*. New York: Doubleday, 1990.

Stall, Ron, Maria Ekstrand, Lance Pollack, Leon McKusick, and Thomas J. Coates. "Relapse from Safer Sex: The Next Challenge for AIDS Prevention Efforts." *Journal of Acquired Immune Deficiency Syndromes* 3, no. 12 (1990): 1181–87.

Stanford, Anthony. *Homophobia in the Black Church: How Faith, Politics, and Fear Divide the Black Community*. Santa Barbara, Calif.: Praeger, 2013.

Stein, Marc. *City of Sisterly and Brotherly Loves: Lesbian and Gay Philadelphia, 1945–1972*. Chicago: University of Chicago Press, 2000.

———, ed. *Encyclopedia of Lesbian, Gay, Bisexual, and Transgender History in America*. Gale Virtual Reference Library. New York: Charles Scribner's Sons, 2004.

Steward, Douglas. "Saint's Progeny: Assotto Saint, Gay Black Poets, and Poetic Agency in the Field of the Queer Symbolic." *African American Review* 33, no. 3 (Autumn 1999): 507–18.

Thomas, Karen Kruse. *Deluxe Jim Crow: Civil Rights and American Health Policy, 1935–1954*. Athens: University of Georgia Press, 2011.

Thomas, Stephen B., and Sandra Crouse Quinn. "The Tuskegee Syphilis Study, 1932 to 1972: Implications for HIV Education and AIDS Risk Education Programs in the Black Community." *American Journal of Public Health* 81, no. 11 (November 1991): 1498–1505.

Thompson, Heather Ann. "Why Mass Incarceration Matters: Rethinking Crisis, Decline, and Transformation in Postwar American History." *Journal of American History* 97, no. 3 (December 2010): 703–34.

Tiemeyer, Phil. *Plane Queer: Labor, Sexuality, and AIDS in the History of Male Flight Attendants*. Berkeley: University of California Press, 2013.

Treichler, Paula A. *How to Have Theory in an Epidemic: Cultural Chronicles of AIDS*. Durham: Duke University Press, 1999.

Turner, Patricia A. *I Heard It through the Grapevine: Rumor in African-American Culture*. Berkeley: University of California Press, 1994.

Turner, Richard Brent. *Islam in the African-American Experience*. Bloomington: Indiana University Press, 1997.

Valdisseri, Ronald O., Terry V. Aultman, and James W. Curran. "Community Planning: A National Strategy to Improve HIV Prevention Programs." *Journal of Community Health* 20, no. 2 (April 1995): 87–100.

Wailoo, Keith. *Dying in the City of the Blues: Sickle Cell Anemia and the Politics of Race and Wealth*. Studies in Social Medicine. Chapel Hill: University of North Carolina Press, 2001.

Wallace, Deborah, and Rodrick Wallace. *A Plague on Your Houses: How New York Was Burned Down and National Public Health Crumbled*. London: Verso, 1998.

Wallace, Rodrick. "Social Disintegration and the Spread of AIDS: Thresholds for Propagation along 'Sociogeographic' Networks." *Social Science and Medicine* 33, no. 10 (1991): 1155–62.

———. "Social Disintegration and the Spread of AIDS—II." *Social Science and Medicine* 37, no. 7 (October 1993): 887–96. https://doi.org/10.1016/0277-9536(93)90143-R.

———. "Urban Desertification, Public Health and Public Order: 'Planned Shrinkage,' Violent Death, Substance Abuse and AIDS in the Bronx." *Social Science and Medicine* 31, no. 7 (1990): 801–13. https://doi.org/10.1016/0277-9536(90)90175-R.

Wallace, Rodrick, and Mindy Thompson Fullilove. "AIDS Deaths in the Bronx 1983–1988: Spatiotemporal Analysis from a Sociogeographic Perspective." *Environment and Planning A* 23, no. 12 (1991): 1701–23. https://doi.org/10.1068/a231701.

Wallace, Rodrick, Mindy Thompson Fullilove, Robert Fullilove, Peter Gould, and Deborah Wallace. "Will AIDS Be Contained within U.S. Minority Urban Populations?" *Social Science and Medicine* 39, no. 8 (October 1994): 1051–62. https://doi.org/10.1016/0277-9536(94)90376-X.

Wallace, Rodrick, and Kristin McCarthy. "The Unstable Public-Health Ecology of the New York Metropolitan Region." *Environment and Planning A* 39 (2007): 1181–92.

Watkins-Hayes, Celeste. *Remaking a Life: How Women Living with HIV/AIDS Confront Inequality*. Oakland: University of California Press, 2019.

White, Monica M. *Freedom Farmers: Agricultural Resistance and the Black Freedom Movement*. Chapel Hill: University of North Carolina Press, 2018.

Whorton, James C. *Nature Cures: The History of Alternative Medicine in America*. New York: Oxford University Press, 2002.

Wiggins, Daphne C. *Righteous Content: Black Women's Perspectives of Church and Faith*. New York: NYU Press, 2004.

Wilentz, Sean. *The Age of Reagan: A History, 1974–2008*. New York: Harper, 2008.

Wimbush, Vincent L. *The Bible and African Americans: A Brief History*. Minneapolis: Fortress Press, 2003.

Wolfinger, James. *Philadelphia Divided: Race and Politics in the City of Brotherly Love*. Chapel Hill: University of North Carolina Press, 2011.

Wolpe, Harold. "Capitalism and Cheap Labour-Power in South Africa: From Segregation to Apartheid." *Economy and Society* 1, no. 4 (1972): 425–56. http://ccs.ukzn.ac.za/files/Wolpe%20Economy%20&%20Society%201972.pdf.

Woodyard, Jeffrey Lynn, John L. Peterson, and Joseph P. Stokes. "'Let Us Go into the House of the Lord': Participation in African American Churches among Young African American Men Who Have Sex with Men." *Journal of Pastoral Care* 54, no. 4 (Winter 2000): 451–60.

Woubshet, Dagmawi. *The Calendar of Loss: Race, Sexuality, and Mourning in the Early Era of AIDS*. Baltimore: Johns Hopkins University Press, 2015.

Young, Rebecca M., and Ilan H. Meyer. "The Trouble with 'MSM' and 'WSW': Erasure of the Sexual-Minority Person in Public Health Discourse." *American Journal of Public Health* 95, no. 7 (July 2005): 1144–49. https://doi.org/10.2105/AJPH.2004 .046714.

## Newspapers and Periodicals

*Afro-American Red Star*
*American Prospect*
*Atlanta Inquirer*
*Atlanta Journal-Constitution*
*Au Courant*
*Bay State Banner (Boston)*
*Big Red News*
*Black/Out*
*BLK*
*Boston Globe*
*Call and Post (Cincinnati)*
*Chicago Citizen*
*Chicago Tribune*
*City Sun (Brooklyn)*
*Critical Path*
*Essence*
*Final Call*
*Fort Lauderdale Sun-Sentinel*
*Gay Community News*
*The Guardian*
*Harper's Magazine*
*Inter Press Service*
*Los Angeles Sentinel*
*Los Angeles Times*
*Michigan Citizen (Detroit)*
*Milwaukee Journal*
*Morning Call (Allentown, Penn.)*
*Nature*
*Newsday*
*New York Amsterdam News*
*New York Native*
*New York Times*

*New Yorker*
*The Observer*
*OutWeek*
*Palm Beach Post*
*Philadelphia City Paper*
*Philadelphia Daily News*
*Philadelphia Gay News*
*Philadelphia Inquirer*
*Philadelphia Inquirer Magazine*
*Philadelphia Magazine*
*Philadelphia Tribune*
*Philadelphia Weekly*
*PI Perspective*
*Plus*
*Positive Nation (UK)*
*Post and Courier (Charleston, S.C.)*
*POZ*
*Reuter News Reports*
*Reuter News Service*
*Reuters*
*Sacramento Observer*
*San Francisco Chronicle*
*Seattle Times*
*The Standard (Kenya)*
*Tri-State Defender*
*Village Voice*
*Wall Street Journal*
*Washington Blade*
*Washington City Paper*
*Washington Informer*
*Washington Post*
*Weekly Review (Kenya)*

## Oral Histories

Abdul-Khabeer, Rashidah. Interview by author, Philadelphia, April 11, 2012, African American AIDS Activism Oral History Project, http://afamaidshist.fiu.edu /omeka-s/s/african-american-aids-history-project/item/2549.

Anderson, Wesley. Interview by author, Clifton Heights, Penn., November 13, 2015, African American AIDS Activism Oral History Project. Not yet available online.

Bell, John. Interview by Pascal Emmer and Jessica Rodriguez, Philadelphia, n.d.

Burnette, Linda. Interview by author, Philadelphia, May 15, 2012, African American AIDS Activism Oral History Project. Not yet available online.

Credle, James. Interview by Candace Bradsher, Newark, N.J., February 15, 2015, Queer Newark Oral History Project, Rutgers University–Newark, https://queer.newark .rutgers.edu/interviews/james-credle.

Davids, JD Interview by author, New York, September 28, 2012, African American AIDS Activism Oral History Project. Not yet available online.

de Marco, Jose. Interview by author, Philadelphia, September 4, 2012, African American AIDS Activism Oral History Project. Not yet available online.

Diallo, Dázon Dixon. Interview by Loretta Ross, April 4, 2009, Voices of Feminism Oral History Project, Sophia Smith Collection, Smith College.

———. Interview by Christina White, August 10, 2010, Remembering AIDS Oral History Project, Emory University Archives.

Driscoll, Earl. Interview by author, Philadelphia, June 12, 2012, African American AIDS Activism Oral History Project. Not yet available online.

Fair, David. Interview by author, Philadelphia, April 13, 2012, African American AIDS Activism Oral History Project. Not yet available online.

Feeback, Steve. Interview by Douglas Noble, Palmdale, Calif., April 3, 2008, Audiovisual Collection, ONE National Gay and Lesbian Archives, Los Angeles.

Flunder, Yvette. Phone interview by Monique Moultrie, February 28, 2011, LGBTQ Religious Archives Network, https://lgbtqreligiousarchives.org/oral-histories /yvette-flunder.

Garner, Darlene. Phone interview by Monique Moultrie, October 27, 2010, LGBTQ Religious Archives Network, https://lgbtqreligiousarchives.org/oral-histories /darlene-garner.

Hayes, Roy. Interview by author, Philadelphia, June 7, 2012, African American AIDS Activism Oral History Project. Not yet available online.

Hinson, Michael. Interview by author, Philadelphia, February 19, 2013, African American AIDS Activism Oral History Project, http://afamaidshist.fiu.edu/omeka-s/s /african-american-aids-history-project/item/2546.

Krauss, Kate. Interview by author, Philadelphia, September 4, 2012, African American AIDS Activism Oral History Project. Not yet available online.

Levine, Debra. Interview by Sarah Schulman, Brooklyn, December 21, 2010, ACT UP Oral History Project, http://www.actuporalhistory.org/interviews/images/levine .pdf.

McGovern, Terry. Interview by Sarah Schulman, New York, May 25, 2007, ACT UP Oral History Project, http://www.actuporalhistory.org/interviews/images /mcgovern.pdf.

McGruder, Kevin. Interview by author, Washington, D.C., January 3, 2014, African American AIDS Activism Oral History Project. Not yet available online.

Milano, Mark. Interview by Sarah Schulman, New York, May 26, 2007, ACT UP Oral History Project, http://www.actuporalhistory.org/interviews/images/milano.pdf.

Minns, Daniel. Interview by Douglas Noble, Washington, D.C., April 28, 2003, Audiovisual Collection, ONE National Gay and Lesbian Archives, Los Angeles.

Morrow-Hall, Gavin. Interview by Douglas Noble, Kansas City, Mo., July 25, 2003, Audiovisual Collection, ONE National Gay and Lesbian Archives, Los Angeles.

Pressley, Joey. Interview by author, Brooklyn, October 8, 2013, African American AIDS Activism Oral History Project. Not yet available online.

Ross, Loretta. Interview by Joyce Follet, Northampton, Mass., November 3–5 and December 1–3, 2004, and February 4, 2005, Voices of Feminism Oral History Project, Sophia Smith Collection, Smith College.

Seele, Pernessa. Interview by author, Richmond, Va., October 11, 2012, African American AIDS Activism Oral History Project. Not yet available online.

Shabazz-El, Waheedah. Interview by author, Philadelphia, June 5 and 7, 2012, African American AIDS Activism Oral History Project. Not yet available online.

Smith, Tyrone. Interview by author, Philadelphia, May 7, 2012, African American AIDS Activism Oral History Project. Not yet available online.

Sowell, Val. Interview by author, Philadelphia, June 15, 2012, African American AIDS Activism Oral History Project. Not yet available online.

Wadlington, Curtis. Interview by author, Philadelphia, May 9, 2012, African American AIDS Activism Oral History Project, http://afamaidshist.fiu.edu/omeka-s/s/african-american-aids-history-project/item/2545.

Wilson, Phill. Interview by author, Los Angeles, November 26, 2012, African American AIDS Activism Oral History Project, http://afamaidshist.fiu.edu/omeka-s/s/african-american-aids-history-project/item/2547.

Wolfe, Maxine. Interview by Jim Hubbard, Brooklyn, February 19, 2004, ACT UP Oral History Project, http://www.actuporalhistory.org/interviews/images/wolfe.pdf.

Young, Terence. Interview by author, Philadelphia, May 23, 2012, African American AIDS Activism Oral History Project. Not yet available online.

## Theses and Dissertations

Maskovsky, Jeff. "'Fighting for Our Lives': Poverty and AIDS Activism in Neoliberal Philadelphia." Ph.D. diss., Temple University, 2000.

Norris, Mackie Lyvonne Harper. "The Black Church Week of Prayer for the Healing of AIDS: An Exploratory Analysis." Ph.D. diss., Emory University, 1996.

Petty, Mary Stuart. "Divine Interventions: Art in the AIDS Epidemic." Ph.D. diss., University of Pennsylvania, 2000.

Sobolewski, Curt. "A Study of the 1993 AIDS Surveillance Definition Revision." M.A. thesis, Baylor University, 1996.

Wise, Janet Marie Bell. "Changing Clergy and Lay Leader Attitudes about HIV/AIDS: The Effectiveness of AIDS Education." Ed.D. diss., North Carolina State University, 1997.

## Documentary Films

Biagiotti, Lisa, dir. *deepsouth*. 2012. Film.

*Breaking the Bank*. New York: Deep Dish Television, 2000. Film. https://archive.org /details/ddtv_187_breaking_the_bank.

Cross, June, dir. *Wilhelmina's War*. 2015. New York: Women Make Movies, 2015. DVD, 53 min.

Everett, Karen, dir. *I Shall Not Be Removed: The Life of Marlon Riggs*. 1996. Film. https:// www.youtube.com/watch?time_continue=1622&v=ku0jQyysroI.

France, David, dir. *How to Survive a Plague*. 2012. Film.

Hirshorn, Harriet, dir. *Nothing without Us: The Women Who Will End AIDS*. New York: Women Make Movies, 2017. DVD, 67 min.

Hubbard, Jim, dir. *United in Anger: A History of ACT UP*. 2012. Film.

Riggs, Marlon, dir. *Tongues Untied*. 1989; San Francisco: Frameline, 2008. DVD, 55 min.

# INDEX

*Page numbers in italics refer to illustrations.*

www.ingramcontent.com/pod-product-compliance
Lightning Source LLC
Chambersburg PA
CBHW031604090725
29363CB00025B/236